Mastitis in Dairy Cows

Guest Editor

PAMELA L. RUEGG, DVM, MPVM

VETERINARY CLINICS OF NORTH AMERICA: FOOD ANIMAL PRACTICE

www.vetfood.theclinics.com

Consulting Editor
ROBERT A. SMITH, DVM, MS

July 2012 • Volume 28 • Number 2

SAUNDERS an imprint of ELSEVIER, Inc.

W.B. SAUNDERS COMPANY
A Division of Elsevier Inc.

1600 John F. Kennedy Boulevard • Suite 1800 • Philadelphia, PA 19103-2899

http://www.vetfood.theclinics.com

VETERINARY CLINICS OF NORTH AMERICA: FOOD ANIMAL PRACTICE Volume 28, Number 2
July 2012 ISSN 0749-0720, ISBN-13: 978-1-4557-3954-7

Editor: John Vassallo; j.vassallo@elsevier.com
Developmental Editor: Teia Stone

Veterinary Clinics of North America: Food Animal Practice (ISSN 0749-0720) is published in March, July, and November by Elsevier Inc., 360 Park Avenue South, New York, NY 10010-1710. Subscription prices are $215.00 per year (domestic individuals), $296.00 per year (domestic institutions), $100.00 per year (domestic students/ residents), $243.00 per year (Canadian individuals), $387.00 per year (Canadian institutions), $307.00 per year (international individuals), $387.00 per year (international institutions), and $153.00 per year (international and Canadian students/ residents). To receive student/resident rate, orders must be accompanied by name of affiliated institution, date of term, and the signature of program/residency coordinator on institution letterhead. *Clinics* subscription prices. All prices are subject to change without notice. **POSTMASTER:** Send address changes to *Veterinary Clinics of North America: Food Animal Practice,* Elsevier Health Sciences Division, Subscription Customer Service, 3251 Riverport Lane, Maryland Heights, MO 63043. Customer Service (orders, claims, online, change of address): Elsevier Health Sciences Division, Subscription Customer Service, 3251 Riverport Lane, Maryland Heights, MO 63043. Tel: 1-800-654-2452 (U.S. and Canada); 314-447-8871 (ouside U.S. and Canada). Fax: 314-447-8029. E-mail: journalscustomerservice-usa@elsevier.com (for print support); journalsonlinesupport-usa@elsevier.com (for online support).

Reprints. For copies of 100 or more, of articles in this publication, please contact the Commercial Reprints Department, Elsevier Inc., 360 Park Avenue South, New York, NY 10010-1710. Tel.: 212-633-3812; Fax: 212-462-1935; E-mail: reprints@elsevier.com.

Veterinary Clinics of North America: Food Animal Practice is covered in *Current Contents/Agriculture, Biology and Environmental Sciences, MEDLINE/PubMed (Index Medicus),* and *Excerpta Medica.*

Printed and bound by CPI Group (UK) Ltd, Croydon, CR0 4YY

Transferred to Digital Print 2012

Contributors

CONSULTING EDITOR

ROBERT A. SMITH, DVM, MS
Diplomate, American Board of Veterinary Practitioners; Veterinary Research and Consulting Services, LLC, Greeley, Colorado

GUEST EDITOR

PAMELA L. RUEGG, DVM, MPVM
Diplomate, American Board of Veterinary Practitioners (Dairy Practice); Professor, Department of Dairy Science, College of Agricultural and Life Sciences, University of Wisconsin, Madison, Madison, Wisconsin

AUTHORS

ALLAN M. BRITTEN, DVM, MPVM
Director, Udder Health Systems, Inc, Boise, Idaho

MATT CHUFF, DVM
Quality Milk Production Services, Cornell University, Ithaca, New York

R.J. ERSKINE, DVM, PhD
Professor, Department of Large Animal Clinical Sciences, College of Veterinary Medicine, Michigan State University, East Lansing, Michigan

LAWRENCE K. FOX, MS, PhD
Professor of Veterinary Clinical Sciences, Department of Veterinary Clinical Sciences, College of Veterinary Medicine, Washington State University, Pullman, Washington

ABHIJIT GURJAR, DVM, PhD
Quality Milk Production Services, Cornell University, Ithaca, New York

JOE HOGAN, PhD
Professor and Associate Chair, Ohio Agricultural Research and Development Center, The Ohio State University, Wooster, Ohio

JOLANDA JANSEN, MSc, PhD
Communication Consultant, Wageningen UR Livestock Research, Lelystad, The Netherlands

GREG KEEFE, DVM, MSc, MBA
Professor and Research Chair, Department of Health Management, Atlantic Veterinary College, University of Prince Edward Island, Charlottetown, Prince Edward Island, Canada

THEO J.G.M. LAM, DVM, PhD
Director of the Dutch Udder Health Centre UGCN, GD Animal Health Service, Deventer; Department of Farm Animal Health, Faculty of Veterinary Medicine, Utrecht University, Utrecht, The Netherlands

KENNETH E. LESLIE, DVM, MSc
Department of Population Medicine, University of Guelph, Guelph, Ontario, Canada

GRAEME A. MEIN, BAgrSc, MAgrSc, PhD
Werribee South, Victoria, Australia

PAOLO MORONI, DVM, PhD
Quality Milk Production Services, Cornell University, Ithaca, New York; Department of
Veterinary Pathology, Hygiene and Public Health, Università degli Studi di Milano,
Milan, Italy

SHELTON E. MURINDA, PhD
Associate Professor of Animal and Veterinary Sciences, Animal and Veterinary Sciences
Department; Director, Center for Antimicrobial Research and Food Safety, California
State Polytechnic University, Pomona, California

STEPHEN P. OLIVER, PhD
Professor of Animal Science, Department of Animal Science; Assistant Dean and
Assistant Director, UT AgResearch, The University of Tennessee, Knoxville, Tennessee

JOSÉ C.F. PANTOJA, MV, MS, PhD
Assistant Professor, Departamento de Higiene Veterinária e Saúde Pública, Faculdade
de Medicina Veterinária e Zootecnia, Universidade Estadual Paulista, Botucatu,
São Paulo, Brazil

CHRISTINA S. PETERSSON-WOLFE, MSc, PhD
Department of Dairy Science, Virginia Tech, Blacksburg, Virginia

DOUGLAS J. REINEMANN, PhD
Professor of Biological Systems Engineering, University of Wisconsin, Madison,
Madison, Wisconsin

DAVID A. RHODA, DVM
Farm and Industry Short Course Instructor, College of Agriculture and Life Sciences,
University of Wisconsin-Madison, Madison, Wisconsin

JERRY R. ROBERSON, DVM, PhD
Diplomate, American College of Veterinary Internal Medicine; Associate Professor,
Department of Large Animal Clinical Sciences, College of Veterinary Medicine,
University of Tennessee, Knoxville, Tennessee

PAMELA L. RUEGG, DVM, MPVM
Diplomate, American Board of Veterinary Practitioners (Dairy Practice); Professor,
Department of Dairy Science, College of Agricultural and Life Sciences, University of
Wisconsin, Madison, Madison, Wisconsin

CARLOS SANTISTEBAN, DVM
Quality Milk Production Services, Cornell University, Ithaca, New York

YNTE SCHUKKEN, DVM, PhD
Quality Milk Production Services, Cornell University, Ithaca, New York

K. LARRY SMITH, PhD
Emeritus Professor, Ohio Agricultural Research and Development Center, The Ohio
State University, Wooster, Ohio

FRANK WELCOME, DVM, MBA
Quality Milk Production Services, Cornell University, Ithaca, New York

RUTH ZADOKS, DVM, PhD
Quality Milk Production Services, Cornell University, Ithaca, New York; Moredun
Research Institute, Penicuik, Midlothian, Scotland

Contents

Preface: Mastitis in Dairy Cows   xi

Pamela L. Ruegg

New Perspectives in Udder Health Management   149

Pamela L. Ruegg

> The nature of mastitis is changing, and environmental mastitis pathogens cause most cases of mastitis on many modern dairy farms. These pathogens often cause mild cases but can become host adapted and behave similar to contagious pathogens. Clinical mastitis is often more difficult to monitor than subclinical disease, and successful control programs are based on effective detection, proper diagnosis, and identification of cow-level risk factors that influence treatment outcomes. Barriers to improvement of milk quality are often related to failure to motivate farm personnel. Development of integrated udder health plans and increased involvement in udder health programs are potential growth areas for veterinary practitioners.

Antimicrobial Resistance of Mastitis Pathogens   165

Stephen P. Oliver and Shelton E. Murinda

> Antibiotics are used in the dairy industry for the prevention and control of mastitis and other diseases affecting dairy cows. Scientific evidence does not support widespread, emerging resistance among mastitis pathogens to antibacterial drugs even though many of these antibiotics have been used in the dairy industry for treatment and prevention of disease for several decades. However, it is clear that use of antibiotics in dairy cows can contribute to increased antimicrobial resistance. The use of antibiotics at times when animals are susceptible to new infection is a sound management decision and a prudent use of antibiotics on the farm.

The Role of Diagnostic Microbiology in Mastitis Control Programs   187

Allan M. Britten

> The dairy practitioner has a special opportunity to influence both the types and quality of mastitis microbiology diagnostic services to support his or her practice. Recommended good laboratory practices, including rigorous use of secondary confirmation testing, specialty selective culture media, and strategic use of enhancement techniques, can significantly impact both sensitivity and specificity of mastitis pathogen detection. Natural variation in shedding patterns of various mastitis pathogens from infected quarters will influence these choices. Bulk tank culture, routine monitoring for contagious pathogens at

freshening, and culture based treatment decisions, should be standard service recommendations for all dairymen.

Update on Control of *Staphylococcus aureus* and *Streptococcus agalactiae* for Management of Mastitis   203

Greg Keefe

The primary method of spread for *S agalactiae* and *S aureus* is from cow to cow. Control is accomplished by decreasing new infections, primarily by milking-time management, and reducing the reservoir of infection in the herd. Adherence to NMC protocols including pre- and post-milking teat disinfection and blanket dry cow therapy will decrease prevalence. There is growing evidence that use of milking gloves is an integral part of contagious mastitis control and the production of high-quality milk. Herds should be closed or have rigorous biosecurity protocols to prevent introduction of novel strains of contagious mastitis pathogens.

Managing Environmental Mastitis   217

Joe Hogan and K. Larry Smith

Environmental mastitis pathogens are the primary agents of infectious mastitis in most well-managed dairy herds. Coliforms and environmental streptococci reside virtually everywhere in the cows' environment, with bedding and manure among the primary point sources of these bacteria. Rates of new infections caused by environmental mastitis pathogens are greatest during the dry period and early lactation. The thrust of herd management strategies for controlling environmental mastitis should focus on reducing intramammary infections during the dry period and early to peak lactation by reducing the exposure of cows to the pathogens and enhancing the ability of cows to combat the infections.

***Mycoplasma* Mastitis Causes, Transmission, and Control**   225

Lawrence K. Fox

Mycoplasma sp are emerging mastitis pathogens. The increase in prevalence of *Mycoplasma* mastitis has been marked over the past decade and appears to be related to increasing herd size and the associated importation of cattle into herds. Evidence points to the importance of asymptomatic carriage as part of the transmission of this disease and nasal discharges are implicated as a major component of transmission. Control strategies are strict milking time hygiene and teat dip. Monitoring the herd prevalence of *Mycoplasma* mastitis through bulk tank cultures is advocated, although a test and slaughter method to control this disease may not be necessary.

The "Other" Gram-Negative Bacteria in Mastitis: *Klebsiella, Serratia,* and More   239

Ynte Schukken, Matt Chuff, Paolo Moroni, Abhijit Gurjar, Carlos Santisteban, Frank Welcome, and Ruth Zadoks

A number of emerging pathogens appear to increase in importance for bovine mastitis. *Klebsiella* spp are considered opportunistic pathogens for humans and animals. *Klebsiella* spp have also been reported as an increasingly important cause of clinical mastitis in the United States and other countries. Clinical mastitis due to *Klebsiella* infection results in high milk loss and high mortality of the affected cows. Prevention of infections through reduction of exposure has been the cornerstone of *Klebsiella* mastitis control on dairy farms. However, contagious behavior of *Klebsiella* spp intramammary infections may occur. Similarly, there has been an increase in other persistent gram-negative infections.

Vaccination Strategies for Mastitis   257

R.J. Erskine

Prevention of exposure is the foundation of infectious disease control programs, including mastitis. The tenets of mastitis prevention are maintaining cows in a clean, dry, comfortable environment and ensuring that recommended milking practices are consistently followed. Under the proper circumstances, vaccination can augment a herd mastitis control program. However, vaccination is essentially an insurance policy to mitigate losses. Thus, veterinarians who counsel dairy producers on mastitis vaccination programs should be able to assess the need, evaluate the available vaccines that could help resolve the problem, and establish a program that balances applied immunology with logistical reality of the dairy operation.

Treatment of Clinical Mastitis   271

Jerry R. Roberson

Decision making in clinical mastitis management requires determining the severity level of each case. Treatment decisions should be based on culture results, and such results can be obtained within 1 day. Making treatment decisions based on culture results allows the practitioner the most justified and judicious use of animal medications. Nearly 50% of all clinical mastitis cases are treated inappropriately or unnecessarily. Although there are many treatments for clinical mastitis, good scientific studies demonstrating the efficacy of most treatments are lacking.

Assessment and Management of Pain in Dairy Cows with Clinical Mastitis   289

Kenneth E. Leslie and Christina S. Petersson-Wolfe

Clinical mastitis has severe detrimental effects on the animal and negative economic impacts for dairy producers. However, pain associated with clinical mastitis, generally, is not measured and not treated.

New technologies may allow dairy producers to identify clinical mastitis in its very early stages, or even before clinical changes occur. With this opportunity for very early detection of infection, there is a potential for early intervention. As the health and well-being of dairy cattle continue to be scrutinized by consumer groups, it is essential that the alleviation of any perceived pain or discomfort associated with clinical mastitis be addressed.

The Role of the Milking Machine in Mastitis Control

Graeme A. Mein

307

Most new infections (NIs) are caused by factors other than the milking machine. Direct and indirect milking machine effects may account for up to 20% of NIs in some herds and about 10% in most herds. Mastitis risk is reduced by keeping bacterial numbers low. Healthy teat-ends reduce the infection risk. NI rates are reduced by pulsation characteristics which provide effective teat massage. Poor machine settings or management conditions can increase the risk of NIs. New research has shown there is no need to leave clusters on cows in an attempt to empty the udder completely at every milking.

Stray Voltage and Milk Quality: A Review

Douglas J. Reinemann

321

This article provides a comprehensive review of research conducted to investigate the effects of electrical exposure (stray voltage) on mastitis, milk composition, and dairy cow health. Although the perception that stray voltage can result in increased somatic cell count (SCC) and incidence of mastitis and suppress dairy cows' immune system, these outcomes have not been observed in a large number of controlled studies with exposures exceeding 8 V. This body of research confirms the 1991 conclusion of a group of national experts who agreed that while exposure to stray voltage at levels of 2 V to 4 V may be a mild stressor to some dairy cows, it will not contribute to increased SCC or incidence of mastitis or reduced milk yield.

Using Mastitis Records and Somatic Cell Count Data

David A. Rhoda and José C.F. Pantoja

347

On-farm records are essential for managing mastitis in dairy herds. Mastitis records are a useful tool for caring for an individual cow, to monitor compliance of farm personnel working with groups of animals, to understand the epidemiology of mastitis in the herd, to ensure responsible drug utilization, and to document accountability in care of the cow. Herds have become larger and more people are involved with individual animal care. This article describes a records plan that can be used to monitor mastitis at the herd level, aid in decision-making processes for individual cows, and improve drug use on dairy herds.

The Role of Communication in Improving Udder Health   **363**

Jolanda Jansen and Theo J.G.M. Lam

This article gives insight into farmers' behavior and mindset toward mastitis management and into the way these can be affected by communication strategies. Elements of farmer mindset are important determining factors in executing mastitis control, including perceived severity and perceived efficacy of mastitis management measures. Veterinary practitioners can be important intermediaries in communication about udder health, provided that they are aware of their role as proactive advisor and apply the accompanying communication skills. Prevention of complex diseases such as mastitis requires customized communication strategies as well as an integrated approach between various stakeholders and different scientific disciplines.

Index   **381**

VETERINARY CLINICS: FOOD ANIMAL PRACTICE

FORTHCOMING ISSUES

November 2012
Diagnostic Pathology
Vicki Cooper, DVM, PhD,
Guest Editor

March 2013
Pain Management
Hans Coetzee, BVSc, PhD, MRCVS,
Guest Editor

RECENT ISSUES

March 2012
Evidence-Based Veterinary Medicine for the Bovine Veterinarian
Sébastien Buczinski, Dr Vét, DÉS, MSc,
and Jean-Michel Vandeweerd, DMV, MS,
Guest Editors

November 2011
Johne's Disease
Michael T. Collins, DVM, PhD,
Guest Editor

July 2011
Ruminant Toxicology
Gary D. Osweiler, DVM, MS, PhD,
Guest Editor

RELATED INTEREST

Veterinary Clinics of North America: Equine Practice
April 2011 (Vol. 27, No. 1)
Endocrine Diseases
Ramiro E. Toribio, DVM, MS, PhD, *Guest Editor*

THE CLINICS ARE NOW AVAILABLE ONLINE!

Access your subscription at:
www.theclinics.com

Preface
Mastitis in Dairy Cows

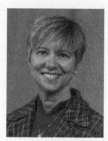

Pamela L. Ruegg, DVM, MPVM
Guest Editor

On a daily basis, veterinarians work with dairy producers to implement preventive health care programs that will ensure the well-being of cows, minimize the use of antimicrobials, and result in the production of safe, high-quality dairy products. Meeting these objectives cannot be achieved without sufficient attention directed toward mastitis control. Virtually all dairy farms have cows that develop mastitis and, on most farms, this disease is the most prevalent and costly disease of adult dairy cows. Veterinary involvement in mastitis control is vital as many studies have shown that treatment and prevention of mastitis are the most common reasons that antimicrobial treatments are administered. The occurrence of mastitis reduces milk production, increases the amount of milk discarded, and increases premature culling and production costs. Additionally, both clinical and subclinical mastitis have been demonstrated to reduce reproductive efficiency. Thus, control of mastitis remains an important facet of veterinary practice and delivery of milk quality programs is an opportunity for veterinarians to positively impact both animal well-being and dairy farm profitability.

Mastitis is a bacterial disease that occurs in individual animals but mastitis control programs must be implemented at the herd level. Mastitis control is a result of the cumulative effect of consistent adoption of best management practices. For many herds, improved milking management, comprehensive use of intramammary antimicrobial dry cow therapy, and improvements in milking machines have resulted in control of mastitis caused by *Staphylococcus aureus* and *Streptococcus agalactiae*. However, on many farms the role of the veterinarian in implementing mastitis control programs is even more important because mastitis is increasingly caused by a diverse group of pathogens that require herd-specific control strategies.

Successful control of mastitis is dependent on effective detection, accurate diagnosis, evaluation of appropriate treatment options, and implementation of preventive practices that address herd-specific risk factors associated with exposure to mastitis pathogens. The topics included in this issue provide practitioners with a comprehensive source of up-to-date information about each of these key aspects of

Vet Clin Food Anim 28 (2012) xi–xii
http://dx.doi.org/10.1016/j.cvfa.2012.04.003
0749-0720/12/$ – see front matter © 2012 Elsevier Inc. All rights reserved.

mastitis control. The contributing authors are well-recognized experts who provided evidence-based practical recommendations. I am grateful for the effort and contributions of each of the authors as they are busy people who took time from their normal activities to prepare these articles. I am impressed with their efforts and confident that the information contained within this issue will be useful in daily veterinary practice.

Pamela L. Ruegg, DVM, MPVM
Department of Dairy Sciences
College of Agricultural and Life Sciences
University of Wisconsin, Madison
282 Animal Science Building
1675 Observatory Drive
Madison, WI 53706-1284, USA

E-mail address:
plruegg@wisc.edu

New Perspectives in Udder Health Management

Pamela L. Ruegg, DVM, MPVM

KEYWORDS

- Mastitis • Udder health • Milk quality • Dairy

KEY POINTS

- The nature of mastitis is changing, and environmental mastitis pathogens cause most cases of mastitis on many modern dairy farms. These pathogens often cause mild cases of clinical mastitis, but some can become host adapted and behave similar to contagious pathogens.
- Clinical mastitis is often more difficult to monitor than subclinical disease, and successful control programs are based on effective detection, proper diagnosis, and identification of cow-level risk factors that influence treatment outcomes.
- Barriers to improvement of milk quality are often related to failure to motivate farm personnel rather than lack of technical knowledge or skills. Development of integrated udder health plans and increased involvement in udder health programs are potential growth areas for veterinarians.

Ensuring production of high-quality milk from healthy cows is the primary objective of many veterinarians who work with dairy farmers. However, despite decades of implementation of control programs, mastitis continues to be the most frequent and economically challenging disease of dairy cows. Mastitis is a unique disease because it directly affects the mammary gland, reducing both the quantity and the quality of milk. Among diseases of dairy cows, mastitis is the only disease that can result in reduced value of the milk, and many processors pay significant monetary premiums to encourage production of high-quality milk. Control of mastitis has been influenced by changes in the dairy industry. Structural shifts in the US dairy industry have resulted in dramatic changes in the way that dairy cows are housed and managed. In 2009, dairy farms housing more than 500 cows contained 56% of cows and produced almost 60% of all milk produced in the United States.[1] These shifts in farm structure have resulted in management changes that have impacted the distribution of mastitis pathogens. While *Staphylococcus aureus* remains a significant cause of mastitis in

The author has nothing to disclose.
Department of Dairy Sciences, College of Agricultural and Life Sciences, University of Wisconsin, Madison, 282 Animal Science Building, 1675 Observatory Drive, Madison, WI 53706–1284, USA
E-mail address: plruegg@wisc.edu

Vet Clin Food Anim 28 (2012) 149–163
http://dx.doi.org/10.1016/j.cvfa.2012.03.001
0749-0720/12/$ – see front matter © 2012 Elsevier Inc. All rights reserved.

some countries,[2,3] widespread adoption of the "5-point plan" (1: post-milking teat disinfection, 2: universal administration of dry cow therapy, 3: appropriate treatment of clinical cases, 4: culling of chronically infected cows, and 5: regular milking machine maintenance) has resulted in significant reductions in prevalence of mastitis caused by contagious pathogens (*Streptococcus agalactiae* and *S aureus*).[4-6] These trends are especially evident when reviewing microbiological results of milk samples obtained from cows with cases of clinical mastitis (**Table 1**). Studies conducted outside of the United States tend to report greater prevalence of clinical mastitis caused by *S aureus* compared to US studies (see **Table 1**). Recovery of the "traditional" mastitis pathogens such as *S agalactiae* or *S aureus* tends to more frequent in regions that are populated by a greater proportion of smaller herds in which tie stall facilities are used[2] or herds in which the use of well-known preventive strategies such as comprehensive use of intramammary antimicrobials at dry off have not been implemented.[14]

In response to the changing distribution of pathogens, udder health programs are increasingly focused on prevention of mastitis caused by environmental pathogens. The term "environmental pathogen" is used to refer to mastitis caused by opportunistic bacteria that reside in the environment of the cows. Common environmental mastitis pathogens include both gram-negative bacteria (such as *Escherichia coli* and *Klebsiella* spp) and gram-positive bacteria (such as *Streptococcus uberis* and *Streptococcus dysgalactia*). Environmental pathogens tend to be less adapted to survival in the udder, and intramammary infection often triggers an immune response that results in mild to moderate clinical symptoms. The duration of infection with environmental pathogens varies among pathogens[15] and can be associated with the degree of host adaptation of the pathogen. Some environmental pathogens (such as most *E coli*) are truly opportunistic and the immune response is often successful in eliminating these pathogens after a brief period of mild clinical disease. Other environmental pathogens (such as many intramammary infections caused by streptococci or *Klebsiella* spp) seem to have become more host adapted and may present as mild clinical cases that erroneously appear to resolve when in actuality the case has returned to a subclinical state. Control of mastitis caused by environmental pathogens can be more complex than control of mastitis caused by contagious bacteria. Bedding materials, moisture, mud, and manure in cow housing areas are common reservoirs for these pathogens, and the standard udder health programs have been expanded into a 10-point plan that includes management procedures that focus on reducing exposure to these pathogens.[16] The purpose of this review is to present new developments in udder health programs and explore ways to strengthen veterinary involvement.

UDDER HEALTH AND MOLECULAR METHODOLOGIES IN THE ERA OF ENVIRONMENTAL PATHOGENS

The classification of mastitis as "contagious" or "environmental" has traditionally been based on the primary reservoir and most likely mode of transmission of mastitis pathogens. Using the traditional classification, the udder of cows with subclinical infections serves as the primary reservoir for contagious pathogens. Transmission of contagious pathogens occurs when teats of healthy cows are exposed to organisms present in milk that originated from infected udders. The most common point of exposure is bacteria present in milk droplets on teat contact surfaces such as milking inflations. In the United States, the most common contagious mastitis pathogens are *S aureus* and *Mycoplasma bovis* but a few herds may still experience problems with *S agalactiae*.[17] However, transmission via a "contagious route" is possible for any

Table 1
Typical Distribution of pathogens causing clinical mastitis in modern dairy herds from selected studies[a]

Study	Year	Country	Cases	S agalactiae[b] or S aureus	CNS	Env streptococci	Coliform	Other	No Growth
Nash et al[7]	2002	US	686 cases in 7 herds	6%	19%	32%	17%	11%	19%
Hoe & Ruegg[8]	2005	US	217 cases in 4 herds	0%	14%	24%	25%	8%	29%
Tenhagen et al[9]	2006	Germany	1261 cases in 10 herds	12%	24%	14%	12%	15%	23%
Bar et al[10]	2007	US	5 herds	5%	3%	21%	40%	10%	21%
Bradley et al[6]	2007	UK	480 samples from 90 farms	3%	13%	25%	21%	11%	27%
McDougall et al[11]	2007	New Zealand	1359 quarters	19%	6%	44%		4%	26%
Olde Riekerink et al[2]	2008	Canada	2850 cases in 106 herds	11%	6%	16%	15%	5%	47%
Unnerstad et al[3]	2009	Sweden	1008 isolates from 51 vet clinics	23%	6%	30%	22%	8%	11%
Lago et al[12]	2011	US	422 cases in 8 herds	7%	9%	14%	23%	13%	34%
Pinzon & Ruegg[13]	2011	US	143 cases in 4 herds	1%	3%	18%	18%	18%	42%
Oliveira & Ruegg, unpublished	2011	US	791 cases from 51 herds	4%	7%	13%	34%	12%	31%

[a] Results characterized as contaminated were excluded from denominators.
[b] S agalactiae was found only by Nash et al[7] and Oliveira & Ruegg, 2011.

microorganism that can cause persistent subclinical mastitis and shed sufficient colonies in milk to establish an infective dose.

The classification of pathogens as contagious or environmental gained widespread use prior to the advent of molecular characterization of bacteria. The use of DNA fingerprinting and other molecular methodologies has resulted in sometimes surprising results relative to how mastitis bacteria appear to behave on farms.[18] Some studies have reported a fairly large diversity within farms of strains of supposedly contagious pathogens such as S aureus.[19] Likewise, the occurrence of host-adapted gram-negative environmental pathogens sometimes occurs on specific farms.[18] Some researchers have reported a wide diversity of strains of environmental mastitis pathogens such as Klebsiella,[20] while other researchers have reported dominant strains that appear to be transmitted among cows.[21] As use of molecular methodologies becomes more commonplace, it is likely that our understanding of how mastitis pathogens are acquired and transmitted among cows will progress and preventive udder health programs will need to be focused on multiple potential routes of exposure regardless of how pathogens happen to be classified. When faced with a herd mastitis problem, veterinarians will need to use epidemiologic skills to investigate risk factors for transmission on each individual farm rather than relying on traditional classifications of expected modes of transmission.

Environmental mastitis problems often present as increased number of cases of clinical mastitis rather than increased bulk milk somatic cell counts (SCC). These clinical mastitis problems are often less obvious to the veterinary practitioner and are more difficult to investigate because many farms lack adequate recording systems for clinical mastitis.[22] Managing exposure to environmental pathogens can be complicated because different groups of cattle may have different abilities to withstand environmental challenges. For example, the disproportionate occurrence of clinical mastitis in early lactation is a hallmark of mastitis caused by environmental pathogens. While exposure to potential environmental pathogens occurs throughout the lactation cycle, periparturient cows are less able to withstand exposure because of immune suppression. Veterinarians should be focused on prevention of the first case of mastitis in a cow because the occurrence of clinical mastitis is a strong predictor of future risk of mastitis in both the present and future lactations.[13,23,24] In a study that followed 218 cows, multiparous cows that experienced a clinical case of mastitis in the previous lactation were 4.2 times more likely to have a case in the first 120 days of the next lactation compared to cows that had completed the previous lactation without a case.[23] This occurred even when the affected quarter had been microbiologically negative in the post-calving period.

Reducing exposure to environmental mastitis pathogens may be difficult because of structural limitations of cattle housing areas. Intensification of dairy farm management often results in exposure to a greater variety of potential mastitis pathogens. Manure handling, type of bedding, stall design, and animal density can all have major impacts on exposure to potential mastitis pathogens. The amount of moisture and bacteria that are present in cow bedding is especially important.[25-27] Organic bedding materials tend to support more bacterial growth as compared to inorganic bedding but significant exposure to streptococci and Klebsiella may also occur when sand bedding is used. A linear relationship between the rate of clinical mastitis and the number of gram-negative bacteria in bedding has been demonstrated.[25] This relationship is especially evident for Klebsiella as increased cases of clinical mastitis caused by this pathogen have been noted as the number of colonies per gram of bedding increased (**Fig. 1**).

As farms increase in size and society looks to them to reduce their environmental impact, it is probable that udder health management programs will need to adapt to

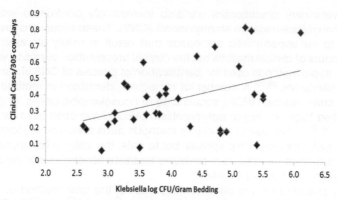

Fig. 1. Relationship between number of colonies of Klebsiella in bedding and rate of clinical mastitis cases (*Data from* Hogan JS, Smith KL, Hoblet KH, et al. Bacterial counts in bedding materials used on nine commercial dairies. J Dairy Sci 1989;72:250–8.)

changing etiologies of mastitis pathogens. Exposure of teats to organic bedding materials is likely to continue to increase as some larger farms adopt the use of anaerobic digesters to process manure. Anaerobic digester solids are usually almost sterile when they are removed from the digester. However, the solids are an excellent media to support growth of enteric organisms. The use of anaerobic digester solids for cow bedding results in direct exposure of cow teats to bacteria that are adapted to living in the nutrient rich organic matter. On some farms, the use of anaerobic digester solids as cattle bedding can result in a large diversity of pathogens causing subclinical and clinical mastitis (**Fig. 2**). Treatment protocols for many of these pathogens are not well defined, nor are there well-known strategies for recommendations about how to best manage digester solids to minimize microbial growth.

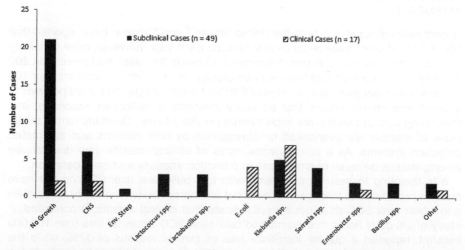

Fig. 2. Distribution of pathogens recovered from quarters with subclinical mastitis (n = 49 cases) and clinical mastitis (n = 17 cases)in April 2010 on a 700 cow WI dairy farm using anaerobic digester solids as bedding.

Modern veterinary practitioners are also increasingly confronted with mastitis caused by coagulase-negative staphylococci (CNS). These organisms are generally considered to be opportunistic pathogens that result in mildly elevated SCC and occasional bouts of clinical mastitis but the clinical presentation seems to vary among farms. Phenotypic methods used for identification of species of CNS are known to be somewhat inaccurate.[28,29] A number of molecular identification methods such as polymerase chain reaction (PCR), sequencing of housekeeping genes, or genotyping using amplified fragment length polymorphism (AFLP) have been used for identification of CNS.[28,30,31] The use of genotypic methods adds precision in identification of CNS and is useful for research purposes, but to date, the utility of enhanced precision may not be apparent for veterinary clinicians because species-based recommendations for control are not well defined.[32]

Veterinary practitioners are often confused about the best method of controlling mastitis caused by CNS. Most researchers agree that mastitis caused by CNS usually results in high rates of spontaneous cure and acceptable responses to antimicrobial treatment,[33] but defining potential differences in pathogenicity among species of CNS is an area of active research. While there are more than 50 identified species of CNS, few consistent differences in mastitis outcomes have been identified among them.[31,33-35] Some research initially suggested that virulence varied based on species,[36,37] but more recent research has reported only minimal or no difference in virulence among species.[38] One study that used both species identification and AFLPs for identification of CNS reported that there was no association between species and production of β-lactamase, severity of the case, or response to antimicrobial treatment.[38] Likewise, there was no statistical difference in bacterial cure based on AFLP cluster,[38] In another study, the same CNS species and isolates with similar AFLP patterns were found in persistent and transient cases of mastitis.[31] It is believed that CNS are usually acquired from both the cow's environment and some contagious transmission from infected or colonized cattle.[39] For most farms, general mastitis control principles continue to be recommended to control mastitis caused by this group of organisms.[40]

DIAGNOSTIC AND TREATMENT ISSUES IN THE ERA OF ENVIRONMENTAL PATHOGENS

Recent national surveys in both the United States[17] and Canada[2] have reported that about 16% of cows experience clinical mastitis each year; however, great variability among farms was noted. A recent survey of 40 herds that each had more than 200 lactating cows reported that there was an average of 40 mastitis treatments per 100 lactating cows per year, with a range of 6 to 90 treatments per 100 cows per year.[41] Veterinarians should ensure that adequate methods of detection, recording, and monitoring clinical mastitis are implemented on dairy farms. On many farms, subtle signs of mastitis are overlooked or disregarded by both humans and automated detection systems. As a consequence, rates of clinical mastitis vary dramatically among studies because of differences in detection intensity and case definition.

It is tempting to assume that herds with low bulk tank milk SCC do not have mastitis problems but that assumption is not always accurate. The ability to maintain a low bulk tank SCC does not always indicate that clinical mastitis is controlled. A study of UK dairy herds that maintained bulk tank SCC values of less than 100,000 cells/mL reported a quarter incidence rate of clinical mastitis of 37%, while the average proportion of the herd affected was 23%.[42] In an older study conducted in the United States, herds with SCC of less than 150,000 cells/mL experienced 4.2 cases of clinical mastitis per 100 cows per month.[43] It is important to recognize that bulk tank SCC values are reflective only of the milk that enters the market chain and can be easily manipulated. Dairy farmers who use pasteurizers to feed milk to calves often divert high SCC milk for this purpose. Bulk tank SCC values can be kept artificially low by drying off high SCC quarters or by diverting milk using quarter milkers. To fully understand the state of mastitis control programs, veterinarians need to review records of clinical mastitis and understand which bulk tank milk SCC management strategies are used on each farm.

Veterinarians should actively communicate with milking technicians and farm managers to be sure that the definition of clinical mastitis and intensity of detection are consistent with farm goals. While clinical mastitis is technically defined as the production of abnormal milk with or without secondary symptoms, the working definition of clinical mastitis varies greatly among farm personnel. On large farms, detection of mastitis is usually dependent on the observational skills of the milking technicians and communication may be impeded by language barriers. As veterinarians became more involved in monitoring clinical mastitis, systems to evaluate detection intensity and case definition are useful. Case definitions should be simple and easily understood by all farm personnel. Use of a 3-point scale based on clinical symptoms is practical, intuitive, and simply recorded and can be an important way to assess detection intensity.[44] In this system, a mastitis severity score of 1 (mild) is assigned when abnormal milk is the only symptom, and severity score of 2 (moderate) is assigned with the abnormal milk is accompanied by udder symptoms such as swelling or redness. Severity score 3 (severe) is assigned when systemic symptoms such as fever, anorexia, or rumen stasis or a large decrease in milk production is observed. Most cases of clinical mastitis are severity score 1 (mild) or 2 (moderate) **(Tables 2** and **3)**. When the proportion of severe cases exceeds about 5% to 20%, it is a signal that detection intensity and case definition should be investigated. Few veterinarians routinely examine or diagnose mild or moderate cases of clinical mastitis, and review of severity scores is also a useful way for veterinarians to gain a better understanding of the full spectrum of mastitis cases occurring on a dairy. While there is a common perception that mastitis caused by gram-negative pathogens is usually severe in nature, assessment of pathogen-specific severity scores collected from 622 cases of clinical mastitis occurring on 52 Wisconsin dairy farms **(Fig. 3**; L. Oliveira and P.L. Ruegg, personal communication, 2011), indicates that systemic involvement occurs at most in only about 30% of cases caused by *E coli* and *Klebsiella* spp, in contrast to less than 20% of cases caused by gram-positive pathogens and in almost no cases that are microbiologically negative. This type of information should be used in the development of mastitis treatment protocols.

Interpretation of treatment outcomes can be confusing because most cases of mastitis caused by environmental pathogens present with mild or moderate clinical signs. In these instances, clinical signs will often abate within about 4 to 6 days with or without treatment, but disappearance of clinical signs does not always indicate that the quarter has been successfully cured. While the milk appears normal, some of these cases may have regressed to a subclinical state and remain bacteriologically positive and at risk for recurrence and transmission to other cows. This is especially true for many gram-positive pathogens and perceptions of treatment success may be distorted if clinical signs are the only outcome indicator used to assess treatments.

Detection and treatment of most mastitis are often performed by farm personnel who milk the cows. The involvement of veterinarians in the development and monitoring of mastitis treatment protocols can only occur if sufficiently useful treatment records are maintained. While the most accurate clinical mastitis records are at the quarter level, farmers usually make decisions about cows, so veterinarians

Table 2
Reported distribution of severity scores for clinical mastitis from selected studies

Severity Score	Case Severity	Clinical Symptom	Study 1[a] (N = 686)	Study 2[b] (N = 622)	Study 3[c] (N = 212)	Study 4[d] (N = 266)	Coliform Cases Only[e] (N = 144)
1	Mild	Abnormal milk only	75%	49%	52%	65%	48%
2	Moderate	Abnormal milk and abnormal udder	20%	37%	41%	27%	31%
3	Severe	Abnormal milk, abnormal udder, and sick cow	5%	14%	7%	8%	22%

[a] From Nash et al, 2002.[7]
[b] From Oliveira & Ruegg, 2011, personal communication.
[c] From Rodrigues et al, 2009.[57]
[d] From Pinzon & Ruegg, 2011.[13]
[e] From Wenz et al, 2001[44] (different but equivalent scoring system used).

Table 3
Calculation of key performance indicators for clinical mastitis[a]

Indicator	Calculation[b]	Suggested Goal
Incidence Rate	Sum of first cases occurring in the appropriate time period[a] divided by average number of lactating cows in the same time period[c]	< 25 new cases per 100 cows per year
Proportion of cases scored 3 (severe)	Number of severity score 3 cases occurring divided by the total number of cases occurring	5%–20% of total cases
Proportion of cases that die	Number of cows experiencing mastitis cases that resulted in death divided by the total number of cows experiencing mastitis	2%[d]
Proportion of cases requiring treatment changes	Number of cases that have the initial treatment protocol changed or supplemented because of nonresponse divided by the total number of detected cases[f]	<20%[e]
Proportion of cases that are recurrent (second or greater treatment)	Number of cows with second or greater case of mastitis occurring >14 days post treatment divided by the total number of cases of mastitis	<30%
Proportion of cows with >1 quarter affected	Number of cases with 2+ quarters affected divided by the total number of cases	<20%[d]
Number of days milk discarded (per case)	Sum of the number of discard days for the time period divided by the total number of cases	Dependent on recommended treatment protocol
Percent of herd milking with <4 quarters	Number of cows milking with <4 quarters[g] divided by the number of lactating cows	<5%

[a] A case is defined as the occurrence of mastitis in 1 or more quarters of a cow (cow-level definition).
[b] Numerators and denominators in all indices should include the statement "in the appropriate time period." The appropriate time period will vary depending on herd size. Smaller herds may need to calculate indices less frequently.
[c] A more correct denominator would exclude cows that had previously experienced a clinical case within that lactation, the inclusion of cows with previous cases produces a more conservation estimate.
[d] Estimated based on 15% of clinical mastitis cases grade 3 (severe) and 15% of those result in death (from Erskine et al[46]).
[e] From Olde Riekerink et al.[14]
[f] Cases that are detected but do not receive initial antimicrobial treatments should be included in this calculation.
[g] Herds that use quarter milkers to discard milk from selected quarters should include those cows in the numerator.

may find it easier to assess outcomes of mastitis treatments at the cow level. At a minimum, farmers should be encouraged to record case severity, drug used for treatment, number of days treated, probable diagnosis (probable pathogen or Gram status), date that meat and milk are suitable for marketing, and follow-up information such as date culled or date of recurrence. Routine monitoring of several key performance indicators for mastitis can allow veterinarians to increase their involvement in evaluating mastitis treatment outcomes (**Table 3**[45]).

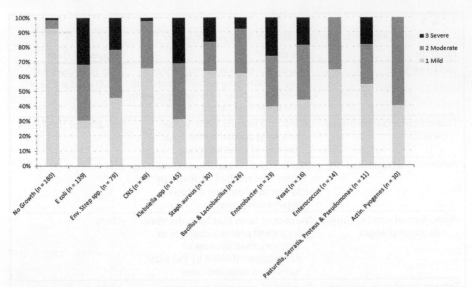

Fig. 3. Distribution of severeity scores by pathogen for 622 cases of clinical mastitis collected from large 52 Wisconsin dairy farms. Each farm contributed < 17 cases of mastitis.

Parity is an important risk factor for clinical mastitis, and veterinary practitioners should assess parity specific incidence and treatment outcomes. Most data demonstrate that older cows are at greater risk for both contagious mastitis and environmental mastitis.[15] Older cows have greater risk of mastitis and a greater risk of recurrence[13] and typically experience fewer bacteriologic and clinical cures.[47] The impact of parity should be considered when making treatment decisions and when evaluating treatment outcomes.

The most effective treatment protocols are based on an accurate diagnosis of the causative pathogen, but an increasing number of milk samples obtained from quarters with subclinical and clinical mastitis are apparently culture negative. No bacteria were isolated from approximately one-third of milk samples submitted to a major mastitis laboratory in Wisconsin between 1994 and 2001, and during that period the proportion of negative results increased from 23% to 50%.[4] In most herds, it is likely that pathogens that caused mastitis in the culture negative samples are similar to the overall distribution of pathogens present in the herd. Current microbiological laboratory methods result in a minimum detection limit for pathogens in milk of about 100 colony-forming units/mL. Potential reasons for negative results from milk samples include a decrease in the amount of mastitis caused by organisms that are known to shed in greater quantities (such as *S agalactiae*), an increased amount of mastitis caused by organisms that do not grow using routine laboratory procedures (such as *Mycoplasma bovis*) and the use of insensitive sampling methods and laboratory techniques (selective media, etc).

At least one PCR method for diagnosis of bovine mastitis pathogens is commercially available and is technically able to accurately detect the presence of bacterial DNA of 11 major mastitis pathogens in aseptically collected milk.[48] In one study, the use of real-time PCR (rtPCR) resulted in identification of bacterial DNA of potential mastitis pathogens in 43% of culture-negative milk samples.[49] However, use of rtPCR for udder health management is not well defined. Just as the occurrence of a few colonies of CNS or *E coli* on a blood agar plate would not be sufficient evidence to indicate that a treatment for CNS or *E coli* mastitis is indicated, the identification of bacterial DNA from milk is not sufficient evidence on which to base a treatment protocol or control program. Decision making for mastitis management using results of rtPCR is also complicated because DNA from dead bacteria is detected. Decision rules for when to initiate treatment or how to determine if an effective cure has occurred after treatment are lacking for all diagnostic systems based on the use of molecular techniques, and veterinarians will need to be aware of new research that will help define the best ways to use these methodologies.

Diagnostic tests are most useful in production medicine programs when results are closely linked to management decisions that result in improved economic outcomes. The development of rapid on-farm culture (OFC) programs has provided a way to link microbiological test results to important mastitis treatment decisions. The use of OFC to direct treatment of clinical mastitis gives farmers the opportunity to make better treatment decisions and reduce costs associated with milk discard and treatment of microbiologically negative cases.[50] OFCs are often used to target intramammary antimicrobials toward appropriate cases and to help determine the appropriate duration of therapy. In general, on diagnosis of a clinical case of mastitis, the cow is examined by farm personnel and a milk sample is obtained. If the case is scored as a grade 1 or 2 (the cow is not demonstrating systemic signs), then no antimicrobial treatment is given until the results of OFC are known (generally 24 hours). Alternatively, some farms initiate treatment immediately but modify treatment duration or drug after receiving the preliminary diagnosis after 24 hours of incubation. Development and oversight of an OFC program are ideal ways for the dairy veterinarian to increase involvement in mastitis control programs and improve treatment protocols. Some veterinary practices increase their involvement in udder health programs by offering complete technical support for OFC systems. Veterinary technicians may visit farms to restock supplies, train farm personnel, and provide oversight and quality control. In areas that have many small herds, it is possible for veterinary clinics to provide a similar system by having the producer promptly drop off milk samples at the clinic and withhold treatments until the microbiological results are known. After 24 hours, the culture result and appropriate treatment protocol can be faxed or e-mailed to the producer. The use of OFC to better target antimicrobial therapy is economically beneficial and can reduce unnecessary antimicrobial therapy by allowing antimicrobial to be administered to cases that are bacteriologically positive and will benefit from therapy. A positively controlled clinical trial evaluating OFC demonstrated that there were no significant differences in either long-term or short-term outcomes for animals with a case of mastitis that received treatment based on results of OFC compared to cases treated immediately without regard to diagnosis.[12,51] In this study, antimicrobials were not administered to cases that were culture negative or gram negative; thus the use of intramammary antimicrobials was reduced by approximately 50% compared to cases that were treated without prior diagnosis.

IMPLEMENTING UDDER HEALTH PROGRAMS

There are numerous reasons for veterinarians to become more involved in udder health programs. The occurrence of mastitis results in reduced milk production and increased milk discard and can result in premature culling, reduced reproductive efficiency, and increased production costs.[10,52-55] The objective of many dairy veterinarians is to prevent animal disease, improve animal well-being, reduce unnecessary treatments, and help ensure the profitability of the dairy business. Mastitis is a bacterial disease that occurs in individual animals, but udder health programs must be implemented at the herd level and must involve significant managerial resources. Successful udder health programs are dependent on effective detection, accurate diagnosis, evaluation of appropriate treatment options, and implementation of herd-specific preventive practices associated with exposure to mastitis pathogens. Veterinarians who wish to be involved in udder health programs should regularly review herd SCC records and help develop and monitor and rates of clinical mastitis and evaluate key performance indicators relative to herd goals. Enough data should be collected so that it is easy to evaluate cow, environmental, and milking machine factors that can contribute to exposure to mastitis pathogens. The involvement of the local veterinarian in the development of annual udder health plans is key to achieving milk quality goals. Milk quality goals should be reviewed annually and be supported by a plan that defines specific action items with clear delineation of responsibility for execution.

It is well known that mastitis can be controlled by the prevention of new infections and the elimination of existing infections, but dairy farms are complex systems and implementation of an udder health plan can be difficult unless all key influencers are in agreement. Surveys of veterinarians and other professionals who work with dairy producers indicate that barriers to improvement of milk quality are primarily related to motivation and implementation rather than to lack of technical knowledge or skills.[56,57] Increased involvement in the design and implementation of mastitis control programs is a potential growth area for many veterinary practices.

REFERENCES

1. US Department of Agriculture. 2010. Overview of the United States Dairy Industry. Natl Agric Stat Serv Available at: www.nass.usda.gov. Accessed November 15, 2011.
2. Olde Riekerink RGM, Barkema HW, Kelton DF, et al. Incidence rate of clinical mastitis on Canadian dairy farms. J Dairy Sci 2008;91:1366–77.
3. Unnerstad HE, Lindberg A, Waller KP, et al. Microbial aetiology of acute clinical mastitis and agent-specific risk factors. Vet Microsc 2009;137:90–7.
4. Makovec JA, Ruegg PL. Characteristics of milk samples submitted for microbiological examination in Wisconsin from 1994 to 2001. J Dairy Sci 2003;86:3466–72.
5. Pitkala A, Haveri M, Pyorala S, et al. Bovine mastitis in Finland 2001—prevalence, distribution of bacteria, and antimicrobial resistance. J Dairy Sci 2004;87:2433–41.
6. Bradley AJ, Leach KA, Breen JE, et al. Survey of the incidence and aetiology of mastitis on dairy farms in England and Wales. Vet Rec 2007;160:253–8.
7. Nash DL, Rogers GW, Cooper JB, et al. Relationship among severity and duration of clinical mastitis and sire transmitting abilities for somatic cell score, udder type traits, productive life, and protein yield. J Dairy Sci 2002;85:1273–84.
8. Hoe FGH, Ruegg PL. Relationship between antimicrobial susceptibility of clinical mastitis pathogens and treatment outcomes. J Am Vet Med Assoc 2005;227: 1461–8.
9. Tenhagen BA, Koster G, Wallman J, et al. Prevalence of mastitis pathogens and their resistance against antimicrobial agents in dairy cows in Brandenburg, Germany. J Dairy Sci 2006;89:2542–51.
10. Bar D, Gröhn YT, Bennett G, et al. Effect of repeated episodes of generic clinical mastitis on milk yield in dairy cows. J Dairy Sci 2007;90:4643–53.
11. McDougall S, Arthur DG, Bryan MA, et al. Clinical and bacteriological response to treatment of clinical mastitis with one of three intramammary antimicrobials. N Z Vet J 2007;55:161–70.

12. Lago A, Godden SM, Bey R, et al. The selective treatment of clinical mastitis based on on-farm culture results. I: Effects on antibiotic use, milk withholding time and short-term clinical and bacteriological outcomes. J Dairy Sci 2011;84:4441–56.
13. Pínzon-Sanchéz C, Ruegg PL. Risk factors associated with short-term post-treatment outcomes of clinical mastitis. J Dairy Sci 2011;94:3397–410.
14. Olde Riekerink RGM, Barkema HW, Scholl DT, et al. Management practices associated with the bulk-milk prevalence of Staphylococcus aureus in Canadian dairy farms. Prev Vet Med 2010;97:20–8.
15. Smith KL, Todhunter DA, Schoenberger PS. Environmental mastitis: cause, prevalence, prevention. J Dairy Sci 1985;68:1531–53.
16. NMC. 2009. NMC recommended mastitis control program. Available at: http://www.nmconline.org/docs/NMCchecklistInt.pdf. Accessed November 15, 2011.
17. US Department of Agriculture. 2008. Prevalence of contagious mastitis pathogens on U.S. dairy operations, 2007. Available at: http://www.aphis.usda.gov/animal_health/nahms/dairy/downloads/dairy07/Dairy07_is_ContMastitis.pdf. Accessed November 15, 2011.
18. Zadoks RN, Middleton JR, McDougall S, et al. Molecular epidemiology of mastitis pathogens of dairy cattle and comparative relevance to humans. J Mammary Gland Biol Neoplasia 2011;16:357–72.
19. Oliveira L, Rodrigues ACO, Hulland C, et al. Toxin production, toxin genes and genetic diversity of Staphylococcus aureus recovered from cases of bovine subclinical mastitis. Am J Vet Res 2011;72:1361–8.
20. Paulin-Curlee GG, Singer RS, Sreevatsan S, et al. Genetic diversity of Mastitis-associated Klebsiella pneumonia in dairy cows. J Dairy Sci 2007;90:3681–9.
21. Munoz M, Welcome FL, Schukken YH, et al. Molecular epidemiology of two Klebsiella pneumoniae mastitis outbreaks on a dairy farm in New York State. J Clin Microsc 2007;45:3964–71.
22. Hoe FGH, Ruegg PL. Opinions and practices of Wisconsin dairy producers about biosecurity and animal well-being. J Dairy Sci 2006;89:2297–308.
23. Pantoja JCF, Hulland C, Ruegg PL. Dynamics of somatic cell counts and intramammary infections across subsequent lactations. Prev Vet Med 2009;90:43–54.
24. Pantoja JCF, Hulland C, Ruegg PL. Somatic cell count status across the dry period as a risk factor for the development of clinical mastitis in subsequent lactations. J Dairy Sci 2009;92:139–48.
25. Hogan JS, Smith KL, Hoblet KH, et al. Bacterial counts in bedding materials used on nine commercial dairies. J Dairy Sci 1989;72:250–8.
26. Hutton CT, Fox LH, Hancock DD. Mastitis control practices: differences between herds with high and low milk somatic cell counts. J Dairy Sci 1990;73:1135–43.
27. Zdanowicz M, Shelford JA, Tucker CB, et al. Bacterial populations on teat ends of dairy cows housed in free stalls and bedded with either sand or sawdust. J Dairy Sci 2004;87:1694–701.
28. Bes M, Guérin-Faublée V, Meugnier H, et al. Improvement of the identification of Staphylococci isolated from bovine mammary infections using molecular methods. Vet Microbiol 2000;71:287–94.
29. Zadoks RN, Watts JL. Species identification of coagulase-negative staphylococci: genotyping is superior to phenotyping. Vet Microsc 2009;134:20–6.
30. Stepanović S, Dakic I, Morrison D, et al. Identification and characterization of clinical isolates of members of the Staphylococcus sciuri group. J Clin Microsc 2005;43:956–8.
31. Taponen S, Koort J, Björkroth J, et al. Bovine intramammary infections caused by coagulase-negative staphylococci may persist throughout lactation according to amplified fragment length polymorphism-based analysis. J Dairy Sci 2007;90:3301–7.

32. Ruegg PL. The quest for the perfect test: phenotypic versus genotypic identification of coagulase negative staphylococci associated with bovine mastitis. Vet Microsc 2009;134:15–9.

33. Apparao DJ, Oliveira L, Ruegg PL. Relationship between in vitro susceptibility test results and treatment outcomes for gram-positive mastitis pathogens following treatment with pirlimycin hydrochloride. J Am Vet Med Assoc 2009;234:1437–46.

34. Wilson DJ, Gonzalez RN, Case KL, et al. Comparison of seven antibiotic treatments with no treatment for bacteriological efficacy against bovine mastitis pathogens. J Dairy Sci 1999;82:1664–70.

35. Thorberg BM, Danielsson-Tham ML, Emanuelson U, et al. Bovine subclinical mastitis caused by different types of coagulase-negative staphylococci. J Dairy Sci 2009;92: 4962–70.

36. Myllys V. Staphylococci in heifer mastitis before and after parturition. J Dairy Res 1995;62:51–60.

37. Aarestrup FM, Jensen NE. Prevalence and duration of intramammary infection in Danish heifers during the peripartum period. J Dairy Sci 1997;80:307–12.

38. Taponen S, Simojoki H, Haveri M, et al. Clinical characteristics and persistence of bovine mastitis caused by different species of coagulase-negative staphylococci identified with API or AFLP. Vet Microbiol 2006;115:199–207.

39. Piessens V, Van Coillie E. Verbist B, et al. Distribution of coagulase-negative Staphylococcus species from milk and environment of dairy cows differs between herds. J Dairy Sci 2011;94:2933–44.

40. Sears PM, McCarthy KK. Management and treatment of staphylococcal mastitis. Vet Clin North Am Food Anim Pract 2003;19:171–85.

41. Oliveira L, Ruegg PL. Treatments for clinical mastitis and other diseases in large dairy herds in Wisconsin. J Dairy Sci 2011;94:66.

42. Peeler EJ, Green MJ, Fitzpatrick JL, et al. Risk factors associated with clinical mastitis in low somatic cell count British dairy herds. J Dairy Sci 2000;83:2464–72.

43. Erskine RJ, Eberhart RJ, Hutchinson LJ, et al. Incidence and types of clinical mastitis in dairy herds with high and low somatic cell counts. J Am Vet Med Assoc 1988;192: 766–8.

44. Wenz JR, Barrington GM, Garry FB, et al. Use of systemic disease signs to assess disease severity in dairy cows with acute coliform mastitis. J Am Vet Med Assoc 2001;218:567–72.

45. Ruegg PL. Managing mastitis and producing high quality milk. In Risco CA, Retamal PM, editors. Dairy production medicine. West Sussex (UK): Wiley Blackwell; 2011. p. 207–32.

46. Erskine RJ, Bartlett PC, VanLente JL, et al. Efficacy of systemic ceftiofur as a therapy for severe clinical mastitis in dairy cattle. J Dairy Sci 2002;85:2571–5.

47. Deluyker HA, Chester ST, van Oye SN. A multilocation clinical trial in lactating dairy cows affected with clinical mastitis to compare the efficacy of treatment with intra-mammary infusions of a lincosin/neomycin combination with an ampicillin/cloxacillin combination. J Vet Pharmacol Therap 1999;22:274–82.

48. Koskinen MT, Holopainen J, Pyorala S, et al. Analytical specificity and sensitivity of a real-time polymerase chain reaction assay for identification of bovine mastitis pathogens. J Dairy Sci 2009;92:952–9.

49. Taponen S, Salmikivi L, Simojoki H, et al. Real-team polymerase chain reaction-based identification of bacteria in milk samples from bovine clinical mastitis with no growth in conventional culturing. J Dairy Sci 2009;92:2610–7.

50. Neeser NL, Hueston WD, Godden SM, et al. Evaluation of the use of an on-farm system for bacteriologic culture of milk from cows with low-grade mastitis. J Am Vet Med Assoc 2006;228:254–60.
51. Lago A, Godden SM, Bey R, et al. The selective treatment of clinical mastitis based on on-farm culture results. II: Effects on lactation performance including, clinical mastitis recurrence, somatic cell count, milk production and cow survival. J Dairy Sci 2011; 94:4457–67.
52. Fetrow J. Mastitis: an economic consideration. In Proceedings of the 39th Annual Conference National Mastitis Council; Atlanta (GA). Madison (WI): NMC; February 13–16, 2000. p. 3–4.
53. Barker AR, Schrick FN, Lewis MJ, et al. Influence of clinical mastitis during early lactation on reproductive performance of Jersey cows. J. Dairy Sci 1998;81:1285–90.
54. Schrick FN, Hockett ME, Saxton AM, et al. Influence of subclinical mastitis during early lactation on reproductive parameters. J Dairy Sci 2001;84:1407–12.
55. Santos JE, Cerri RL, Ballou MA, et al. Effect of timing of first clinical mastitis occurrence on lactational and reproductive performance of Holstein dairy cows. Anim Repro Sci 2004;80:31–45.
56. Rodrigues ACO, Ruegg PL. Actions and outcomes of Wisconsin dairy herds completing milk quality teams. J Dairy Sci 2005;88:2672–80.
57. Rodrigues ACO, Roma CL, Amaral TGR, et al. On-farm culture and guided treatment protocol. Proceedings of the 48th Annual Meeting of the NMC; Charlotte (NC). Madison (WI): NMC; January 25 –28, 2009. p. 148–9.

Antimicrobial Resistance of Mastitis Pathogens

Stephen P. Oliver, PhD[a],*, Shelton E. Murinda, PhD[b]

KEYWORDS

- Antibiotics • Antimicrobial resistance • Bovine mastitis • Mastitis pathogens
- Milk

KEY POINTS

- Antibiotics are used in the dairy industry for the prevention and control of mastitis and other diseases affecting dairy cows.
- Scientific evidence does not support widespread, emerging resistance among mastitis pathogens to antibacterial drugs even though many of these antibiotics have been used in the dairy industry for treatment and prevention of disease for several decades.
- However, it is clear that use of antibiotics in dairy cows can contribute to increased antimicrobial resistance.
- The use of antibiotics at times when animals are susceptible to new infection is a sound management decision and a prudent use of antibiotics on the farm.
- As the debate on the use of antibiotics in animal agriculture continues, we need to consider the consequences of "What would happen if antibiotics are banned for use in the dairy industry and in other food-producing animals?" This question should be an important aspect in this ongoing and controversial debate!

The production of maximum quantities of high-quality milk is an important goal of every dairy producer. High-quality milk tastes better, is more nutritious, and has a longer shelf-life. On the other hand, poor- or reduced-quality milk affects all segments of the dairy industry, ultimately resulting in milk with decreased manufacturing properties and dairy products with reduced shelf-life. Mastitis is the most important factor associated with reduced milk quality.

Mastitis is an inflammation of the udder that affects a high proportion of dairy cows throughout the world. Mastitis differs from most other animal diseases in that several

---

The authors have nothing to disclose.

[a] Department of Animal Science and UT AgResearch, The University of Tennessee, 2621 Morgan Circle Drive, 103 Morgan Hall, Knoxville, TN 37996, USA; [b] Animal and Veterinary Sciences Department and Center for Antimicrobial Research and Food Safety, California State Polytechnic University, 3801 West Temple Avenue, California State Polytechnic University, Pomona, CA 91768, USA
* Corresponding author.
E-mail address: soliver@utk.edu

Vet Clin Food Anim 28 (2012) 165–185
http://dx.doi.org/10.1016/j.cvfa.2012.03.005
0749-0720/12/$ – see front matter © 2012 Elsevier Inc. All rights reserved.

diverse bacteria are capable of infecting the udder. These pathogens invade the udder, multiply there, and produce harmful substances that result in inflammation, reduced milk production, and altered milk quality.[1] Because mastitis can be caused by many different pathogens, control can be difficult and economic losses due to mastitis can be immense. The National Mastitis Council estimates that mastitis costs dairy producers in the United States more than $2 billion annually.[2] Thus, mastitis continues to be one of the most significant limiting factors, if not the most significant, to profitable dairy production in the United States and throughout the world.

CONTROL OF MASTITIS

Mastitis is a difficult disease to control because many different bacteria are capable of infecting the udder and producing the disease. Microorganisms that most frequently cause mastitis can be divided into 2 broad categories: contagious pathogens (*Streptococcus agalactiae*, *Staphylococcus aureus*, and *Mycoplasma* spp), which are spread from cow to cow primarily during the milking process, and environmental pathogens (*Streptococcus uberis*, *Streptococcus dysgalactiae* subsp *dysgalactiae*, and coliforms including *Escherichia coli* and *Klebsiella* spp), which are found throughout the habitat of dairy cows.[2]

MASTITIS AND ANTIBIOTIC THERAPY

Despite mastitis control measures such as pre- and post-milking teat disinfection and good milking-time hygiene, cows that develop mastitis often require antibiotic intervention. The term "antibiotic" in this review is used to encompass all antimicrobials used in control of mastitis in dairy cows. Antibiotic therapy of clinical mastitis involves (1) detection of the infected quarter, (2) prompt initiation of treatment, (3) administration of the full series of recommended treatments, (4) maintaining a set of treatment records, (5) identification of treated cows, and (6) ensuring the milk is free of antibiotic residues before adding to the bulk tank.

Dry Cow Antibiotic Therapy

A classic study by Neave and colleagues[3] demonstrated that udders were markedly susceptible to new intramammary infection (IMI) during the early dry (nonlactating) period. The rate of new IMI during the first 21 days of the dry period was over 6 times higher than the rate observed during the previous lactation. Studies have also shown that udders are highly susceptible to new IMI near calving.[4–8] Increased susceptibility to new IMI is likely associated with physiologic transitions of the mammary gland either from or to a state of active milk production.[8] Many IMIs that occur at this time persist throughout the dry period and are often associated with clinical mastitis after calving. Thus, the early and late portions of dry period were identified as extremely important times for the control of mastitis in dairy cows.

Most dairy advisors recommend that all mammary quarters of all cows be infused with antibiotics approved for use in dry cows following the last milking of lactation. The objectives of dry cow therapy are 2-fold: (1) to eliminate infections present during late lactation and (2) to prevent new infections during the early dry period when mammary glands are highly susceptible to new IMI. Antibiotic therapy at drying off plays an important role in the control of mastitis during the dry period.

Some Issues Associated with Antibiotic Use in Dairy Cows

Antibiotics are used extensively in food-producing animals to combat disease and to improve animal performance. On dairy farms, antibiotics such as penicillin, cephalosporin, streptomycin, tetracycline, and many others are used for treatment and prevention of mastitis caused by a variety of gram-positive and gram-negative bacteria. Antibiotics are often administrated routinely to entire herds to prevent mastitis during the dry period. Benefits of antibiotic use include healthier, more productive cows; lower disease incidence; reduced morbidity and mortality; decreased pathogen loads; and production of abundant quantities of nutritious, high-quality milk for human consumption. In contrast to these benefits, however, are suggestions that agricultural use of antibiotics may be partly (largely) responsible for the emergence of antimicrobial-resistant bacteria, which in turn may impact treatment of diseases affecting the human population that require antibiotic intervention. In addition, milk from cows treated for mastitis is associated with a higher incidence of antibiotic residues in milk.[9] The risk of antibiotic residues in raw milk is not only a public health and food safety issue but an important economic factor for the producer who gets penalized for adulterated milk and for the milk processing plant that jeopardizes the manufacture of dairy foods by processing adulterated milk. Readers are encouraged to read reviews that have been published on the topic of antimicrobial use in food-producing animals and development of antimicrobial resistance.[10–14]

Data from the US Department of Agriculture (USDA) National Animal Health Monitoring System (NAHMS) Dairy 2007 study conducted in 17 major dairy US states in 79.5% of dairy operations and 82.5% of dairy cows revealed that the percentage of farms that treated cows with any antibiotic was 85.4% for mastitis, 58.6% for lameness, 55.8% for respiratory, 52.9% for reproduction, 25.0% for diarrhea or other digestive problems, and 6.9% for all other categories.[15] The percentage of cows treated with antibiotics was 16.4% for mastitis, 7.4% for reproduction, 7.1% for lameness, 2.8% for respiratory, and 1.9% for diarrhea or other digestive problems.[15] Antibiotics are also used frequently on dairy farms for disease prevention. Over 90% of dairy farms practiced antibiotic dry cow therapy.[15,16] Approximately 80% of farms that practiced antibiotic dry cow therapy treated all cows on the farm.

Several antibiotics are used for treatment and prevention of diseases of dairy cows. Mastitis continues to be the most commonly treated disease of dairy cows. Cephalosporin was the most widely used antibiotic for treatment of mastitis; 53.2% of cows were treated with cephalosporin. Other antibiotics used frequently to treat cows with mastitis included lincosamide (19.4% of cows), and 19.1% of cows were treated with noncephalosporin β-lactam antibiotics. Penicillin G/dihydrostreptomycin and cephapirin were the 2 most commonly used antibiotics for dry cow therapy.[15]

Results from the NAHMS Dairy 2007 study regarding antibiotic use and types of antibiotics used were consistent with results from the NAHMS Dairy 2002 study. Antibiotic use in adult cattle on dairy farms remained mostly unchanged. Mastitis continues to be the most common disease where antibiotics are used; about 85% of dairy farms use antibiotics to treat cows with mastitis and approximately 90% of dairy farms use antibiotics at drying off. Most cows with mastitis are treated by intramammary infusion of the antibiotic. Cephalosporin continued to be the most commonly used antibiotic for the treatment of mastitis.[15,16]

RESISTANCE PATTERNS OF MASTITIS PATHOGENS ISOLATED FROM DAIRY COWS

According to the National Mastitis Council's Expert Group, currently available scientific evidence does not support widespread, emerging antimicrobial drug resistance among mastitis pathogens.[17] Although resistance to antimicrobial drugs among mastitis pathogens has been well documented for nearly 4 decades, evidence has not been presented to suggest that this is either an emerging or a progressing phenomenon. Inferences on development of resistance in relation to antimicrobial

Table 1
Antimicrobial resistance of *S aureus* from bovine mastitis in the United States and Chile

Antibiotic	% Resistant			
Amox-Clav[a]	—[b]	—	—	38.1
Ampicillin	49.6	10.8/14.3[c]	6.5/2.4[d]	26
Ceftiofur	0.2	2.4	43.1/44.7	6.1
Cephalothin	0.2	2.4/0	0/1.2	—
Erythromycin	6.9	—	28.9/25.9	—
Gentamicin	1.1	—	—	3.3
Oxacillin	0.6	3.6/1.8	1.9/0	—
Oxytetracycline	—	—	—	6.8
Penicillin	49.6	26.5/39.3	11.8/2.4	28.8
Pirlimycin	2.1	3.6/7.1	23.1/5.9	8.3
Sulfatrimethoprim	0.6	—	—	6.9
Tetracycline	8.5	—	5.8/3.6	—
Country	USA	USA	USA	Chile
Duration of study	7 y	16 mo	1 y	2 y
Reference	Erskine et al[19]	Rajala-Schultz et al[20]	Pol and Ruegg[18]	San Martin et al[21]

[a] Amoxacilin-clavulinic acid.
[b] —, not tested.
[c] First lactation versus older cows.
[d] Organic versus conventional dairying.

drug therapy are confounded by lack of science-based evidence that presents comparative antibiograms that demonstrate resistance trends over time, before and after drug administration.[17] Except for a report by Pol and Ruegg,[18] studies that quantified antimicrobial usage at the farm or cow level are also lacking.

A summary of some of the pertinent literature on the antimicrobial resistance of *S aureus*[18–27] (**Tables 1** and **2**), coagulase-negative *Staphylococcus* (CNS) sp[18,20,22–26,28,29] (**Tables 3** and **4**), environmental *Streptococcus* sp[28–30] (**Table 5**), *E coli*[19,21,24,25,29] (**Table 6**), other gram-negative bacteria[19,20,28,31] (**Table 7**), *S uberis*[19,22,23,26,30,32] (**Table 8**), *S dysgalactiae*[19,22,26,32,34] (**Table 9**), *S agalactiae*[19,22,30] (**Table 10**), and esculin-positive *Streptococcus* and *Entero-coccus* spp[18,20,21,32] (**Table 11**) isolated in milk from cows with mastitis worldwide is presented. Importantly, only data from studies that were conducted over a period of 6 months and greater were considered. The most extensive available data were from a 7-year study by Erskine and colleagues[19] and a 6-year study by Nam and colleagues.[31]

TREND STUDIES ON RESISTANCE PATTERNS OVER TIME IN RESPONSE TO ANTIBIOTIC USE

Very few studies have amply demonstrated long-term effects or trends (eg, over 3–7 years[19,30–32]) regarding the use of antibiotics on antimicrobial susceptibility of mastitis pathogens from dairy cows. Most studies referenced in this review conducted studies over a shorter time-frame of 6 months to 2 years.[18,20–26]

In the longest trends that were reported, from a 7-year study of Michigan dairy herds that included gram-positive (see **Tables 1** and **8–10**) and gram-negative (see

Table 2						
Antimicrobial resistance of *S aureus* from bovine mastitis in Europe and Iran						
Antibiotic			% Resistant			
Amox-Clav[a]	—[b]	—	—	—	—	—
Ampicillin	59.5	—	—	—	0/0[d]	64
Ceftiofur	—	—	—	—	2.2/0	—
Cephalothin	3.8	—	—	—	—	—
Chloramphenicol	—	—	—	—	19.6/6.1	—
Clindamycin	18.1	—	—	—	4.3/0	22
Erythromycin	4.8	3.1/1.0[c]	0	1.9	8.7/0	—
Gentamicin	6.8	0.8/2.4	0	0.5	10.9/6.1	0
Oxacillin	—	—	0	0	6.5/0	0
Oxytetracycline	—	—	—	—	—	—
Penicillin	61.4	14.1/17	4	7.1	13.0/3	56
Pirlimycin	—	—	—	—	—	—
Sulfatrimethoprim	3.4	—	—	0	—	2
Tetracycline	4.1	1.6/1.4	3	—	2.2/0	22
Vancomycin	—	0/0	—	—	0/0	—
Country	Estonia	Germany	Sweden	Sweden	Switzerland	Iran
Duration of study	2 y	2 y	1 y	1 y	1 y	6 mo
Reference	Kalmus et al[22]	Botrel et al[23]	Persson[24]	Bengtsson et al[25]	Roesch et al[26]	Sahebekhtiari et al[27]

[a] Amoxacilin-clavulinic acid.
[b] —, not tested.
[c] Clinical versus subclinical cows.
[d] Organic versus conventional dairying.

Tables 6 and **7**) mastitis pathogens, the proportion of bacterial isolates susceptible to antibiotics did not change for the majority of tests.[19] On the other hand, Rajala-Schultz and colleagues[20] conducted a 16-month study on antimicrobial susceptibility of mastitis pathogens isolated from first lactation and older dairy cows (see **Tables 1, 4, 7,** and **11**). Their results appear to support the notion that use of antibiotics is a main factor in development of antibiotic resistance. The study targeted CNS, esculin-positive streptococci, and gram-negative pathogens (*E coli, Serratia* spp, *Klebsiella* spp, *Citrobacter* spp, and *Enterobacter* spp). Most resistance was observed against penicillin, with 39% and 26% of CNS isolates from older cows and first lactation cows, respectively, demonstrating resistance to this antimicrobial. Differences in proportions of resistant isolates between the 2 groups were not statistically significant.[20]

Conclusions from 14 short-term to long-term studies (**Table 12**) that reported resistance in mastitis pathogens over a period of 6 months to 7 years suggest that most mastitis pathogens are generally susceptible to antibiotics used for treatment of mastitis.[17,18,23–27] A few of these studies indicated increased resistance. For example, *S aureus* has demonstrated heightened resistance particularly to penicillin[21,22,24,25,27] and ampicillin.[21,27] Rajala-Schultz and colleagues[20] indicated CNS resistance was associated with antimicrobial usage in the study herd. Although generally susceptible to most antibiotics,[21] *E coli* has demonstrated increased

Table 3
Antimicrobial resistance of CNS from bovine mastitis in Europe

Antibiotic	% Resistant				
Amox-Clav[a]	—[b]	—	—	—	0/0[d]
Ampicillin	38.5	—	—	—	—
Ceftiofur	—	—	—	—	0/0
Cephalothin	3.6	—	0	—	—
Chloramphenicol	—	—	0	0	10.5/0
Clindamycin	17.6	—	—	—	5.3/5.3
Erythromycin	14.5	13.8/7.3[c]	0	3.6	0/5.3
Gentamicin	1.4	1.2/1.5	0	1.8	5.3/0
Oxacillin	—	—	0	0	26.3/42.1
Oxytetracycline	—	0/0	—	—	—
Penicillin	34.5	40/30.7	4	12.5	31.6/47.4
Pirlimycin	—	—	—	—	—
Sulfatrimethoprim	2.6	—	—	7.2	—
Tetracycline	11.6	—	3	5.4	1/0
Vancomycin	—	—	—	0/0	0/0
Country	Estonia	Germany	Sweden	Sweden	Switzerland
Duration of study	2 y	2 y	1 y	1 y	1 y
Reference	Kalmus et al[22]	Botrel et al[23]	Persson et al[24]	Bengtsson et al[25]	Roesch et al[26]

[a] Amoxacilin-clavulinic acid.
[b] —, not tested.
[c] Clinical versus subclinical cows.
[d] Organic versus conventional dairying.

resistance[21,31] to some antibiotics, such as tetracycline[31] and β-lactam agents and lincomycin.[23]

One of the more consistent uses of antibiotics in dairy herds is in dry cow mastitis therapy programs in which every mammary quarter of every cow is treated at the end of the lactation period.[15,16] Over a 1-year study, during a dry cow mastitis program, therapeutic antibiotic treatment with intramammary administration of large doses of penicillin/dihydrostreptomycin had little or no effect on drug resistance to *E coli* in the dairy herd and its immediate environment.[33]

RESISTANCE OF MASTITIS PATHOGENS FROM CONVENTIONAL AND ORGANIC DAIRY FARMS

One way to assess the effect of antimicrobial use on antimicrobial resistance is to compare and contrast systems that use different production strategies—such as "organic" dairies, which use little to no antibiotics, and "conventional dairies," where antibiotics are used in all categories of dairy animals.[34] Pol and Ruegg[18] analyzed relationships between antimicrobial use at the farm level and compared organic and conventional dairies and antimicrobial susceptibility of *Staphylococcus* (see **Table 1**), CNS (see **Table 4**), and esculin-positive *Streptococcus* and *Enterococcus* spp (see **Table 11**) bacterial isolates collected from 1994 through 2000 in the United States. Contrary to expectations, more IMIs were present in organic than conventional herds.

Table 4 Antimicrobial resistance of CNS from bovine mastitis in the United States and other countries				
Antibiotic	**% Resistant**			
Ampicillin	10.8/14.3[a]	1.3/6.4[c]	16.67/57.14[c]	—
Ceftiofur	2.4/0	16.7/12	—	—
Cephalothin	2.4/0	0.6/3	—	—
Chloramphenicol	—[b]	16.7/12	—	0
Clindamycin	—	0.6/3	—	—
Erythromycin	4.8/12.5	17/14.3	—	42.86
Gentamicin	—	—	33.33/100	14.29
Oxacillin	3.6/1.8	1.3/0	—	—
Oxytetracycline	—	—	—	42.86
Penicillin	26.5/39.3	19.6/9.7	16.67/28.57	42.86
Pirlimycin	3.6/7.1	33.1/3.7	—	—
Sulfadimethoxine	12/12.5	52.5/61.5	—	—
Sulfatrimethoprim	—	—	16.67/57.14	—
Tetracycline	13.2/8.9	18.1/7	—	—
Country	USA	USA	Thailand	Iran
Duration of study	1 y	l y	8 mo	2 seasons[d]
Reference	Rajala-Schultz et al[20]	Pol and Ruegg[18]	Suriyasathaporn[20]	Ebrahimi et al[29]

[a] First lactation versus older cows.
[b] —, not tested.
[c] Organic versus conventional dairying.
[d] Assumed to translate to ~8 mo.

In fact, all isolates (ie, CNS, *Streptococcus* spp *S aureus* and *S agalactiae,* except coliforms) were more prevalent in organic herds.

Roesch and colleagues[26] indicated that antibiotic resistance in mastitis pathogens (ie, *S aureus* [see **Table 2**], non-aureus staphylococci [see **Table 3**], *S uberis* [see **Table 8**], and *S dysgalactiae* [see **Table 9**]) from organic and inorganic farms was not different. The authors suggested that this discrepancy necessitates a study of the factors accounting for the absence of reduced resistance in organic farms. A study that investigated antimicrobial susceptibility of *S aureus* in bulk tank milk in organic and conventional farms in Denmark and the United States reported small differences between organic (8.8%) and conventional (14%) farms. Penicillin resistance against CNS isolated from subclinically infected mammary quarters was 48.5% in conventional versus 46.5% in organic herds.[35]

Methicillin-Resistant S aureus (MSRA) and Bovine Mastitis

MRSA is an important human pathogen, but it can also colonize and cause infection in a variety of animal species including dairy cows. High levels of resistance to β-lactams conferred by the *mecA* gene encoding a modified penicillin-binding protein was first observed in the early 1960s.[36] MRSA have been implicated in both hospital-acquired infections (HA-MRSAs) and community-acquired infections (CA-MRSAs), including a small number of human mastitis cases and outbreaks due to

Table 5
Antimicrobial resistance of environmental *Streptococcus* species from bovine mastitis

Antibiotic	% Resistant		
Ampicillin	5.88/43.48[a]	—	—
Cephalothin	—[b]	—	11.3
Chloramphenicol	—	6.67	—
Cloxacillin	5.88/4.35	—	—
Colistin	—	46.67	—
Enrofloxacin	—	0	—
Erythromycin	—	40	0–30.7
Furazolidone	—	33.34	—
Gentamicin	29.41/26.09	13.34	28.9
Kanamycin	—	20	—
Lincomycin	—	—	52.8
Lincospectine	—	0	—
Oxacillin	—	—	39.28
Oxytetracycline	—	80	—
Penicillin	17.65/8.70	73.34	0–8.7
Streptomycin	35.29/30.43	20	—
Tetracycline	—	—	62.2
Sulfatrimethoprim	35.29/30.43	—	—
Country	Thailand	Iran	Korea, Republic
Duration of study	8 mo	2 seasons[c]	4 y 5 mo
Reference	Suriyasathaporn[28]	Ebrahimi et al[29]	[d]Nam et al[30]

[a] Organic versus conventional.
[b] —, not tested.
[c] Assumed to translate to ~8 mo.
[d] Includes *Streptococcus* spp, *S bovis*, *S oralis*, *S salivarius*, and *S intermedius*; all except *S oralis* are esculin positive.

CA-MRSA. In Europe, there have been reports of bovine mastitis caused by ST398 MRSA. Emergence of MRSA in dairy cattle may be associated with contact with other host species of animals (eg, pigs or humans) or bacterial host species such as CNS that often carry antimicrobial resistance determinants that could be transferred to coagulase-positive *S aureus* associated with mastitis.[36]

Several studies worldwide have established low levels of MRSA associated with bovine mastitis, such as in Korea,[37] Germany,[38] Switzerland,[39] Japan,[40] Turkey,[41] and Belgium.[42] Characteristics of MRSA isolates are summarized in **Table 13**. Of note, the prevalence of MRSA in *S aureus* isolates obtained from bovine mastitis ranged from 1.1% to 17.3%. It appears that certain MRSA genotypes, notably V, t001, and ST398, are widespread in Europe.[38,39,42] In some instances, bovine mastitis and human MRSA were indistinguishable.[37,38] MRSA pathogens appear to be emerging in bovine mastitis. This has great implications in animal husbandry. On the other hand, studies done on bulk tank milk (BTM) in Switzerland[39] and the United States[43] did not yield any MRSA isolates from BTM samples. The conclusions were that BTM is not a common source of MRSA. It is reasonable to assume that MRSA could cause future treatment problems in both humans and animals, including bovine mastitis due to

Table 6
Antimicrobial resistance of *E coli* from bovine mastitis worldwide

Antibiotic	% Resistant						
Ampicillin	7.4	5.9	15.7	—	—	31.3	—
Cefoperazone	—a	—	—	—	3.6	0	0.8
Ceftiofur	0	0	4.6	—	11.2	—	0.8
Cephalothin	—	—	25.5	—	—	—	0.7
Chloramphenicol	1.8	0	—	0	—	—	—
Erythromycin	—	—	—	88.24	—	—	—
Gentamicin	0	0	2	70.59	15.7	5.7	0.7
Oxytetracycline	—	—	—	88.24	20.6	—	0.8
Penicillin	—	—	—	88.24	—	—	—
Streptomycin	11	5.9	—	88.24	—	21.4	13.4
Sulfatrimethoprim	—	—	2.8	—	0	15.7	—
Tetracycline	4.9	5.9	33.2	—	—	22.2	10.4
Country	Sweden	Sweden	USA	Iran	Chile	Estonia	Germany
Duration of study	1 y	2 y	7 y	2 seasonsb	2 y	2 y	2 y
Reference	Bengtsson et al[25]	Persson et al[24]	Erskine et al[19]	Ebrahimi et al[29]	San Martin et al[21]	Kalmus et al[22]	Botrel et al[23]

a —, not tested.
b Assumed to translate to ~8 mo.

their inherent multiantibiotic resistance (**Table 13**). Genetic analysis of MRSA isolated from humans and bovine mastitis has indicated that horizontal genetic transfer between human and animal pathogens can occur.[44] It is therefore necessary to establish monitoring systems for trend analysis in bovine mastitis since it appears MRSA are an emerging pathogen in this sector.[37–42]

IMPACT OF CESSATION OF ANTIBIOTIC USE IN DAIRY COWS ON ANTIBIOTIC RESISTANCE

Complete cessation of antibiotic use for treatment of clinical mastitis may result in increased clinical mastitis incidence and increased expense in the long term.[45] Although there seems to be a consistent association between organic management and lower prevalence of antimicrobial resistance, resistant bacteria persist on organic farms even after years of antimicrobial-free management, suggesting that factors other than antimicrobial use play an important role in long-term persistence of antimicrobial resistance.[34]

Antibiotic resistance is equally likely to diminish in prevalence when antibiotic use is decreased or discontinued. Although individual bacterial strains may retain resistance genes, they are often (gradually) replaced by susceptible strains when the selective pressure is removed (reviewed by Phillips and colleagues[12]). An 8-month study was conducted in Thailand to investigate the effects of antimicrobial-resistant patterns of mastitis pathogens during an experimental farm's 6-month transition from conventional to organic farming[28] Antimicrobial resistance of mastitis pathogens in the before (conventional) and after (organic) transition periods were compared for 7 antimicrobial drugs used to treat mastitis. **Tables 4**, **5**, and **7** summarize data for CNS, environmental *Streptococcus* spp, and gram-negative mastitis bacterial isolates,

Table 7
Antimicrobial resistance of gram-negative bacteria isolated from cows with mastitis

Antibiotic	% Resistant		
Amikacin	—[b]	—	4
Amox-Clav[a]	—	—	19
Ampicillin	15.7/81.1/100[c]	0/50[e]	32.2
Ceftiofur	14.1/2.6/100	—	—
Cephalothin	4.2/98.7/98.1	—	15
Chloramphenicol	14.1/2.6/100	—	18.4
Cloxacillin	—	0/0	—
Erythromycin	100	—	—
Gentamicin	0/0/0	0/100	10.3
Kanamycin	—	—	30
Oxacillin	100	—	—
Penicillin	100	0/0	—
Pirlimycin	100	—	—
Streptomycin	—	0/0	52.8
Sulfatrimethoprim	3.7/5/98.1	0/0	—
Tetracycline	33/97.5/96.2	—	47.3
Trimethoprim	—	—	14.6
Country	USA	Thailand	Korea, Republic
Duration of study	16 mo	8 mo	6 y
Reference	Rajala-Schultz et al[20]	Suriyasathaporn[28]	[d]Nam et al[31]

Antibiotic	% Resistant	
Amikacin	—	
Amox-Clav[a]	—	
Ampicillin	0/100[f]	
Ceftiofur	—	
Cephalothin	—	
Chloramphenicol	—	
Cloxacillin	0/0	
Erythromycin	—	
Gentamicin	75/100	
Kanamycin	—	
Oxacillin	—	
Penicillin	25/0	
Pirlimycin	—	
Streptomycin	0/0	
Sulfatrimethoprim	0/0	
Tetracycline	—	
Trimethoprim	—	
Country	Thailand	
Duration of study	8 mo	
Reference	Suriyasathaporn[28]	

[a] Amoxacillin-clavulinic acid.
[b] —, not tested.
[c] *Klebsiella pneumonia, Serratia marcescens,* and *Pseudomonas aeruginosa,* respectively.
[d] The most commonly observed gram-negative bacteria were *E coli, Pseudomonas fluorescens, Klebsiella pneumonia, Enterobacter cloacae, Acinetobacter Iwaoffiljunii, Pseudomonas aeruginosa,* and *Serratia marcescens.*
[e] *Alcaligenese pyogenes* isolates; organic versus conventional.
[f] *Corynebacterium bovis* isolates; organic versus conventional.

Table 8
Antimicrobial resistance of *S uberis* isolates from bovine mastitis

Antibiotic	% Resistant					
Ampicillin	2.1	0/0[b]	—	7.5	0.4	0/0[c]
Ceftiofur	0	—	—	6.8	—	—
Cephalothin	0.2	0/09	1	2.8	0.4	—
Chloramphenicol	—[a]	15.8/11.1	—	—	—	—
Clindamycin	—	10.5/0	—	—	8	—
Enrofloxacin	—	42.1/22.2	—	3.8	—	0.5/1.2
Erythromycin	31.9	10.5/0	34.3	48.1	10.4	16.5/12.9
Gentamicin	34.2	52.6/33.3	42.4	—	28.1	0.5/0
Lincomycin	—	—	41.4	49.6	—	15.4/14.1
Oxacillin	41.7	—	33.3	3.8	—	12.6/12.9
Penicillin	5.5	5.3/11.1	8.1	49.6	0.4	—
Pirlimycin	20.1	—	—	39.1	—	—
Spiramycin	—	—	—	—	—	17/12.9
Streptomycin	—	—	—	—	—	17.1/18.8
Sulfatrimethoprim	4.4	—	—	—	4.1	—
Tetracycline	45.2	0/0	57.6	72.9	20.1	7.2/12.9
Vancomycin	—	0/0	—	—	—	0/0
Country	USA	Switzerland	Korea, Republic	USA	Estonia	Germany
Duration of study	7 y	1 y	4 y 5 mo	3 y	2 y	2 y
Reference	Erskine et al[19]	Roesch et al[26]	Nam et al[30]	Rossitto et al[32]	Kalmus et al[22]	Botrel et al[23]

[a] —, not tested.
[b] Organic versus conventional.
[c] Clinical versus Subclinical.

respectively. Generally, percentages of antimicrobial resistance before (conventional) were significantly higher than after (organic) the transition. Overall, percentages of antimicrobial resistant mastitis pathogens decreased after 6 months operating as an organic farm system.[28]

WHAT ARE THE CONSEQUENCES OF NOT USING ANTIBIOTICS?

Antibiotics are used in food-producing animals to combat disease and to improve animal performance. Benefits of antibiotic use include decreased pathogen loads, a lower incidence of disease, and a better quality food product for human consumption. Mastitis was previously reported as the most common disease requiring antibiotic treatment in lactating dairy cows and it continues to be a predominant practice.[15,16,46] According to the 2002 and 2007 NAHMS studies, which respectively represented 82.9% and 79.5% of the US dairy operations and 85.5% and 82.5% of US dairy cows, and 17 and 21 major dairy states, 16.4% and 15% of cows with mastitis were treated with antibiotics by 85% of operations (ie, 85.4% in 2002 and 84.3% in 2007). Additionally, approximately 95% of these operations used intramammary antibiotics in cows at dry-off.[15,16] The use of antibiotics in the dairy industry is therefore a sound and ethical management practice that takes the welfare of the animals and humans into consideration. It reduces the suffering of animals and

Table 9
Antimicrobial resistance of *S dysgalactiae* isolates from bovine mastitis

Antibiotic			% Resistant		
Amox-Clav[a]	—[b]	0/0[c]	0	—	—
Ampicillin	0.8	—	0	0	0/0[d]
Ceftiofur	0	0/0	0.7	—	—
Cephalothin	0.3	—	0	0	—
Chloramphenicol	—	0/0	—	—	—
Clindamycin	—	0/50	—	7.8	—
Erythromycin	16	0/50	6.6	11.7	4.1/5.5
Gentamicin	3.2	—	—	11.4	0
Lincomycin	—	—	—	—	4.1/4.3
Oxacillin	1.9	22.2/25	1.1	—	1.4/1.0
Penicillin	5.5	0/25	2	0	—
Pirlimycin	11	—	7.9	—	—
Rifampicin	—	—	—	—	5.5/3.3
Spiramycin	—	—	—	—	4.1/4.4
Streptomycin	—	—	—	—	5.5/2.2
Sulfatrimethoprim	3.5	—	—	1	—
Tetracycline	60.2	55.6/100	71.7	51.1	42.5/35.2
Vancomycin	—	0/0	—	—	0/0
Country	USA	Switzerland	USA	Estonia	Germany
Duration of study	7 y	1 y	3 y	2 y	14 mo
Reference	Erskine et al[19]	Roesch et al[26]	Rossitto et al[32]	Kalmus et al[22]	Botrel et al[23]

[a] Amoxacillin-clavulinic acid.
[b] —, not tested.
[c] Organic versus conventional.
[d] Clinical versus subclinical.

prevents pathogenesis in humans via consumption of milkborne/foodborne mastitis pathogens that are potential human pathogens.[47]

ARE THERE VIABLE ALTERNATIVES TO THE USE OF ANTIBIOTICS?

A variety of physical, chemical, and biological approaches, and combinations thereof, are continuously under investigation for the control of mastitis. Ironically, alternative approaches for the prevention and control of bovine diseases, including mastitis, have achieved only limited success. Interventions currently under investigation for mastitis disease control include improvements in housing, management systems and feed formulation, and the development of more vaccines, probiotics, and competitive exclusion products. However, it will always be necessary to have available a range of antibiotics for therapeutic use in animals. Established veterinary steps to prevent or control infectious diseases include improved husbandry practices, quarantines and other biosecurity measures, and vaccinations. Other interventions include genetic selection to enhance disease resistance, uses of antiseptics such as teat dipping to prevent mastitis, vector control, and use of probiotics or other competitive microorganisms to exclude pathogens. Moreover, control of viral and other infections can

Table 10		
Antimicrobial resistance of *S agalactiae* isolates from bovine mastitis		
Antibiotic	**% Resistant**	
Ampicillin	2.6	—	0
Ceftiofur	0	—	0
Cephalothin	0	0	0
Erythromycin	15.4	0	3.9
Gentamicin	76.9	20	36.4
Lincomycin	—[a]	60	—
Oxacillin	3.8	40	—
Penicillin	3.9	20	0
Pirlimycin	7.1	—	—
Sulfatrimethoprim	50.5	—	6.4
Tetracycline	46.2	60	21.9
Country	USA	Korea, Republic	Estonia
Duration of study	7 y	4 y 5 mo	2 y
Reference	Erskine et al[17]	Nam et al[30]	Kalmus et al[22]

[a] —, not tested.

lessen secondary bacterial infections, thus reducing the need for antimicrobial therapy.[14,47]

PRUDENT USE OF ANTIBIOTICS FOR THE TREATMENT OF MASTITIS

The prudent use of antimicrobials is an approach that takes into consideration the optimal selection of the antibiotic and the dose and duration of treatment, accompanied by reduced inappropriate and excessive use that will result in slowing the emergence of antimicrobial resistance.[48] Reviews and committees in many countries have highlighted the need for better control of licensing of antibiotics and codes for prudent use of antibiotics by veterinary practitioners and farmers.[49,50] International agencies including the Food and Agricultural Organization (FAO), World Health Organization, and World Organization for Animal Health (OIE)[51] have stressed the need to find alternative approaches to address the issue of antimicrobial use in food animal production and its effect on the emergence of antimicrobial resistance in human pathogens. In the United States, growing demand from human health organizations, nongovernment agencies, and consumers on curtailing the use of antimicrobials in food animal production has resulted in the development of programs and policies that favor judicious use of antimicrobials.[46,52]

The American Association of Bovine Practitioners (AABP) and other groups have taken proactive measures through education and outreach programs for veterinarians such that they can work effectively with their clientele on the "judicious" or "prudent" use of antimicrobials. Production of safe and wholesome animal products for human consumption is a primary goal of members of the AABP. The AABP provided prudent drug usage guidelines for dairy and beef cattle.[53]

There are several guidelines developed and used for judicious use of antimicrobials in bovine medicine (reviewed by Oliver and colleagues[46]) of which the best documented evidence is that of use of antimicrobials for dry cow therapy. Dry cow therapy

Table 11
Antimicrobial resistance of esculin-positive *Streptococcus* and *Enterococcus* spp isolated from bovine mastitis

Antibiotic	% Resistant				
Ampicillin	77.3	21.6	0	34.9	7.1/9.4[b]
Ceftiofur	63.6	13.5	—	14.2	4.8/1.9
Cephalothin	63.6	10.8	60	—	4.8/0
Erythromycin	59.1	18.9	60	—	85.7/90.6
Oxacillin	36.4	24.3	77.5	—	4.8/0
Oxytetracycline	—[a]	—	—	27.5	—
Penicillin	90.9	43.2	2.5	36.7	9.5/9.4
Pirlimycin	50	21.6	—	10.1	35.7/7.0
Spiramycin	—	—	—	—	—
Sulfadimethoxine	86.4	73	97.5	—	42.9/60.4
Sulfatrimethoprim	—	—	—	17.4	—
Tetracycline	68.2	37.8	22.5	—	48.8/16.7
Country	USA	USA	USA	Chile	USA
Duration of study	16 mo	3 y	3 y	2 y	1 y
Reference	Rajala-Schultz et al[20]	Rossitto et al[32]	Rossitto et al[32]	San Martin et al[21]	Pol & Ruegg[18]

[a] —, not tested.
[b] Organic versus conventional dairying.

has been in practice for almost 4 decades. To date, all of the investigations done thus far show clearly that β-lactam antimicrobials and other classes of antimicrobials used for dry cow therapy are as effective since their first use for treating dry cows. This demonstrates that guidelines for judicious use of antimicrobials for dry cow therapy that were developed in consensus with the industry and academia are effective at preventing the emergence of antimicrobial resistance of bovine mastitis pathogens.

The use of a particular antimicrobial should also take into consideration the relative importance of the antimicrobial in human medicine[54] and the regulations that are placed for a class of antimicrobials being considered for therapy.[55] Guidelines for antimicrobial use serve as the first effective approach toward the judicious use of antimicrobials. The guidelines should be able to lead the veterinarian to select the optimal antimicrobial therapy that takes into account the drugs or the drug class for the therapy of specific diseases, such as clinical mastitis. The sole purpose of the guidelines should be to minimize inappropriate use of antibiotics, and considerations should include the type of drug used and dosage and duration of treatment. It is recommended that guidelines should be developed in consultation with a variety of individuals including veterinarians, microbiologists, epidemiologists, those in the pharmaceutical industry, state and federal regulatory agents, and members of nonprofit organizations such as the National Mastitis Council, American Veterinary Medical Association, and AABP.

Although it did not pass, a recent bill in the 111th Congress (2009–2010), HR 1549: Preservation of Antibiotics for Medical Treatment Act of 2009 had 109 co-sponsors on the bill (http://www.govtrack.us/congress/bill.xpd?bill=h111-1549). Several organizations such as the Union of Concerned Scientists, The Pew Trust, and the American

Table 12
Conclusions from short- to long-term studies on the effect of antibiotics on resistance of mastitis pathogens worldwide

Reference	Country	Comment
Bengtsson et al[25]	Sweden	Bacteria associated with acute mastitis for the most part were susceptible to antibiotics used in therapy, but resistance to penicillin in *S aureus* is not uncommon.
Botrel et al[23]	France	The overall proportion of antibiotic resistance was low, except for penicillin G in staphylococci, as well as for macrolides and tetracycline in streptococci.
Ebrahimi et al[29]	Iran	Results indicated the world hazard of increased resistance by environmental mastitis pathogens. *E coli* resistance (71%–88% for 5 of 11 antibiotics) was most pronounced.
Erskine et al[19]	USA	Analysis for linear trends indicated increased susceptibility by some pathogens to some antibiotics. Overall, there was no indication of increased resistance of mastitis isolates to antibacterials that are commonly used in dairy cattle mastitis.
Kalmus et al[22]	Estonia	Antimicrobial resistance was highly prevalent, especially penicillin resistance in *S aureus* and CNS.
Nam et al[30]	Korea	Wide differences in the prevalence of resistance were apparent among individual *Streptococcus* spp. Some were 100% susceptible, but others showed varying rates of resistance.
Nam et al[31]	Korea	There was no significant change in the prevalence of bacterial and the proportion of antimicrobial resistance among gram-negative bacteria isolates during a 6-y period. A relatively high resistance to tetracycline was observed.
Persson et al[24]	Sweden	*S aureus* and CNS were the most frequently isolated pathogens. Whereas, 45% of *S aureus* isolates and 35% of the CNS isolates were resistant to penicillin G. Resistance to other antimicrobials was uncommon.
Pol & Ruegg[18]	USA	Most isolates of *S aureus*, CNS, and *Streptococcus* spp were inhibited at the lowest dilution of most antimicrobial drugs tested. Exposure to most antimicrobial drugs commonly used for prevention and treatment of mastitis was not associated with resistance.
Rajala-Schultz et al[20]	USA	Differences in the proportions of resistant isolates of CNS between first lactation and older cows were not statistically significant. Resistance patterns of the CNS isolated during the study were concordant with antimicrobial usage in the study herd.
Roesch et al[26]	Switzerland	Antibiotic resistance in mastitis pathogens (*S aureus,* non-aureus staphylococci, *S dysgalactiae, S uberis*) from organic and conventional dairy farms was not different.
Rossitto et al[32]	USA	*Enterococcus* spp were the most resistant organisms tested. Environmental streptococci are a diverse group of organisms composed of several different genera and species and their identification to species level is needed for targeted control methods.

(continued on next page)

Table 12
(continued)

Reference	Country	Comment
Sahebekhtiari et al[27]	Iran	All *S aureus* isolates were susceptible to ciprofloxacin, gentamicin, imipenem, minocycline, oxacillin, and vancomycin and demonstrated highest resistance to ampicillin (64%) and penicillin (56%), and median resistance to other antimicrobials.
San Martin et al[21]	Chile	*E coli* was sensitive to most antimicrobials. CNS demonstrated greatest resistance (26.8%–56.9%) to antibiotics. *S aureus* showed the highest level of resistance (24.7%–38.9%) to five antibiotics. Streptococcal strains were highly resistant to lincomycin (61.9%).
Suriyasathaporn[28]	Thailand	Percentages of antimicrobial resistant bacteria (CNS, environmental streptococci, *A pyogenes*, *C bovis*) at a former organic farm decreased after 6 mo operating as an organic farm system.

Medical Association have called for stricter regulation or "phasing out" use of antimicrobials in food animal practice, starting with antimicrobials used in livestock feed for prophylactic purposes. The primary contention of these organizations is that use of antimicrobials is not regulated and antibiotics are used extensively in food animal

Table 13
Characteristics of bovine mastitis–associated MRSA strains isolated worldwide

			MRSA Isolates			
Prevalence	6.2%	N/A	1.4%	1.1%	17.2%	9.3%
PVL[a] gene	—[g]	—	—	—	—	—
SCC*mec* types[b]	IV, IVa	IV, V	V	II, IIIa	III, IV	IVa, V
spa[c] types	t286, t324, Untypable	t011, t034, t2576	t011	t002, t375, t5266	t190, t030	t011, t567
SE[d]	N/A[h]	—	A, D	N/A	N/A	N/A
MLST[e]	ST1, ST72	ST398	ST398	ST5, ST89	ST8, ST239	ST398
MDR[f]	+[i]	+	+	+	+	+
Country	Korea	Germany	Switzerland	Japan	Turkey	Belgium
Reference	Nam et al[37]	Fessler et al[38]	Huber et al[39]	Hata et al[40]	Turkiylmaz et al[41]	Vanderhaeghen et al[42]

[a] PLV, Panton-Valentin leukocidin gene.
[b] SCC*mec* types, *Staphylococcus* cassette chromosomal methicillin gene types.
[c] *spa*, staphylococcal toxin gene.
[d] SE, *Staphylococcus* enterotoxin.
[e] MLST, multilocus sequence typing.
[f] MDR, multiple drug resistance.
[g] —, negative.
[h] N/A, data not available.
[i] +, positive for multiple drug resistance.

practice, and this has led to and continues to lead to the rise of antimicrobial-resistant bacteria in the human population. On the other hand, the AVMA is of the opinion that science-based data and decisions should be considered before any legislative action is called for. To address the issue of antimicrobial resistance, prudent drug use guidelines developed by the AVMA state that "Prophylactic or metaphylactic use of antimicrobials should be based on a group, source, or production unit evaluation rather than be utilized as standard practice."[55(p16)]

In the European Union, there is growing pressure to evaluate the use of antibiotics in livestock based on the Precautionary Principle. In fact, several European Union countries have instituted restrictions on use of antibiotic growth promoters in food animals, with varying degrees of success.[56] The premise of the Precautionary Principle is that use of an antibiotic in livestock production should be halted if there is any future possibility that it could lead to the development of resistant bacteria that could threaten human health.[57] On the other hand, according to Phillips and colleagues,[12] the banning of antibiotic use in animals based on the Precautionary Principle in the absence of a full quantitative risk assessment is likely to be wasted at best and even harmful to both animal and human health.

SUMMARY

Antibiotics are used extensively in the dairy industry to combat disease and to improve animal performance. Antibiotics such as penicillin, cephalosporin, strepto-mycin, and tetracycline are used for the treatment and prevention of diseases affecting dairy cows caused by a variety of gram-positive and gram-negative bacteria. Antibiotics are often administrated routinely to entire herds to prevent mastitis during the dry period. An increase in the incidence of disease in a herd generally results in increased use of antimicrobials, which in turn increases the potential for antibiotic residues in milk and the potential for increased bacterial resistance to antimicrobials. Continued use of antibiotics in the treatment and prevention of diseases of dairy cows will continue to be scrutinized. It is clear that strategies employing the prudent use of antimicrobials are needed. This clearly illustrates the importance of effective herd disease prevention and control programs.

Based on studies published to date, scientific evidence does not support wide-spread, emerging resistance among mastitis pathogens to antibacterial drugs even though many of these antibiotics have been used in the dairy industry for treatment and prevention of disease for several decades. However, it is clear that use of antibiotics in dairy cows can contribute to increased antimicrobial resistance. While antimicrobial resistance does occur, we are of the opinion that the advantages of using antibiotics for the treatment of mastitis far outweigh the disadvantages. The clinical consequences of antimicrobial resistance of dairy pathogens affecting humans appear small. Antimicrobial resistance among dairy pathogens, particularly those found in milk, is likely not a human health concern as long as the milk is pasteurized. However, there are an increasing number of people who choose to consume raw milk. Transmission of an antimicrobial-resistant mastitis pathogen and/or foodborne pathogen to humans could occur if contaminated unpasteurized milk is consumed, which is another important reason why people should not consume raw milk. Likewise, resistant bacteria contaminating meat from dairy cows should not be a significant human health concern if the meat is cooked properly.

Prudent use of antibiotics in the dairy industry is important, worthwhile, and necessary. Use of antibiotics at times when animals are susceptible to new infection such as the dry period is a sound management decision and a prudent use of antibiotics on the farm. Strategies involving prudent use of antibiotics for treatment encompass identification of the pathogen causing the infection, determining the susceptibility/resistance of the pathogen to assess the most appropriate antibiotic to use for treatment, and a sufficient treatment duration to ensure effective concentrations of the antibiotic to eliminate the pathogen.

As the debate on the use of antibiotics in animal agriculture continues, we need to consider the consequences of, "What would happen if antibiotics are banned for use in the dairy industry and in other food-producing animals?" The implications of this question are far reaching and include such aspects as animal welfare, health, and well-being and impacts on food quantity, quality, and food costs. This question should be an important aspect in this ongoing and controversial debate!

REFERENCES

1. Oliver SP, Calvinho LF. Influence of inflammation on mammary gland metabolism and milk composition. 2nd Intl. Workshop on Biology of Lactation in Farm Animals. J Anim Sci 1995;(Suppl 2)73:18–33.
2. Hogan JS, Berry E, Hillerton E, et al. Current concepts of bovine mastitis. 5th edition. Verona (WI): National Mastitis Council; 2011.
3. Neave FK, Dodd FH, Henriques E. Udder infections in the "dry period." J Dairy Res 1950;17:375.
4. Smith KL, Todhunter DA, Schoenberger PS. Environmental pathogens and intramammary infection during the dry period. J Dairy Sci 1985;68:402–17.
5. Smith KL, Todhunter DA, Schoenberger PS. Environmental mastitis-cause, prevalence, prevention. J Dairy Sci 1985;68:1531–53.
6. Oliver SP. Frequency of isolation of environmental mastitis-causing pathogens and incidence of new intramammary infection during the nonlactating period. Am J Vet Res 1988;49:1789–93.
7. Oliver SP, Mitchell BA. Susceptibility of bovine mammary gland to infections during the dry period. J Dairy Sci 1983;66:1162–6.
8. Oliver SP, Sordillo LM. Udder health in the periparturient period. J Dairy Sci 1988;71: 2584–606.
9. Ruegg PL. Relationship between bulk tank milk somatic cell count and antibiotic residues. In: Proceedings of the National Mastitis Council. Verona (WI): National Mastitis Council; 2005; pp. 28–35.
10. van den Bogaard AE, Stobberingh EE. Epidemiology of resistance to antibiotics: Links between animals and humans. Intl J Antimicrobial Agents 2000;14:327–35.
11. McEwen SA, Fedorka-Cray PJ. Antimicrobial use and resistance in animals. Clin Infect Dis 2002;34:S93–106.
12. Phillips I, Casewell M, Cox T, et al. Does the use of antibiotics in food animals pose a risk to human health? A critical review of published data. J Antimicrob Chemother 2004;53:28–52.
13. Mathew AG, Cissell R, Liamthong S. Antibiotic resistance in bacteria associated with food animals: a United States perspective of livestock production. Foodborne Pathog Dis 2007;4:115–33.
14. Oliver SP, Murinda SE. Interventions to improve the safety of milk production. In Callaway T, Edrington T, editors. Advances in food safety and food microbiology: on-farm strategies to control foodborne pathogens. New York: NOVA Science Publishers; 2012, in press.
15. USDA APHIS. United States Department of Agriculture, Animal Plant Health Inspection Service National Animal Health Monitoring System. Antibiotic use on U.S. dairy operations, 2002 and 2007. Available at: http://nahms.aphis.usda.gov/dairy/index. htm#dairy2007. Accessed October 2, 2011.

16. USDA APHIS. United States Department of Agriculture, Animal Plant Health Inspection Service National Animal Health Monitoring System. Highlights of Dairy 2007, part III: reference of dairy cattle health and management practices in the United States, 2007. Available at: http://nahms.aphis.usda.gov/dairy/index.htm#dairy2007. Accessed April 23, 2010.

17. Erskine R, Cullor J, Schaellibaum M, et al. Bovine mastitis pathogens and trends in resistance to antibacterial drugs. National Mastitis Council Research Committee Report. In: Proceedings of the National Mastitis Council. Verona (WI): National Mastitis Council; 2004. p. 400–14.

18. Pol M, Ruegg PL. Relationship between antimicrobial drug usage and antimicrobial susceptibility of gram-positive mastitis pathogens. J Dairy Sci 2007;90:262–73.

19. Erskine RJ, Walker RD, Bolin CA, et al. Trends in antibacterial susceptibility of mastitis pathogens during a seven-year period. J Dairy Sci 2002;85:1111–8.

20. Rajala-Schultz PJ, Smith KL, Hogan JS, et al. Antimicrobial susceptibility of mastitis pathogens from first lactation and older cows. Vet Microbiol 2004;102:33–42.

21. San Martín B, Kruze J, Morales MA, et al. Antimicrobial resistance in bacteria isolated from dairy herds in Chile. Int J Appl Res Vet Med 2003;1. Available at: http://www.jarvm.com/articles /Vol1Iss1/SANMAJVM.htm. Accessed March 15, 2012.

22. Kalmus P, Aasmae B, Karssin A, et al. Udder pathogens and their resistance to antimicrobial agents in dairy cows in Estonia. Acta Vet Scand 2011;53:4.

23. Botrel MA, Haenni M, Morignat E, et al. Distribution and antimicrobial resistance of clinical and subclinical mastitis pathogens in dairy cows in Rhône-Alpes, France. Foodborne Pathog Dis 2010;7:479–87.

24. Persson Y, Nyman AK, Gronlund-Andersson U. Etiology and antimicrobial susceptibility of udder pathogens from cases of subclinical mastitis in dairy cows in Sweden. Acta Vet Scand 2011;53:36.

25. Bengtsson B, Unnerstad H, Ekman E, et al. Antimicrobial susceptibility of udder pathogens from cases of acute clinical mastitis in dairy cows. Vet Microbiol 2009;136: 142–9.

26. Roesch M, Perreten V, Doherr MG, et al. Comparison of antibiotic resistance of udder pathogens in dairy cows kept on organic and on conventional farms. J Dairy Sci 2006;89:989–97.

27. Sahebekhtiari N, Nochi Z, Eslampour MA, et al. Characterization of *Staphylococcus aureus* strains isolated from raw milk of bovine subclinical mastitis in Tehran and Mashhad. Acta Microbiol Immunol Hung 2011;58:113–21.

28. Suriyasathaporn W. Milk quality and antimicrobial resistance against mastitis pathogens after changing from a conventional to an experimentally organic dairy farm. Asian Austral J Anim Sci May 1, 2010. Available at: http://www.thefreelibrary.com/Milk+quality+and+antimicrobial+resistance+against+mastitis+pathogens. . .-a0225314875. Accessed March 15, 2012.

29. Ebrahimi A, Kheirabadi KH, Nikookhah F. Antimicrobial susceptibility of environmental bovine mastitis pathogens in west central Iran. Pak J Biol Sci 2007;10:3014–6.

30. Nam HM, Lim SK, Kang HM, et al. Prevalence and antimicrobial susceptibility of gram-negative bacteria isolated from bovine mastitis between 2003 and 2008 in Korea. J Dairy Sci 2009;92:2020–6.

31. Nam HM, Lim SK, Kang HM, et al. Antimicrobial resistance of streptococci isolated from mastitic bovine milk samples in Korea. J Vet Diagn Invest 2009;21:698–701.

32. Rossitto PV, Ruiz L, Kikuchi Y, et al. Antibiotic susceptibility patterns for environmental streptococci isolated from bovine mastitis in central California dairies. J Dairy Sci 2002;85:132–8.

33. Rollins LD, Pocurull DW, Mercer HD, et al. Use of antibiotics in a dairy herd and their effect on resistance determinants in enteric and environmental *Escherichia coli*. J Dairy Sci 1974;57:944–50.
34. Call DR, Davis MA, Sawant AA. Antimicrobial resistance in beef and dairy cattle production. Anim Health Res Rev 2008;9:159–67.
35. Sato K, Bennedsgaard TW, Bartlett PC, et al. Comparison of antimicrobial susceptibility of *Staphylococcus aureus* isolated form bulk tank milk in organic and conventional dairy herds in midwestern United States and Denmark. J Food Prot 2004;67:1104–10.
36. Holmes MA, Zadoks RN. Methicillin resistant *S. aureus* in human and bovine mastitis. J Mammary Gland Biol Neoplasia 2011. DOI: http://dx.doi.org/10.1007/s10911-011-9237-x.
37. Nam HM, Lee AL, Jung SC, et al. Antimicrobial susceptibility of *Staphylococcus aureus* and characterization of methicillin-resistant *Staphylococcus aureus* isolated from bovine mastitis in Korea. Foodborne Pathog Dis 2011;8:231–8.
38. Fessler A, Scott C, Kadlec K, et al. Characterization of methicillin-resistant *Staphylococcus aureus* ST398 from cases of bovine mastitis. J Antimicrob Chemother 2010;65:619–25.
39. Huber H, Koller S, Giezendanner N, et al. Prevalence and characteristics of methicillin-resistant *Staphylococcus aureus* in humans in contact with farm animals, in livestock, and in food of animal origin, Switzerland, 2009. Euro Surveill 2010;15:pii: 19542.
40. Hata E, Katsuda K, Kobayashi H, et al. Genetic variation among *Staphylococcus aureus* strains from bovine milk and their relevance to methicillin-resistant isolates from humans. J Clin Microbiol 2010;48:2130–9.
41. Turkyilmaz S, Tekbiyik S, Oryasin E, et al. Molecular epidemiology and antimicrobial resistance mechanisms of methicillin-resistant *Staphylococcus aureus* isolated from bovine milk. Zoon Public Health 2010;57:197–203.
42. Vanderhaeghen W, Cerpentier T, Adriaensen C, et al. Methicillin-resistant *Staphylococcus aureus* (MRSA) ST398 associated with clinical and subclinical mastitis in Belgian cows. Vet Microbiol 2010;144:166–71.
43. Virgin JE, Van Slyke TM, Lombard JE, et al. Short communication: methicillin-resistant *Staphylococcus aureus* detection in US bulk tank milk. J Dairy Sci 2009;92:4988–91.
44. Brody T, Yavatkar AS, Lin Y, et al. Horizontal gene transfers link a human MRSA pathogen to contagious bovine mastitis bacteria. PLoS One 2008;3:e3074.
45. Morin DE, Shanks RE, McCoy GC. 1998. Effectiveness of antibiotic therapy for treatment of mastitis. Available at: http://www.livestocktrail.uiuc.edu/dairynet/paper Display.cfm? Content ID=179. Accessed October 3, 2011.
46. Oliver SP, Murinda SE, Jayarao BM. Impact of antibiotic use in adult dairy cows on antimicrobial resistance of veterinary and human pathogens: a comprehensive review. Foodborne Pathog Dis 2011;8:337–55.
47. Oliver SP, Boor KJ, Murphy SC, et al. Food safety hazards associated with consumption of raw milk. Foodborne Pathog Dis 2009;7:793–806.
48. Shlaes DM, Gerding DN, John JF, et al. Society for Healthcare Epidemiology of America and Infectious Diseases Society of America Joint Committee on the Prevention of Antimicrobial Resistance: guidelines for the prevention of antimicrobial resistance in hospitals. Infect Control Hosp Epidemiol 1997;8:275–91.
49. Cattaneo AA, Wilson R, Doohan D, et al. Bovine veterinarian's knowledge, beliefs, and practices regarding antibiotic resistance on Ohio dairy farms. J Dairy Sci 2009;92:3494–502.
50. FDA. United States Food and Drug Administration. FDA issues order prohibiting extralabel use of cephalosporin antimicrobial drugs in food-producing animals. 2008. Available at: www.fda.gov/AnimalVeterinary/NewsEvents/CVMUpdates/ucm054431.htm. Accessed October 10, 2011.

51. FAO/WHO/OIE 2007. Report of the Joint FAO/WHO/OIE expert meeting on critically important antimicrobials. Rome, Italy. November 26–30, 2007. Available at: http://www.who.int/foodborne_disease/resources/Report%20joint%20CIA%20Meeting.pdf. Accessed October 1, 2010.

52. Torrence ME. Activities to address antimicrobial resistance in the United States. Prev Vet Med 2001;51:37–49.

53. American Association of Bovine Practitioners Prudent Drug Usage Guidelines for Cattle 2000. Available at: http://www.avma.org/issues/policy/jtua_cattle.asp. Accessed October 7, 2011.

54. WHO. World Health Organization. Critically important antibacterial agents for human medicine for risk management strategies of non-human use: report of a WHO working group consultation; Canberra, Australia; February 15–18, 2005. Available at: http://www.who.int/foodbornedisease/resources/FBD_CanberraAntibacterial_FEB2005.pdf. Accessed October 10, 2011.

55. DHHS:FDA:CVM. Department of Health and Human Services Food and Drug Administration Center for Veterinary Medicine 2000. Judicious use of antimicrobials for dairy cattle veterinarians. Available at: http://www.fda.gov/downloads/AnimalVeterinary/SafetyHealth/AntimicrobialResistance/JudiciousUseofAntimicrobials/UCM095571.pdf. Accessed October 6, 2011.

56. Cogliani C, Goossens H, Greko C. Restricting antimicrobial use in food animals: lessons from Europe. Microbe 2011;6:274–9.

57. McAllister TA, Yanke LJ, Inglis GD, et al. Is antibiotic use in dairy cattle causing antibiotic resistance? Adv Dairy Technol 2001;13:229–47.

The Role of Diagnostic Microbiology in Mastitis Control Programs

Allan M. Britten, DVM, MPVM

KEYWORDS

- Mastitis • Microbiology • Laboratory • Diagnostics • Culture

KEY POINTS

- The scope and quality of microbiological laboratory services can profoundly enhance the effectiveness of mastitis control programs.
- Appropriate use of culture enhancement methods can significantly increase sensitivity of detection of mastitis organisms in milk.
- Targeted use of selective media offers significant improvements in sensitivity in composite cow samples and bulk tank milk culture.
- Practitioners should recommend zero tolerance of the three major contagious mastitis pathogens Staph. aureus, Strep ag. and Mycoplasma with routine bulk tank culture and fresh cow and fresh heifer culture.
- Practitioners should be aware of the need to utilize Level 3 microbiological laboratory services to diagnose important major environmental pathogens such as Pseudomonas aeruginosa, Klebsiella pneumonia and Prototheca.
- On farm culture leading to appropriate intramammary treatment decisions can offer economic benefit to dairymen by reducing therapy costs and discarded milk.
- PCR detection of mastitis pathogens does not necessarily offer advantages in sensitivity or specificity and should be evaluated critically. The clinical relevance of PCR-positive/culture negative results due to dead bacteria detection requires further investigation.

The dairy practitioner can greatly enhance the quality of service to his or her clients by the choice made in the types of mastitis diagnostic services offered or recommended. The primary focus here will be on tools available to practitioners in traditional microbiological culture. In this regard, a variety of decisions will be made as to the features of the culture media used, the strategies for selection of diagnostic tools for different purposes, and the implications of the when and where the testing will take

The author owns and operates Udder Health Systems, Inc, a dairy health diagnostic service and mastitis laboratory supply company.
Udder Health Systems, Inc, PO Box 5776, Boise, ID 83705-0776, USA
E-mail address: allanbritten@yahoo.com

Vet Clin Food Anim 28 (2012) 187–202
http://dx.doi.org/10.1016/j.cvfa.2012.03.006
0749-0720/12/$ – see front matter © 2012 Elsevier Inc. All rights reserved.

place. Finally, some consideration should be given to alternatives to traditional culture services, such as enzyme-linked immunosorbent assay (ELISA) or polymerase chain reaction (PCR) testing, and their potential applications in mastitis control programs.

MASTITIS DIAGNOSTIC SERVICE CONSIDERATIONS

The dairy practitioner has a special opportunity to influence both the types of mastitis control practices and the types of laboratory support for the dairy farms he or she serves. The nature and quality of this laboratory support can profoundly enhance the effectiveness of the mastitis control efforts of the dairy practitioners, and it is the practitioner's responsibility to identify where and how these laboratory tools can best be used. This may include a combination of in-house mastitis diagnostic services, some on-farm testing, and selected out-lab services. A fundamental decision must be made about the relative merits of having an in-house diagnostic service at all. There exists a divergence of business models in North American dairy practice. These range from an in-house mastitis diagnostic service operated by a trained support staff to a solo practitioner who spends part of his or her time performing the laboratory services. Alternatively, practices may choose to out-lab all diagnostic services to a regional specialty mastitis laboratory. This is appropriate if a practice cannot or chooses not to invest in the necessary facilities and/or management oversight necessary to maintain the integrity of an in–house service. As culture media has a limited shelf-life, a practice must secure a sufficiently large enough laboratory business activity to justify keeping fresh media in stock, in order to maintain a quality service. Finally, the merits of an on-farm laboratory service should be weighed on how this effort could bring value to a milk quality program of a client.

The most widely used reference source for culture methods is the National Mastitis Council Laboratory Handbook.[1] For the analyst performing the culture, the recommended standard is to use blood agar as a primary isolation media for the detection of the widest variety of mastitis-causing organisms. Along with this broad scope of detection capability comes a greatly increased burden for the analyst to appropriately differentiate the variety of species that will grow on this media. In standard dairy practice, there is an economic limitation to how much cost the dairy practitioner will be willing to incur to obtain a diagnosis. As a consequence, most service labs will both limit the scope of service and accept some reductions in diagnostic accuracy in order to deliver a quality mastitis management service while maintaining an acceptable level of cost to the end user. The use of bi-plates, tri-plates, and quad-plates may offer some diagnostic conveniences to the analyst. These products typically contain selective media that offer the advantage of simplifying the decision process in identifying the organism. The disadvantage of this multi-agar approach is that it can affect the analysts' ability to detect important mastitis pathogens. Some of these multi-agar products have shorter shelf-lives (expired Edwards agars will lessen the ability to detect Streptococcus agalactia), or they use decision tree recommendations that significantly deviate from recommended practices to detect Staphylococcus aureus (insufficient application of follow-up coagulase testing).

Two terms that are frequently used to describe the quality of a testing method are "sensitivity" and "specificity." The sensitivity of a test is the probability (typically expressed as a percentage) of a test to detect a true positive. The specificity is the probability of a test to correctly identify a true negative. These 2 terms are frequently used to describe the ability of a test method to describe disease presence based on a sample. In mastitis microbiological culture, the goal is to cultivate and identify at least one colony of a single viable organism (colony-forming unit [cfu]). The diagnosis is declared when the identified organism is then said to be the cause of that case of

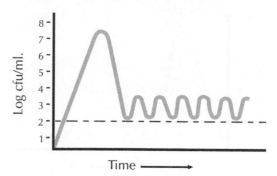

Fig. 1. Typical bacteria shedding pattern from mastitis episode. *Gray line,* bacterial numbers shed per 1 mL over time; *dashed line,* detection limit from culture of 10-μL sample.

mastitis. In any discussion using these terms, it is appropriate to discuss 2 aspects of successful detection separately: (1) the likelihood that a collected sample will contain the target organism and (2) the likelihood that the laboratory method will isolate and correctly identify the target organism.

WILL THE SHEDDING PATTERN ALLOW DETECTION?

Evidence based on shedding patterns of bacteria from experimental mastitis investigations where animals are sampled hourly after artificial inoculation,[2] as well as from natural clinical infections, show a bacterial shedding pattern "idealized" in **Fig. 1**. In many mastitis infection episodes, cfu/mL count increases rapidly early in the course of the infection. Later in the course of infection, largely due to inflammatory antibacterial responses of the cow, the cfu/mL will fall to a lower level of shedding. In many traditional culture methods, as little as 10 μL of a milk sample collected from a cow is cultured. For the culture to successfully detect even a single mastitis organism, there theoretically must be a minimum of 100 cfu/mL in the sample. For the purposes of this discussion, we will call this the detection limit of traditional culture (represented by the dashed gray line in **Figs. 1–5**). If the shedding rate of a mastitis pathogen approaches this detection limit, the presence of even 1 cfu of causative agent in a

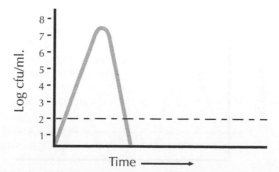

Fig. 2. Bacteria shedding pattern from a mastitis cow followed by a quick recovery. *Gray line,* bacterial numbers shed per 1 mL over time; *dashed line,* detection limit from culture of 10-μL sample.

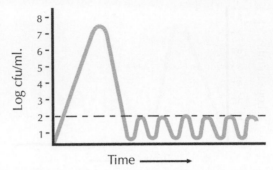

Fig. 3. Low bacteria shedding pattern from subclinical mastitis cow. *Gray line,* bacterial numbers shed per 1 mL over time; *dashed line,* detection limit from culture of 10-µL sample.

10-µL aliquot of the sample is not ensured. Shedding rates for mastitis organisms vary widely. *S aureus* mastitis is an example of an infection that is frequently characterized by relatively low shedding rates. In one study, only 75% of a group of experimentally infected *S aureus* cows showed positive on a single culture.[3] The author attributed this to the great variability in shedding patterns for these staphylococcal infections. Calculating from the data of other workers, the estimated sensitivities for culture from a single milk sample would be greater than 90% for *S aureus*.[4,5] *Mycoplasma* infections have also been shown to have variations in shedding rates above and below detection limits.[6] When pathogen shedding falls below the detection limit in a mastitis infection, the resulting false negatives threaten the success of disease management efforts, which depend on detection and separation of all infected cows to protect healthy cows. A "no growth" laboratory result could be an indication that the cow has recovered (**Fig. 2**). It can also be the case that a cow shedding below the detection limit continues to pose a threat to her herd mates even at this low level of shedding (**Fig. 3**). In the future, the infection may result in additional clinical episodes and intermittent shedding above the detectable limit (**Fig. 4**). It is therefore appropriate that some consideration be given to enhancing detection.

A number of strategies have been suggested to compensate for the detection problem of cows shedding at low levels. One tactic is to simply repeat the culture. This may allow for the detection of infected cows that intermittently shed organisms

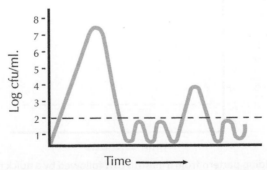

Fig. 4. Intermittent bacteria shedding pattern from chronic mastitis cow. *Gray line,* bacterial numbers shed per 1 mL over time; *dashed line,* detection limit from culture of 10-µL sample.

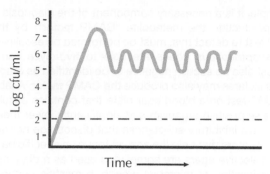

Fig. 5. High bacteria shedding pattern from a "grade buster" cow. *Gray line,* bacterial numbers shed per 1 mL over time; *dashed line,* detection limit from culture of 10-μL sample.

at slightly higher levels or increase the chance of capturing a single cfu. In one investigation, it was shown that sensitivity increased from 75% on a single sample to 94% and 98% with a second and third sampling, respectively.[3] This may be indicated particularly for aggressive contagious mastitis elimination programs, where concern for false negatives is higher. It is suggested that cows with a "no growth" history and persistent elevated somatic cell counts (SCCs) may be better candidates to reveal an organism on a subsequent culture effort.

Another strategy to increase sensitivity is to lower the detection limit by using a increasing the amount of the sample placed on the agar from the traditional 10 μL plated by loop to 100 μL delivered by pipette. It must be mentioned that this greatly enlarged volume will not be easily contained on a quarter section of agar, so this technique requires a larger surface area of agar (such as a half plate) to accommodate this larger volume. A more effective enhancement technique requires re-plating any cultures that initially show no growth after 24-hour incubation from direct plating. This second plating is done with a preincubated milk sample (4 hours at 37°C). This method has been shown to significantly increase culture sensitivity with only a minor increase in overgrowth from contaminants.[7] This enhancement method may be particularly valuable for contagious mastitis like S aureus where successful detection of low shedding infected cows is considered critical to a disease control. At Udder Health Systems laboratory, this method increases sensitivity for S aureus detection about 6%.

The terms "sensitivity" and "specificity" may also describe the ability of a test method to correctly identify an organism, once it has been isolated from a sample. Here the focus is on the components of the identification scheme used by the analyst. It is recommended that all staphylococci showing a large zone of incomplete hemolysis (from β-hemolysin production), should be called S aureus. It is also recommended that all staphylococcal colonies that do not show this hemolysis (nonhemolytic or only narrow complete hemolysis) should be tested for coagulase enzyme. These coagulase-positive strains should also be called S aureus. In our laboratory, in a study of 3018 staphylococcal isolates from milk samples, 316 were classified as S aureus by these criteria. Of these, only 65% showed the incomplete hemolysis (β zone). Hemolysin production from S aureus is highly variable. A laboratory method that fails to routinely coagulase test these non–β-staphylococci in their protocol may suffer a markedly reduced sensitivity. This serious error in methodology can result in underreporting, and it has happened where analysts have failed to diagnose an entire S aureus outbreak because it was caused by a non–β-toxin–producing strain.

In another example, it is a necessary component of the diagnosis of *S agalactia* to demonstrate the production the metabolite "CAMP factor", by the streptococcal isolate. The CAMP test to detect this, must be performed on esculin-containing blood agar plates. All *Streptococcus uberis* are able to hydrolyze esculin. The CAMP positive isolate must also be esculin negative to be identified as *S agalactia*. As many as 15% of *S uberis* isolates may also produce the CAMP factor. A laboratory that fails to perform the CAMP test on a blood agar plate that contains esculin will fail to rule out this possible false positive organism and significantly lower their test specificity.

Selective agars have inhibitory substances that discourage nontarget growth and may also contain indicators that help the analyst focus on specific bacteria groups. As mentioned earlier, selective agars are sometimes used as a diagnostic convenience to simplify the identification of microbial growth in mastitis culture. An even more valuable benefit of the use of selective agars is the opportunity to increase sensitivity. A classic selective agar is MacConkey agar, which only allows for the growth of gram-negative bacteria and also contains a lactose fermentation indicator that allows for easy identification of coliform bacteria. Another very valuable selective agar is modified Edwards media, which can be formulated to be discourage all growth except for streptococci and also contain esculin and CAMP factor indicators for rapid sensitive detection of *S agalactia*. The reduction in nontarget growth also means higher inoculation volume may be used in mixed cultures (composite cow samples, string samples, and bulk tank samples). Smith and colleagues recommended the practice of plating 100 µL onto MacConkey agar to detect low-level shedding from coliform-infected cows.[8] In a study comparing use of blood agar alone with the use of modified Edwards, there was a greater than 400% increase in detection of *S agalactia*–infected cows in 2120 composite samples from 3 problem herds.[9]

BULK TANK CULTURE

One of the simplest and most valuable steps to evaluate the udder health on a dairy is to look at its influence on the quality of milk in the bulk tank. Most dairy practitioners are well aware of the connection between mastitis-infected cows and bulk tank SCC. They may not be as aware that bacteria shed from infected quarters can also influence the total bacteria count. A bulk tank culture (BTC) is a series of laboratory cultures performed on a sample of bulk tank milk to provide counts of mastitis and nonmastitis bacteria that frequently contribute to the total bacteria count. It differs from processor-required quality testing in that it uses the same diagnostic technology used on individual cow milk samples. It can be used in troubleshooting sources of high bacteria count problems and to obtain insight into the variety of mastitis pathogens causing disease in a herd. The confirmation steps used to identify organisms in the mixed culture of bulk tank milk are essentially the same as would be used on individual cows. The challenge presented to the analyst in BTC is picking isolates of importance from the wide variety of strains present from this mixed culture grown on blood agar. Only the most seasoned analysts with significant experience diagnosing these mastitis organisms from individual cow culture are suited to this challenging protocol. BTC also reveals significant presence of nonmastitis strains introduced from teat skin or soil on milk contact surfaces of the milking equipment. **Table 1** lists several categories of organisms that can be found in BTC and their relative association with various herd milk quality and udder health problems. A short discussion follows regarding the likely significance of finding these organisms in BTC.

S aureus, S agalactia, and *Mycoplasma* are all major mastitis pathogens and are highly contagious. These contagious mastitis organisms have the greatest potential to spread to numerous cows, resulting in concurrent high bulk tank SCC. If bulk tank

Table 1
Commonly identified organisms in BTC and their expected contribution to the total bacteria count, association with various milk quality problems, potential for contagious spread, and possible original sources of the organism

Bulk Tank Organisms Chart

Organism	Goal	High Raw	High SCC	High PI	High LPC	Very Contagious	Source
S aureus	0	•	•••			••	Infected quarters
S agalactia	0	•••	••			•••	Infected quarters
E coli	<100	•	•	•			Manure/infected quarters
Klebsiella	0						Bedding/infected quarters
P aeruginosa	0	•				•	Infected quarters/water
Streptococcus spp	<500	•					Infected quarters
E. strep	<500	••	•	•			Infected quarters/skin
Staphylococcus spp	<1000						Skin/infected quarters
Pseudomonas spp	<100			••			Soil/water
Bacillus	0				••		Soil
A pyogenes	0	•					Infected quarters
Serratia	0						Infected quarters/bedding
Yeast	0						Infected quarters
Prototheca	0		••			••	Infected quarters
Mycoplasma	0		•			•••	Infected quarters

The presence of the one or more "•" symbols indicates the relative likelihood of an organisms to be associated with the problem described in the column head.

milk shows their presence, then a search should be initiated to discover and eliminate the source of these organisms. The only reasonable explanation for their detection by BTC is that they were shed from infected cows.

Streptococcus spp, environmental "streps" (E. streps), and *Staphylococcus* spp are all minor mastitis pathogens and are readily found on teat skin. They are commonly found in bulk tank milk and elevated counts may be associated with infected quarters or teat sanitation problems. The most commonly present streptococcal species in BTC are *S dysgalactia*, and many E. streps are *S uberis*. *Streptococcus* spp and E. strep mastitis infections have both occasionally resulted in "grade buster" cows that can cause extremely high bacteria counts for a period of time and elevate the bulk tank bacteria count (see **Fig. 5**). In one investigation that included an attempt to quantify bacterial shedding rates in *S uberis* mastitis cases, more than 10% of the cases had counts between 10^6 and 10^8 cfu/mL.[10]

Escherichia coli, *Klebsiella*, and *Serratia* are commonly found in manure, bedding, and sometimes water supplies in the dairy environment. They can cause acute mastitis but are a less likely cause of high bacteria counts. Contamination of milk by dirty teats or manure more likely explains high bacteria counts of these organisms. Their presence in BTC cannot reliably be assumed to be an indication of mastitis by these organisms.

Prototheca are environmental alga, but some strains can cause mastitis. They are frequently associated with contaminated surface water in the dairy environment. *Prototheca*, although considered an environmental mastitis pathogen, also may spread from cow to cow like contagious mastitis, once chronic infected cows become established in the herd. *Prototheca* mastitis may cause a persistent low level or intermittent shedding of the organism and is significantly underdiagnosed. The presence of this organism in BTC may indicate significant herd infection.

Pseudomonas aeruginosa is relatively rare but very damaging and can be mildly contagious. Its presence in bulk milk is almost certainly from infected quarters. Cows frequently become exposed from a contaminated water source. *P aeruginosa* can localize in biofilms in milking parlor hoses or other parts of the plumbing on the dairy. *Pseudomonas* spp are readily found as a non–disease-causing bacteria in the dairy environment. If there are soil deposits on the stainless or if contaminated water supplies are used in washing equipment, then they will show up in bulk tank milk. They will grow at cool temperatures and may be a cause of high persistent infection (PI) counts.

Arcanobacterium pyogenes is the most common abscess causing bacteria in cattle (uterus, skin, and udder). This is an infrequent cause of mastitis but it produces very abnormal milk and can result in high bacteria counts. Their presence in bulk tank milk indicates poor abnormal milk diversion practices. Yeast are rare fungal causes of mastitis. They are often associated with contaminated udder treatment devices.

Bacillus spp are various types of (usually) non–disease-causing bacteria. Because these organisms are from heat-resistant spores, they can cause a high lab pasteurized test. Although typically introduced into bulk tank milk from contaminated teat skin, they can grow in soil deposits on stainless steel milking equipment.

One of the most valuable uses of BTC is to detect any of the 3 major contagious mastitis pathogens: *S aureus*, *S agalactia,* and *Mycoplasma*. The culture methods used should be designed for low-level detection of these pathogens. A major challenge to their detection is the significant dilution of the bacteria count coming from infected quarters, as well as large numbers of bacteria from other sources such as teat skin and soil. It is strongly recommended that a combination of a larger sample volume in conjunction with selective media be used to increase sensitivity for detecting these organisms. *Staphylococcus*-selective agar,[11] modified Edwards media,[9] and broth-enhanced *Mycoplasma* cultures[6] have been advocated to improve sensitivity for the detection of these organisms. Inoculation volumes of 100 to 200 μL are plated onto a half plate of selective media to provide an indication of lower-level herd infection. More sensitive *Prototheca* detection may also be indicated as this organism is characterized by low shedding levels and contagious spread. Its detection in BTC can be enhanced greatly by use of *Prototheca* isolation media.[12] A more limited BTC service that only reports on the presence of contagious mastitis organisms in bulk tank milk, based solely on the culture results of one or more of these selective agars, can still be a valuable screening service for producers.

SCOPE OF SERVICE

A practical concept to help clarify the objectives of any laboratory service is to define the scope of service. In the case of a mastitis microbiological service, scope of service describes the specific mastitis organism diagnostic capabilities for which the laboratory will provide. Different service levels can be defined that provide an increasing ability to diagnose a larger variety of mastitis organism but are increasingly more expensive to implement and complex to maintain. **Table 2** depicts 4 such proposed groupings of scope of service. A culture service operating at the TNT (treat-no-treat)

Table 2
Organism identification offered by 4 different schemes of laboratory service ordered by degree of complexity

Organism	TNT	Scope of Service Levels Level 1	Level 2	Level 3
Gram positive	•			
Gram negative	•			
S agalactia		•	•	•
Strep non-ag		•		
S aureus		•	•	•
S spp		•	•	•
Mycoplasma		•	•	•
Coliform		•		
Bacillus		•	•	•
E coli			•	•
E. strep		•		
Strep spp		•		
K pneumonia			•	•
Pseudomonas			•	•
A pyogenes			•	•
S uberis				•
S dysgalactia				•
Serratia				•
P aeruginosa				•
Pasteurella				•
Proteus				•
Yeast				•
C bovis				•
Prototheca				•

The "•" in a row indicates that organism category or species will be identified by the laboratory service identified in the column heading.

service level limits its scope to only providing information about presence or absence of gram- or gram-negative growth. This simplest manifestation of a laboratory culture service provides no organism identification but does provide timely information to aid herdsman in making the economically significant intramammary treatment decision. The Level 1 service provides the necessary culture information needed for effective management of the 3 major contagious mastitis pathogens: S aureus, S agalactia, and Mycoplasma. As a narrowly focused basic scope of service, Level 1 will have the broadest practical appeal as a greater percentage of dairy producers will appreciate the economic importance of managing these major contagious mastitis pathogens. Diagnostic service Level 2 or 3 will provide a broader range of detection for mastitis-causing organisms. Many of the pathogens detected at these higher service levels can be economically damaging but may occur less frequently within herds or may affect fewer herds. The practitioner who offers these broader scopes of service is poised to help a larger number of producers with a wider variety of mastitis problems. The disadvantage comes from the increased costs of equipment, diagnostic supplies, and microbiological skills to execute these services.

THE TREATMENT DECISION

The use of antibiotics to treat clinical and subclinical infections has been an important tool for the dairy practitioner and the veterinarian as an aid to cure infected cows and improve milk quality. Since the introduction of intramammary infusion products in the 1960s, mastitis control experts have recommended that all clinical mastitis cases be treated promptly and that intramammary dry cow treatment be used routinely. These practices, along with routine post milking teat dipping and other milking time hygiene practices, have dramatically reduced the prevalence of gram-positive contagious mastitis infections. As a benefit of these control programs, many progressive dairy operations in the 1970s and 1980s became completely free of infections caused by S agalactia, and clinical mastitis caused by S aureus has become very rare. Based on this progress, some of these progressive dairy managers assumed 2 things: that clinical mastitis was entirely caused by environmental mastitis organisms on their dairies and that no benefit could be demonstrated for treating these infections with intramammary antibiotics.[13] From these new conditions came the idea that it was both appropriate and beneficial to use only "nonantibiotic" therapy (eg, oxytocin and/or more frequent milking) to treat clinical mastitis cases. Some dairy managers who used these programs were very satisfied with the outcome.[14] Supporters of this approach claimed benefits, including reduced therapy costs, lack of antibiotic residue fears, cow recoveries that remained about the same even in the absence of intramammary treatment, and continued good bulk tank milk quality. In contrast, others claimed that this lack of intramammary therapy caused an increase in bulk tank SCC and clinical mastitis from Streptococcus spp.[15] Further investigations into the efficacy of intramammary antibiotics continued to show a lack of benefit in treating "no growth" cows or those with gram-negative infections but did show significant benefit for non–S agalactia streptococcal infections.[16]

These experiences led many to conclude that an optimal decision to treat or not to treat cannot be made without knowledge of the bacteriological status of the cow. The widespread assumption of those that wanted the benefit of therapy is that they could not afford to wait for a laboratory result from a diagnostic service. The fear is that any delay in initiating therapy would greatly increase damage to the cow. Some practitioners emphasized the value of rapid culture turnaround times to help dairy practitioners make relatively prompt treatment decisions for those willing to take clinical samples to a laboratory on a daily basis.[17] Others lamented the fundamental "impossibility of establishing and etiologic diagnosis at the time of first treatment,"[18] as frequently veterinary diagnostic services are simply not sufficiently convenient for daily use.

ON-FARM TESTING

One of the simplest, yet very powerful applications for microbiological culture is the real-time use of TNT testing. In this application, an on-farm culture service is set up with a selective culture media service that defines infections as either gram-positive growth, gram-negative growth, or no growth. The strategy here is that for all mild clinical mastitis cases, no treatment decision will be made until the culture results are complete (18–24 hours). If the culture shows gram-positive growth, then intramammary treatment is initiated. An extensive controlled study comparing culture-based selective treatment strategy using the Minnesota Easy Culture System (University of

Minnesota, St Paul, MN, USA), to conventional systematic treatment of *all* mild clinical mastitis cases demonstrated significant economic benefits.[19] Significant reductions in discarded milk and a 50% reduction in antibiotic use were seen in the selective group versus the all treatment group. Despite the necessary delay in initiating treatment of gram-positive infections and no treatment of most of the cows in the culture-based treatment group, there was no significant difference in cure rates between these and the all-treatment group.

On-farm culture has also been promoted for diagnosis of selected mastitis pathogens on the farm and/or even implementing a Level 1 or Level 2 type service. Identification of non–*S agalactia* streptococci may offer an additional benefit of improving the cure rate through focused extended therapy.[20] Similar dramatic reductions in intramammary antibiotic use and smaller hospital pens have been seen in western US herds using the TNT biplate (Udder Health Systems, Inc, Boise, ID, USA). Udder Health Systems actively promotes on-farm laboratory services, and our experience has been that a TNT service will provide immediate benefits with relatively little management oversight. Only a smaller percentage of herds attempt a Level 1–type service on farm. As herd sizes grow along with increased sophistication and academic preparation of middle management, it is likely that the popularity of Level 1 or even Level 2 on-farm diagnostic services will increase.

ZERO TOLERANCE

Zero tolerance is a management attitude that says you will not allow cows with contagious infections to be milked with your clean cows. It means that if a contagious mastitis-infected cow is found, a planned management response will be implemented immediately. Three planned responses include treatment, segregation, or culling. Prompt intramammary treatment will be initiated if there is going to be an attempt to clear the infection. This approach is most suitable for any *S agalactia*–infected cow but is also appropriate for fresh heifers diagnosed with *S aureus*. Unfortunately, with the majority of contagious mastitis cases, treatment should not even be attempted, as with *Mycoplasma* or most *S aureus* cases. If no attempt is going to be made with treatment, then the cow should be milked last. Segregation of all contagious cows and milking them last is a very powerful tool for preventing new infections. In this scheme, it is not effective to simply segregate cows with a high SCC or clinical history. Segregation is about isolating the shedders. For segregation strings to be effective, they must be based on accurate culture information and all the shedders (clinical and subclinical) must be in the quarantined group. This approach has been very successful with *S aureus* mastitis management but is less commonly recommended for *Mycoplasma* mastitis. If these infected cows are not going to be segregated, then they must be culled, and the sooner the better. Culling is the preferred recommendation for *Mycoplasma* mastitis management. Because of the contagious behavior of *Prototheca* mastitis infections, it is recommended that zero tolerance by either segregation or culling be used for this major environmental pathogen.[21] Zero tolerance programs require aggressive monitoring to protect uninfected cows from being milked with contagious mastitis cows. The monitoring should include culture of all fresh cows and heifers, new herd additions, clinical mastitis cows, persistent high SCC cows, as well as monthly BTC. Detecting these contagious mastitis-infected cows for action under a comprehensive zero tolerance program is one of the most powerful applications of a Level 1 service.

ENVIRONMENTAL MASTITIS

A sophisticated Level 2 or Level 3 diagnostic service offers the veterinarian valuable detail on the types of environmental organism that are causing infections for a specific client. By knowing the name of the organism in a mastitis case, a whole spectrum of disease management opportunities open up, as known epidemiologic and pathogenic information about that species can be applied to the disease control plan. Diagnosing an environmental mastitis organism specifically as *S uberis*, *Klebsiella pneumonia*, *Pseudomonas aeruginosa,* or *Prototheca* can be essential to economic survival for the dairy practitioner who suffers from any of these less common mastitis problems. This diagnostic benefit is simply not available at a Level 1 service and the responsible consulting dairy practitioner must be poised to bring these higher levels of service into play. Level 3 services may also include detecting these pathogens in samples such as water, bedding, or contaminated disinfectant products in order to pinpoint environmental sources.

OPPORTUNITIES WITH MILK ELISA AND PCR

Modern diagnostic methodology and laboratory automation are creating new opportunities for animal health testing. Examples of these technologies include ELISA and PCR testing. Commercial testing platforms have been developed and promoted by manufacturers and are increasingly being taken up by private and university laboratories. In addition, there have been some adaptations of these technologies to perform disease testing on cow milk samples. As milk samples are routinely collected on many cows for Dairy Herd Improvement Association (DHIA) monthly testing, this offers a tremendous advantage for access to the dairy population for dairy health programs. Increasingly, we see DHIA organizations expanding their scope of service to take advantage of this access to samples, both to increase revenue and to increase customer service. Veterinary laboratories that are routinely involved in mastitis diagnostic services are also in an excellent position to acquire milk samples from individual cows as part of scheduled mastitis prevention and monitoring programs. The opportunity is there for these laboratories to use these milk samples to provide additional disease testing for those tests services that have been developed for application on milk.

Diseases that have already been successfully adapted to ELISA milk testing include detection of antibody to *Mycobacterium paratuberculosis* for the diagnosis of Johne's disease, detection of antibody to bovine leucosis virus (BLV) for BLV diagnosis, or the direct detection of bovine viral diarrhea (BVD) virus for BVD-PI diagnosis. Services for BVD-PI virus detection by PCR are also available for cow and bulk tank milk. These applications are scientifically defensible and, at least in the case of BLV and Johnes, have received regulatory approval for official government testing programs.

There have also been commercial applications for the detection of mastitis organism by both ELISA and PCR. Widespread application and study of the ProStaph ELISA for detection of specific antibody to *S aureus* (VMRD, Pullman, WA, USA) showed a high sensitivity and specificity for infection detection and a high correlation to culture-based detection.[22] Since this test was looking at antibody instead of the organism itself, the test result would not be expected to always be the same as with culture. Streak canal colonization that can occur with *S aureus* can create a situation where aseptically collected milk samples are repeatedly culture positive, but since the cow's immune system has not detected its presence at this almost external location, she will be ELISA negative. ELISA in this situation will correctly report there is no established infection. The veterinarian may prefer the culture test in this situation as he or she intends to use intramammary treatment to eliminate the colonization or at least re-culture to assess the permanence of this condition. On the other hand, ELISA would reliably report test positive for low and intermittent shedding cows with established *S aureus* infections and bacterial culture may more frequently report the cow as "false negative." The veterinarian in this case would prefer the ELISA-based result to include all the appropriate cows in the quarantine pen. ELISA-based antibody diagnosis for mastitis would be particularly beneficial where culture methods are unreliable due to low and intermittent shedding as is the case with *Prototheca*.[23] One investigator developed an ELISA method for diagnosing the infection and claimed that the pathogen was successfully eradicated from the herd within 2 years by culling antibody-positive cows.[24]

PCR, when used for microorganism detection, offers significant advantages for its speed and its specificity. The speed benefit in the mastitis organism example would be due to its ability to amplify a single strand of any microbial DNA into a signal that can be detected in as little as 4 hours. In microbial culture, it will frequently take at least a day or longer for a single bacterial cell to form a visible colony. Same-day turnaround for results will always appeal to the end user. Applications for PCR diagnosis of *Mycoplasma* mastitis in milk offer dramatically improved turnaround times as traditional culture results can take from 3 to 10 days. The specificity advantage of PCR is a function of the properly designed primer. If the primer generates a product in the thermocycler and hence is "test positive," it means the target organism was in the sample, and misidentification is highly unlikely. Conversely, if the primer does not generate a product, the sample is truly negative for that organism. The question is whether the target will be in the sample. It is sometimes mistakenly assumed that PCR may also offer the advantage of increased sensitivity. PCR methods typically test as little as 1 μL of sample. This sample size is another order of magnitude smaller than the typical 10-μL sample size of conventional culture. This is one reason why PCR is not inherently sensitive. To boost likelihood of detection to allow it to be at least as sensitive as culture, the sample must be enriched, or the target concentrated (DNA extraction), so that the modified 1-μL sample presented to the thermocycler contains at least as much target DNA as 10 μL of the original specimen. One area where PCR is gaining widespread and scientifically defensible application is pathogen testing of food. Certified applications in this arena typically involve preenrichment to increase the cfu count before presenting the specimen to the thermocycler. Even with the extra time associated with sample handling for target enrichment, or target concentration, it is still likely to be faster than culture but it does involve added cost. Each proposed method would have to be critically evaluated to prove increased sensitivity compared to conventional culture.

There are 2 additional issues that must be considered on the topic of PCR sensitivity in milk microbiology. An increase in sensitivity (over conventional blood agar culture) is likely to occur with PCR in cases where the milk sample contains more than 1 species of microorganism. Composite cow samples, bulk tank milk samples, and in-line string samples will all likely contain multiple organism populations. This is similar to the benefit seen with some selective agar cultures (again compared to conventional blood agar), where *only* a narrow range of target organisms is detected and disregards any potential interference from the presence of nontarget organisms. On the other hand, a challenge with PCR is that most methods do not distinguish dead bacteria from live bacteria. For example, in one study, it was shown that a commercially available mastitis detection PCR methodology reported significantly more bacteria positives than conventional culture in a study of 1000 individual quarter clinical and subclinical milk samples.[25] This implication is that PCR is superior to culture due to greater sensitivity. The PCR methodology used in the study uses a significantly larger milk sample (375 μL before extraction) compared to the culture method used (10 μL). Some of the increased detection may be "true positives" related to this initial larger sample size. On the other hand, the authors of the study acknowledge that clinical relevance of PCR-positive/culture-negative results require further investigation. There are likely some "false positives" for infection as PCR may detect dead bacteria from resolved infections. The frequency of occurrence of dead bacteria in bovine mastitis is not well understood. It is reasonable to speculate that phagocytic macrophages that contain dead bacterial DNA may be present in milk samples for days or even weeks after a transient infection has resolved.

Samples for traditional microbiological culture must always be collected aseptically and milk meter–derived samples are never suitable. A separate consideration must be made for the consequence of using samples not aseptically collected with these newer mastitis detection technologies. This issue is variously referred to as signal-to-noise ratio, carry-over, or trailing effect in DHIA samples collected through a milk meter. In the meter, it is expected that a carry-over of a high signal sample will "contaminate" one or more subsequent samples. This signal carry-over is considered acceptable for milk components or somatic cell testing and even for ELISA antibody detection as the "noise" introduced is at such a low level that it does not significantly influence the test value of the subsequent cow samples collected through that meter. Carry-over noise from high ProStaph antibody cows would not result in a "false positive" due to carry-over from contaminated milk meters.

The commercial PathoProof PCR method (Finnzymes Diagnostics, Espoo, Finland) has been promoted as a system suitable to detect mastitis organism from milk collected through a DHIA meter.[26] The signal here is mastitis bacterial DNA. The test will reliably detect the high signal sample from the DHIA meter, but the test may also detect the carry-over signal that will contaminate one or more subsequent samples resulting in "false positives." As is the case with culture where a single cfu of bacteria will cause a test positive, a single strand of bacterial DNA may amplify in the PCR, also resulting in a test positive result. It has been suggested that by internal evaluation of the Ct (cycle threshold) value in the PCR operation, these weak "false positives" from carry-over can be distinguished from the stronger "true positives." As discussed earlier, however, cyclic low-level bacterial shedding can be normal in bovine mastitis. A low-count culture positive or a weak PCR positive may be a valid result. On this basis, it is not possible to reliably separate these "true" weak positives from low-level shedding from the "false" weak positives caused by the carry-over effect of the meter. In one investigation using this commercial platform, the PCR test diagnosed 4 to 7 organisms as present in each of 4 cow milk samples collected through a DHIA meter. Samples collected aseptically from these same 4 cows showed only a pure culture of 1 organism per sample.[27] It would appear that distinguishing carry-over "false positives" and low-count true positives in DHIA meter-derived samples will be an issue with PCR just as it is with culture.

SUMMARY

There are a number of important issues for the dairy practitioner to consider in designing the most appropriate mastitis microbiological service for his or her clients. These include the decision to use enhancement tools or selective agars to optimize sensitivity and specificity. The service should include a monthly BTC service that monitors for the important contagious mastitis organisms: *S aureus, S agalactia,* and *Mycoplasma*. At the cow level, a zero tolerance program to protect healthy cows from exposure to contagious mastitis will require a routine culture service to monitor for these pathogens in new herd additions, clinical cases, and all fresh cows and heifers. A wide variety of additional benefits for maintaining good udder health and the production of quality milk can come from a more comprehensive diagnostic service that looks at both individual cow and bulk tank milk. Finally, more practitioners can help their clients economically by implementation of an on-farm TNT culture service and significantly reducing the use of intramammary therapy.

REFERENCES

1. Hogan JS, Gonzales RN, Harmon RJ, et al. Laboratory handbook on bovine mastitis. Madison (WI): National Mastitis Council; 1999.
2. Schalm OW, Lasmanis J, Carroll EJ. Pathogenesis of experimental coliform (Aerobacter aerogenes) mastitis in cattle. Am J Vet Res 1964;25:75.
3. Sears PM, Smith BS, English PB, et al. Shedding pattern of staphylococcus aureus from bovine intramammary infections. J Dairy Sci 1990;73:2785–9.
4. Dohoo IR, Smith J, Andersen S, et al. Diagnosing intramammary infections: evaluation of definitions based on a single milk sample. J Dairy Sci 2011;94:250–61.
5. Erskine RJ, Eberhart RJ. Comparison of duplicate and single quarter milk samples for the identification of intramammary infections. J Dairy Sci 1988;71:854–6.
6. Biddle MK, Fox LK, Hancock DD. Patterns of mycoplasma shedding in the milk of dairy cows with intramammary mycoplasma infection. J Am Vet Med Assoc 2003; 223:1163–6.
7. Dinsmore RP, English PB, Gonzalez RN, et al. Use of augmented cultural techniques in the diagnosis of the bacterial cause of clinical bovine mastitis. J Dairy Sci 1992;75: 2706–12.
8. Smith KL, Todhunter DA, Schoenberger PS. Environmental mastitis: cause, prevalence, prevention. J Dairy Sci 1985;68:1531–53.
9. Britten A. Use of a selective agar for improving Streptococcus agalactiae detection. Proceedings of the 35th National Mastitis Council at Nashville (TN). February 18, 1996. Madison (WI): National Mastitis Council; 1996. p. 151–2.
10. Britten AM. Is strep mastitis causing high bacteria counts in your bulk tank? National Mastitis Council Regional Meeting at Bellevue (WA). August 20, 1998. Madison (WI): National Mastitis Council; 1998. p. 35–9.
11. Jayarao BM, Wolfgang DR. Bulk-tank milk analysis: a useful tool for improving milk quality and herd udder health. Vet Clin North Am Food Anim Pract 2003;19:75–92.
12. Britten A, Cerar J, Gurajala M. Use of a selective agar for detection of Prototheca in bulk tank and cow milk culture. Proceedings of the 50th National Mastitis Council at Arlington (VA). January 23, 2011. Verona (WI): National Mastitis Council; 2011. p. 140–50.
13. Guterbock WM, Van Eenennaam AL, Anderson RJ, et al. Efficacy of intramammary antibiotic therapy for treatment of clinical mastitis caused by environmental pathogens. J Dairy Sci 1993;76:3437–44.
14. Mellenberger RW. Assessing non-antibiotic therapy for clinical mastitis. Proceedings of the 35th National Mastitis Council at Nashville (TN). Feburary 18, 1996. Madison (WI): National Mastitis Council; 1996. p. 131–4.
15. Cattell MB. An outbreak of Streptococcus uberis as a consequence of adopting a protocol of no antibiotic therapy for clinical mastitis. Proceedings of the 35th National Mastitis Council at Nashville (TN). February 18, 1996. Madison (WI): National Mastitis Council; 1996. p. 123–30.
16. Wilson DJ, Gonzalez RN, Case KL, et al. Comparison of seven antibiotic treatments with no treatment for bacteriological efficacy against bovine mastitis pathogens. J Dairy Sci 1999;82:1664–70.

17. Vandamme DM, Practitioner's approach to mastitis microbiology: acute and subclinical. Proceedings of the 23rd National Mastitis Council at Kansis (MO). February 13, 1984. Arlington (VA): National Mastitis Council; 1984. p. 133–43.
18. Guterbock W. Rational treatment of clinical mastitis. Proceedings of the 33rd National Mastitis Council at Orlando (FL). January 31, 1994. Arlington (VA): National Mastitis Council; 1994. p. 40–50.
19. Lago A, Godden SM, Bey R, et al. The selective treatment of clinical mastitis based on on-farm culture results: I. effects on antibiotic use, milk withholding time, and short-term clinical and bacteriological outcomes. J Dairy Sci 2011;94:4441–56.
20. Hillerton JE, Kliem KE. Effective treatment of Streptococcus uberis clinical mastitis to minimize the use of antibiotics. J Dairy Sci 2002;85:1009–14.
21. Britten A. Epidemiologic aspects of a mastitis outbreak caused by Prototheca sp. on a large dairy herd. Proceedings of the 3rd International Symposium on Mastitis and Milk Quality at Arlington (VA). January 23, 2011. Verona (WI): National Mastitis Council; September 2011.
22. Matsushita T, Dinsmore RP, Eberhart RJ, et al. Performance studies of an enzyme-linked immunosorbent assay for detecting Staphylococcus aureus antibody in bovine Milk. J Vet Diagn Invest 1990;2:163–6.
23. Pore RS, Shahan TA, Pore MD, et al. Occurrence of Prototheca zopfii, a mastitis pathogen in milk. Vet Microbiol 1987;15:315–23.
24. Roesler U, Hensel A. [Eradication of Prototheca zopfii infection in a dairy cattle herd]. Dtsch Tierarztl Wochenschr 2003;110:374.
25. Koskinen MT, Wellenberg GJ, Sampimon OC, et al. Field comparison of real-time polymerase chain reaction and bacterial culture for identification of bovine mastitis bacteria. J Dairy Sci 2010;93:5707–15.
26. High J. Real-time qPCR-based DNA mastitis analysis using the preserved DHIA sample. Proceedings of the 49th National Mastitis Council at Albuquerque (NM). January 31, 2010. Verona (WI): National Mastitis Council; 2010. p. 238–9.
27. Schukken YH, Moroni P, Zadoks R. New technologies to improve milk quality and udder health on dairy farms. Proceedings of the 50th National Mastitis Council at Arlington (VA). January 23, 2011. Verona (WI): National Mastitis Council; 2011. p. 82–92.

Update on Control of *Staphylococcus aureus* and *Streptococcus agalactiae* for Management of Mastitis

Greg Keefe, DVM, MSc, MBA

KEYWORDS

- *Staphylococcus aureus* • *Streptococcus agalactiae* • Bovine • Mastitis • Control
- Biosecurity

KEY POINTS

- The primary method of spread for *Streptococcus agalactiae* and *Staphylococcus aureus* is from cow to cow.
- Control is accomplished by decreasing new infections, primarily by milking-time management, and reducing the reservoir of infection in the herd, by strategic treatment and culling.
- Adherence to NMC protocols including pre- and post-milking teat disinfection and blanket dry cow therapy will decrease prevalence.
- There is growing evidence that use of milking gloves is a integral part of contagious mastitis control and the production of high-quality milk.
- Treatment outcome depends on cow, pathogen, and treatment regimen factors for *S aureus* and is often not successful, whereas cure rates are typically very high for *S agalactiae*.
- Herds should be closed or have rigorous biosecurity protocols to prevent introduction of novel strains of contagious mastitis pathogens.

In countries with a developed dairy industry, mastitis is the most common and costly infectious disease affecting dairy farms. In addition to negatively impacting production efficiency and quality, mastitis is an important animal health and welfare issue. *Streptococcus agalactiae* and *Staphylococcus aureus* are considered major mastitis pathogens because of their large effect on milk quality, production, and cow somatic cell count (SCC). The primary method of spread for these pathogens is contagious (cow to cow) with infected cows within a herd acting as a reservoir of infection. Historically, these pathogens have been grouped together because of their common

The author has nothing to disclose.
Department of Health Management, Atlantic Veterinary College, University of Prince Edward Island, 550 University Avenue, Charlottetown, Prince Edward Island, Canada C1A 4P3
E-mail address: gkeefe@upei.ca

Vet Clin Food Anim 28 (2012) 203–216
http://dx.doi.org/10.1016/j.cvfa.2012.03.010
0749-0720/12/$ – see front matter © 2012 Elsevier Inc. All rights reserved.

epidemiology. However, there are some very important differences in their pathobiology that has resulted in large variations in herd and cow prevalence levels between the 2 pathogens in most developed dairy countries.

Because the primary reservoir of the infection with contagious pathogens is infected cattle, the focus of control is within and between herd biosecurity. Control of contagious pathogens is accomplished by decreasing new infections, primarily by milking time management, and reducing the reservoir of infection in the herd. Adherence to NMC protocols including pre- and post-milking teat disinfection and blanket dry cow therapy will decrease prevalence. There is growing evidence that use of milking gloves is an integral part of contagious mastitis control and the production of high-quality milk. Herds should be closed or have rigorous biosecurity protocols to prevent introduction of novel strains of contagious mastitis pathogens. This article examines biosecurity practices for Streptococcus agalactiae and Staphylococcus aureus that decrease new intramammary infection risk (incidence) and the reservoir of infected cows in the herd (prevalence).

EPIDEMIOLOGY
Source of Infection

S agalactiae is a highly contagious obligate parasite of the bovine mammary gland. It generally does not survive for long periods of time outside of the mammary gland.[1] Conversely, while the mammary gland is a primary site for S aureus, the pathogen is commonly found on skin surfaces, the nares, and the vulva and can be also found in environmental sites.[2] A recent study in Norway found that cows hocks are a common site for S aureus colonization and that the proximity of the hocks to teats when cows are recumbent could be a risk for new intramammary infection (IMI).[3] Despite the ability to recover the organism from the environment, it is more consistently recovered from the mammary gland and other body sites, making these sites the primary herd reservoir.[2] For both pathogens, teat skin and any fomite such as milkers' hands and milking equipment can be heavily contaminated. The teat canal is the only route of entry into the gland for these bacterial pathogens. As a result, the primary method of transmission is via contact between susceptible, uninfected quarters with fomites contaminated with infective milk. Consequently, the milking time is the primary risk period.

Presentation

Both organisms cause a low-grade persistent type of infection that does not have a high self-cure rate.[4] At the cow level, infections are typically subclinical. Somatic cell counts of greater than 1,000,000 are not uncommon for S agalactiae infections, while S aureus SCC is more moderate.[5] In a meta- analysis, Djabri and colleagues found a geometric mean of 357,000 and 857,000 for quarters infected with S aureus and S agalactiae, respectively.[6]

At the herd or bulk tank level, presentation depends on within-herd prevalence. Because of the contagious nature of these pathogens, historically they have had high within-herd prevalence and been associated with greatly elevated bulk tank SCC.[1,7,8] As adoption of within-herd biosecurity has improved, cow prevalence within infected herds has decreased leading to moderation of bulk tank SCC levels. In addition to elevated SCC, herds infected with S agalactiae can also experience very high total bacteria count load in bulk tank milk. Cows infected S agalactiae can shed up to 100 million bacteria/mL.[9] Infected herds will frequently have standard plate counts in the range of 20,000 to 100,000 colony-forming units (cfu)/mL.[10] In New York State, control of *S agalactiae* was found to be an important measure for improving bacterial quality.[11]

Detection

It is difficult to assess the sensitivity and specificity of cultures for *S agalactiae* from individual cows due to the lack of a reference gold standard; however, the level of bacterial shedding and the fact that the test is highly repeatable support a high relative sensitivity and specificity of 95% and 100%, respectively.[1] For an obligate intramammary pathogen like *S agalactiae*, the bovine udder is recognized as the only reasonable source of the organism in the milk. Consequently, isolates in the bulk tank are usually assumed to have come from the udder and specificity approaches 100%.[1] In the past, when a herd is infected with *S agalactiae*, typically there has been a high within-herd prevalence and therefore a substantial pathogen burden in the bulk tank. As a consequence, culture methods similar to those used in individual animals provided adequate sensitivity. As within-herd prevalence drops, the sensitivity of conventional methods decreases and augmented methods are required. These method might include preincubation of samples prior to culture and the use of larger inoculum volumes on highly selective media.[1] More recently, polymerase chain reaction (PCR)-based techniques have become commercially available.[12,13] These methods appear to have high levels of sensitivity both at the cow and bulk tank level, and particularly for an obligate intramammary pathogen like *S agalactiae* retain high specificity.[12,14]

Sensitivity of culture for *S aureus* at the cow level Is lower than that of *S agalactiae*. Cyclical shedding has been observed with the ebb of shedding potentially below the detection limit of conventional culture. Single sample sensitivity was reported to be as low as 75% in an experimental infection model but improved with serial sample collection.[15] A recent field study that used random effects modeling techniques determined that the sensitivity of a single culture could be as high as 90% if all cultures (including mixed growth cultures) were considered positive with a threshold of 1 cfu on standard culture (100 cfu/mL).[16] Specificity of *S aureus* culture at the cow level is very high (approaching 100%) when samples are collected sterilely.[16] These results are in agreement with another study, which found a sensitivity of 91% for a 0.01 mL inoculum and 96% for a 0.1 mL inoculum.[17] Sensitivity of PCR methods appears to be very high with higher recovery rates than conventional methods, but caution must be observed with respect to specificity if samples are not collected in a sterile manner due to the fact that the organism is not restricted to the mammary gland.[2,12]

PREVALENCE OF INFECTION

In countries that have had longstanding extension programs for the control of *S agalactiae,* prevalence has declined dramatically.[18–22] In countries with emerging dairy industries the herd level prevalence can still be quite high. In South America, the herd prevalence has been reported to be 60% in Brazil, 42% in Colombia, and 11% in Uruguay.[23–25]

Eradication is the ultimate goal of an *S agalactiae* control strategy. In Denmark, a national eradication program has been in place for several decades. Despite achieving very low levels in the late 1980s and early 1990s, there has been an apparent rise in the prevalence of infection at the herd level.[26] Additionally, using molecular techniques in the surveillance program has increased the recovery rate of the pathogen from bulk tank samples.[14]

In contrast to *S agalactiae*, *S aureus* remains a very common cause of mastitis on dairy farms. At the herd level, infection with *S aureus* was 43% in a recent US survey and 74% from a Canadian study.[22,27] In a recent study, S aureus was the most commonly isolated pathogen from clinical mastitis samples (13.0%) and the second most commonly isolated pathogen (behind coagulase-negative staphylococci) in subclinical samples (2.4%–3.0%).[28] The cow prevalence of S aureus has been report to be 6.4% in Switzerland and 22.2% in Norway.[19,29] In a recent Dutch study, 3.7% of low-SCC cows and 15.0% of high-SCC cows had S aureus.[30]

Some studies have also identified S aureus as the most commonly recovered pathogen from heifer mastitis cases. A full discussion of the impact of the organism on heifer mastitis can be found in a recent review.[31]

Because the organism is not obligated to live within the mammary gland like S agalactiae, eradication from the herd is very challenging. Despite this, within-herd prevalence can be reduced by systematic adoption of mastitis control programs.[32,33]

PUBLIC HEALTH

Both S agalactiae and S aureus can have public health significance. S agalactiae is a well-known cause of neonatal septicemia and is a common organism in the urogenital tract of women. Human and cattle strains are distinctive with limited risk of transfer from cows to people.[34] With respect to S aureus, there is evidence that cattle and humans can share the same strains, but at this point, because the ability to spread in the non–primary host seems restricted, zoonotic risk is limited.[34] The issue of methicillin-resistant S aureus (MRSA) is an important public health concern. The MRSA that have been found in cattle do not appear to act differently that other strains S aureus; however, the fact that MSRA has been found in cattle raises public health concerns.

Within-Herd Biosecurity

Within herd biosecurity for contagious pathogens can be viewed as methods to reduce the reservoir of infected cows in the herd (prevalence) and transmission from these animals to susceptible herdmates (incidence). The original mastitis control programs, developed more than 40 years ago, were focused on gram-positive organisms, primarily S agalactiae and S aureus. When implemented in a consistent, rigorous fashion, it is clear that the 5-point mastitis control program from the United Kingdom[35] and that later expanded to a 10-point scheme in North America (www.nmconline.org/docs/NMCchecklistNA.pdf) are effective in controlling these organisms.[32]

The basic tenets of the NMC 10-point plan are as follows (1) establishment of goals for udder health, (2) maintenance of a clean, dry, comfortable environment, (3) proper milking procedures, (4) proper maintenance and use of milking equipment, (5) good record keeping, (6) appropriate management of clinical mastitis during lactation, (7) effective dry cow management, (8) maintenance of biosecurity for contagious pathogens and marketing of chronically infected cows, (9) regular monitoring of udder health status, and (10) periodic review of mastitis control program (www.nmconline. org/docs/NMCchecklistNA.pdf).

From the checklist, items 1, 5, 9, and 10 are generally applicable to all herd monitoring programs. As major SCC producers, monitoring and goal setting for S agalactiae and S aureus often revolve around this surveillance tool. Herd goals should be developed with the individual dairy farmer. Achievable goals on well-managed herds are to have bulk tank SCC below 150,000, a prevalence of chronic infections (individual cows repeatedly higher than a 200,000 SCC threshold) of less than 5%, and the incidence of new IMI (cows breaching a 200,000 threshold) of less than 5% on a monthly basis.[36] Participation in dairy herd improvement provides key data for monitoring contagious mastitis programs and uploading these data into herd management software, such as DairyComp (www.vas.com).

REDUCING INCIDENCE THROUGH MILKING PRACTICES

Checklist items 3 and 4 are critical control points for reduction of incidence of new infections with both *S agalactiae* and *S aureus*. A recent systematic review of practices associated with low SCC concluded that proper milking procedures have a consistent association with lower contagious mastitis risk.[37] Among the most reliable predictors of SCC were having annual milking system checks, having an established milking order, wearing gloves during milking, using automatic take-offs, and using post-milking teat disinfection.

A milking equipment evaluation schedule should be established with the equipment dealer, and periodic (yearly) independent system checks should be conducted. The milking machine is an important component of the mastitis prevention strategy. In a study in the United Kingdom, more than 60% of parlors failed annual performance testing.[38]

While general guidelines can be given, customized milking procedures should be standardized and formulated into written operating procedures for each farm. Cows should be milked in a stress-free manner to harvest milk with minimum risk of new IMI. Fore-stripping is recommended to remove bacteria and SCC-laden first milk and to stimulate letdown. Farmers often express concern that fore-stripping may decrease parlor efficiency by prolonging the milking routine. Some research would suggest that total milking time and peak milk flow are actually reduced with fore-stripping, particularly for late-lactation or low-production cows.[39,40] Others have reported, however, that incorporating fore-stripping into a premilking routine that included predipping, teat massage, and wiping produced no significant difference for milk-out time, milk flow rates, and milk yield.[41]

Predipping teats with disinfectant solution has become the standard method for premilking teat disinfection. Predipping was associated with the lowest bacterial burden in milk compared to other methods.[42] Typically, predipping is emphasized for the prevention of environmental infections. A recent Canadian study found that it was also associated with a lower risk for prevalence and incidence of *S aureus*.[43] NMC annually publishes a list of approved premilking and postmilking teat disinfectant products.[44] For a premilking teat disinfection protocol to be most effective, it must have good coverage on the teat and be in contact with the teat skin for 30 seconds. Applying the product as a dip rather than spray is highly recommended because of the challenges of getting adequate coverage with a spray apparatus on a consistent basis.

Cloth towels are the gold standard for drying udders. Towels must be used on a single cow and laundered between use. Cloth towels provide excellent removal of organic matter and disinfectant from the teats and good stimulation of the cow for milk letdown. Organic matter and disinfectant removal is important for quality milk production.[42,45] Maximum stimulation is important for fast milk out, which reduces teat-end stress. Teats should be full and plump when the milking unit is applied, so that the teat-cup sits properly on the teat and milk flow begins immediately. The duration of drying required to maximize letdown will vary from herd to herd but minimum recommendations are 10 seconds of teat and cloth contact time and contact time may be higher in 3-times-a-day milking versus twice-a-day milking. One study found that a drying time of 20 seconds reduced bacterial load on test more than shorter durations.[46] In recognition of the importance of stimulation and having full teats at the start of milking, overall lag time between first contact and applying the milking unit should be 90 to 120 seconds. Indeed some herds may require longer if milk letdown is not sufficient in that time-frame.

A Lactocorder (WMB AG, Balgach, Switzerland) can be used to evaluate the efficiency of preparation and the readiness of cows when the unit is attached. The unit can also evaluate milk flow rates and accuracy of automatic unit removal systems.[47,48] Attachment of the milking unit should be accomplished with a minimum of air intake (see discussion of impacts later).

The recommended order of milking preparation is strip-dip-dry-apply or dip-strip-dry-apply. Both of these methods provide good stimulation by having the fore-stripping early in the procedure and avoid contact between milkers' hands and clean teats.[49]

Gloves should be worn during milking. Research in the Netherlands indicates that bacterial load on milkers' hands is reduced by 75% when gloves are worn, and when the gloves are disinfected periodically bacteria loads, decrease by 98%, compared to bare hands.[50] In a recent Canadian study, gloves were found to be clearly protective with respect to new IMIs with S aureus. When gloves were worn, the odds ratio for new S aureus IMI incidence was 0.43 and the odds of eliminating existing infection was 2.2 times higher for herds where milkers wore gloves.[43] In a separate study, wearing gloves was also found to have a positive net economic benefit.[51]

When friction is lost between the teat skin and the milking unit inflation, liner slips can occur, which allow air to be admitted in an uncontrolled fashion into the milking unit. This results in pressure changes that can cause milk, which may be laden with bacteria, to be propelled against contralateral teats. This phenomenon, known as an impact, can spread pathogens within the udder or, when the claw is contaminated with milk from previous cows, from infected to uninfected cows. These liner slips are associated with higher risk of new IMI.[52] Additionally, within the teat cistern, negative pressures relative to outside the teat canal can be created leading to a reverse pressure gradient. These are most predominant when the teat is empty, at the beginning of milking (prior to letdown) and at the end of milking.[53] These pressure gradients could facilitate transfer of pathogens into the gland. The overall goal for linear slips is less than 5 to 10 per 100 cows milked.[54]

When milk flow slows, units should be removed in a stress free manner, with minimum of air entry to prevent exposure of the teat-end to bacteria when the risk of reverse pressure gradients is high. Exact flow rates at take off depend on type of equipment and herd productivity factors. Removal of the unit in a timing fashion is also important to maintain teat-end integrity. Teat-end lesion score was linearly associated with risk of acquiring a new S aureus infection, with severely affected quarters at 3.7 times the risk of normal teats.[43] Teat end scoring charts are available at the website of the Canadian Bovine Mastitis Research Network (www.mastitisnetwork.org).

After removal of the milking unit, an approved postmilking teat disinfectant should be applied. A large number of studies have demonstrated the effectiveness of the practice, particularly against S aureus and S agalactiae.[44] In a recent Canadian study, 96% of herds used postmilking teat disinfectant.[27] While overall use is high, it is more difficult to quantify the effectiveness of application. Dipping the teats in disinfectant is recommended over spraying because it provides a more consistent teat coverage and is less expensive.[55] Teats should be fully covered to provide milk film breakdown, pathogen disinfection, and teat skin conditioning to all parts of the teat that are in contact with the milking unit. This is particularly important with pathogens that colonize teat skin like S agalactiae and S aureus.

SEGREGATION

Infected animals pose a risk to their uninfected herdmates. In a recent Canadian study, the herd prevalence of *S aureus* was strongly associated with the subsequent odds of acquisition of an IMI. In that study, each 5% increase in the herd initial prevalence was associated with a doubling of incidence risk.[43] Infectious disease control would suggest that physical separation of infectious and susceptible animals should reduce spread. Two methods are used to accomplish this goal. The first is segregation of the infectious cows with a specific milking order that reduces exposure of susceptible cows. The second is back-flushing of the milking unit so that uninfected glands are not exposed to contaminated milking units from infectious cows. In one study, prevalence of *S aureus* infection and SCC decreased much more rapidly in herds that practiced segregation of infected cows than those that did not.[56] An Italian study also found that segregation was an import tool in decreasing prevalence.[57] In a herd that had a novel and particularly virulent strain of *S aureus*, which did not seem to be controlled with standard hygiene practices, segregation was deemed an effective component of the control strategy.[58] The data are not always consistent, however. In one study, there was no significant benefit of segregation and the authors suggested that *S aureus* could be controlled as effectively with other hygiene measures.[59]

The ideal milking order would be to milk healthy, uninfected cows first, followed by cows of unknown status, cows with elevated SCC, and finally known chronic contagious mastitis cows last. Segregation in this manner can be achieved relatively easily in tie stall barns, although care should be taken to update the milking order when new information is available, for example after a dairy herd improvement test. Large free stall herds can also group cows based on infection risk, but it is often difficult to do so in small or moderate-sized herds. In these herds, an alternative is to have certain milking units assigned to milk cows of higher risk. For herds where this is not practical, extra care and attention should be paid to other aspects of the udder health program focused on transmission risk.

The effectiveness of automated disinfectant back-flush systems may depend on the prevalence of contagious pathogens, such as *S aureus*. One study found that both liner bacterial population and risk of new IMIs with *S aureus* were reduced by using a back-flush system.[60] A second study, in a herd with low *S aureus* prevalence, found that liner bacteria numbers were reduced, but the risk of new IMIs was not affected.[61] When using a back-flush system, care should be taken to avoid disinfectant residues in milk.[61] A more recent study found that back-flushing of the milk cluster after milking a cow with clinical mastitis was a cost-effective control strategy.[51]

Heifers can calve with *S aureus*.[31,62] There is not a full understanding of the role of waste milk in the transmission of *S aureus* to young heifer calves.[2] When waste milk is fed, consideration should be given to pasteurization to reduce risk of transmission of mastitis or other pathogens.

REDUCING PREVALENCE

For contagious mastitis pathogens like *S aureus* and *S agalactiae*, incidence risk depends on the pool of infected cows in the herd (prevalence). As a result, a reduction of this pool of animals may be justified to bring R_0 to less than 1. Prevalence reduction can be accomplished by successful treatment or culling. While prevention strategies for *S aureus* and *S agalactiae* are quite similar, treatment programs are markedly different.

Lactational Treatment of S agalactiae

The goal of treatment for S agalactiae is usually eradication from the herd. Antimicrobial susceptibility for S agalactiae remains very high.[63,64] In vivo treatment for S agalactiae is highly successful and eradication is relatively straightforward, if recommendations are followed.[1,35]

Protocols have been developed for a systematic elimination of the pathogen from the herd.[65] The method used will depend on herd circumstances. A rigorous implementation of milking hygiene and universal dry cow therapy, coupled with biosecurity to limit reintroduction, can be expected to drastically reduce or eliminate infection over a few years. If the goal is more-rapid eradication, a test and treatment strategy can be used. In a culture-and-treat protocol, the herd is cultured and infected animals are treated at 3-week intervals until all cows have 2 consecutive negative cultures.[65] Cows that are refractory to treatment (typically <5%) should be culled.

Lactational Treatment of S aureus

The goal of treatment for S aureus is to potentially cure individual cases and reduce the pool of infected cows within the herd. Due to the fact that the organism is not an obligate udder pathogen and cure rates are far lower than S agalactiae, eradication is not an option. In vitro antimicrobial susceptibility for S aureus remains relatively high,[63,64] but in vivo treatment success is much lower. Barkema and colleagues[66] reviewed the probability of cure for S aureus infections and found that it depends on cow, pathogen, and treatment factors. They suggested that the wide discrepancy in reported cure rate between studies may be due to these factors. Using a model, they calculated that expected cure rate for relatively new infections in young animals was approximately 60%, whereas cure rates for older animals with chronic high SCC and multiple quarters infected could be as low as 1%.[66] Examining these cow factors is important before deciding if a cow is worth treating.

S aureus has the ability to survive in neutrophils, form small-colony or L-form variants that are cell wall deficient, invade into mammary epithelial cells, form microabscesses, and promote biofilm formation, all of which make the organism more difficult to treat in vivo. The level of true penicillin resistance appears to vary widely around the world. Penicillin resistant appears to be a marker for in vivo treatment failure, regardless of the antibiotic used.[66] Strain type is associated with cure after antimicrobial treatment with host-adapted strains approximately 2.5 times less likely to cure than non–host-adapted strains.[67] In the same study, no difference in spontaneous cure was observed in untreated control quarters between strains.

A recent systematic review of the literature reported that when similar antibiotics were used cure rates were much higher for longer duration treatment (>5 days) versus short-duration therapy.[68] Despite the increased cure rates, 2 reports recently concluded that on an economic basis, shorter-duration treatment (2–3 days) provided the most expected value for the costs incurred.[69,70] The options for treatment will depend on cow value versus culling and replacement costs.

An approach that has been suggested is to use vaccination as either prevention or as an adjunct to treatment. Prevention of S aureus mastitis with vaccination has proved to be a challenge.[71] A recent review suggests that vaccines based on new technologies may have better efficacy, but there is a lack of large field-based trials to evaluate this claim.[72] Barkema and colelagues reviewed the literature on vaccination as an adjunct to treatment and suggested that the results are encouraging but must be viewed in light of the farm-specific strain. They suggested that more research in this area is warranted.[66]

DRY COW THERAPY FOR *S AGALACTIAE* AND *S AUREUS*

The dry period offers a economical option for therapy, with typically higher cure rates than lactational therapy, particularly for *S aureus*. It is recommended that blanket dry cow therapy of all cows should be performed and a meta-analysis has shown that the risk of IMI in the subsequent lactation is much higher in cows that do not receive blanket dry cow treatment.[73] Despite this fact, a recent study in Canada revealed that only 72% of herds implemented blanket dry cow treatment.[27] This figure was much lower than the adoption rate of postmilking teat disinfection (96%) from the same study. In a study of the cost-effectiveness of standard mastitis control procedures, blanket dry cow therapy was shown to be one of the few measures that consistently showed a positive net economic benefit.[51]

CULLING

Culling can be an important component of management of contagious pathogens. While most *S agalactiae* infections can be cured with appropriate therapy, refractory cases should be culled to eliminate the reservoir of infection from within the herd.[65] As outlined earlier, cure rates for *S aureus* infections are far inferior to those for *S agalactiae*. As a result, culling takes on a much more important role in reduction of new IMI risk in infected herds.

The impact of reducing prevalence through strategic culling can be substantial. The odds of new *S aureus* infection doubled for every 5% increase in the historic herd prevalence of infection.[43] Culling decisions on dairy farms are complex; however, strong emphasis should be placed on culling chronic *S aureus* cows to prevent a cycle of new IMI through this reservoir. Culling should be part of a complete program, which emphasizes all aspects of new IMI incidence reduction, particularly milking time management.

BETWEEN-HERD BIOSECURITY

Biosecurity protocols are important for the prevention of infectious disease transmission among farms. Maintaining a closed herd should be the goal of every biosecurity program. For pathogens that have been eradicated from a particular herd, such as *S agalactiae*, biosecurity take on additional relevance.[74] However, even for pathogens like *S aureus* that are often endemic within herds, introduction of novel strains can result in increased incidence of new IMI.[58,75]

Sometimes maintaining a closed herd is not consistent with the expansion or herd genetic development goals of the dairy farmer. In these situations, protocols should be established to reduce risk from the new herd entrants. The history of both the herd of origin and the specific animal should be examined.

To reduce the overall risk and improve the negative predictive value of prepurchase diagnostics, only low contagious mastitis prevalence herds, as documented by a consistent bulk tank SCC of less than 200,000, should be considered. The herd should be on a regular program of milk culturing with a low number of *S aureus* clinical mastitis cases and no documented *S agalactiae* over several years.

At the cow level, because milking is a risk for transmission, prepartum heifers are often considered the lowest risk animals. However, in a recent Canadian study, 10% of heifers in a convenience sample of herds were found to be infected with *S aureus*.[62] This indicates a need for assessment (next) upon entry into the herd, even for heifers.

With mature animals, assessment should take place at the herd of origin. This assessment should include a complete SCC history for the animal, records of clinical mastitis and previous culture information, and a current quarter culture. Historic SCC should be at minimum less than 200,000 and, for greater certainty of freedom from infection, a 100,000 threshold should be considered. Animals should also be examined for udder and teat-end lesions, which would increase infection risk. When prepurchase evaluation is not available, or in the case of dry cows or prepartum heifers, milk cultures should be conducted as soon as possible after arrival. These animals should be considered potentially infected and segregation procedures (earlier) put in place until results are available.

Communication of expectations between the buyer and seller is important. The Canadian Bovine Mastitis Research Network promotes the use of an udder health status disclosure with clear buyer and seller responsibilities in the TACTIC Udder Health kit (www.mastitisnetwork.org).

ADDITIONAL BIOSECURITY

The risk of transfer of contagious mastitis pathogens from farm to farm by personnel or fomites is not well studied. However, people can be carriers of contagious mastitis pathogens and the risk for transmission for other infectious diseases is well documented. Therefore, farms should develop a protocol to control this exposure in consultation with their herd veterinarian.[74,75]

SUMMARY

The primary method of spread for S agalactiae and S aureus is from cow to cow, so prevention focuses on within and between herd biosecurity to reduce or eliminate the reservoir of infection. S agalactiae is an obligate pathogen of the mammary gland, whereas S aureus is more widespread on other cow body sites and in the environment. Both organisms cause persistent infections, with S agalactiae typically causing higher SCC and bacteria counts in milk.

Conventional methods of detection through culture perform well at the cow level. In bulk tanks, augmented procedures should be considered. PCR methods show promise of high sensitivity and specificity, at both the cow and bulk tank level.

In developed dairy industries, prevalence of infection has decreased dramatically over the past 30 years for S agalactiae. For S aureus, the herd level of infection remains very high, although with rigorous, consistent application of control measures, within-herd prevalence has decreased.

Because the milking time is the primary period for new IMI, it is the focal point of most prevention activities. Premilking and postmilking teat disinfection and proper stimulation and milk-out with adequately functioning equipment are key factors. There is growing evidence that the use of milking gloves is an integral part of contagious mastitis control and the production of high-quality milk.

Treatment success is dramatically different between the 2 pathogens. For S agalactiae, eradication can be completed rapidly through a culture and treatment program with minimal culling. For S aureus, treatment success, particularly during lactation, is often disappointing and depends on cow, pathogen, and treatment factors. These factors should be reviewed prior to initiating any treatment to determine the potential for cure. Blanket dry cow therapy and strategic culling are important control procedures for contagious mastitis pathogens.

Maintaining a closed herd or, at minimum, adhering to clearly defined biosecurity protocols is critical to reduce risk of reintroduction of S agalactiae or the addition of new, potentially more virulent strains of S aureus to endemic herds.

REFERENCES

1. Keefe GP. Streptococcus agalactiae mastitis: a review. Can Vet J 1997;38:429–37.

2. Roberson JR, Fox LK, Hancock DD, et al. Ecology of *Staphylococcus aureus* isolated from various sites on dairy farms. J Dairy Sci 1994;77:3354–64.

3. Capurro A, Aspán A, Ericsson Unnerstad H, et al. Identification of potential sources of *Staphylococcus aureus* in herds with mastitis problems. J Dairy Sci 2010;93:180–91.

4. Farnsworth RJ. Indications of contagious and environmental mastitis pathogens in a dairy herd. Proceedings 26th Annual Meeting of the National Mastitis Council. Orlando (FL). Verona (WI): National Mastitis Council, Inc; 1987;26:151–5.

5. Erskine RJ, Eberhart RJ, Hutchinson LJ, et al. Herd management and prevalence of mastitis in dairy herds with high and low somatic cell counts. J Am Vet Med Assoc 1987;190:1411–6.

6. Djabri B, Bareille N, Beaudeau F, et al. Quarter milk somatic cell count in infected dairy cows: a meta-analysis. Vet Res 2002;33:335–7.

7. Jayarao BM, Pillai SR, Sawant AA, et al. Guidelines for monitoring bulk tank milk somatic cell and bacterial counts. J Dairy Sci 2004;87:3561–73.

8. Eberhart RJ, Hutchinson LJ, Spencer SB. Relationships of bulk tank somatic cell counts to prevalence of intramammary infection to indices of herd production. J Food Prot 1982;45:1125–8.

9. Guterbock WM, Blackmer PE. Veterinary interpretation of bulktank milk. Vet Clin North Am Large Anim Pract 1984;6:257–68.

10. Hogan JS, Smith KL. Using bulk tank milk cultures in a dairy practice. Arlington (VA): National Mastitis Council Mastitis Microbiology Diagnostics Workshop; 1992.

11. Zadoks RN, González RN, Boor KJ, et al. Mastitis-causing streptococci are important contributors to bacterial counts in raw bulk tank milk. J Food Prot 2004;67:2644–50.

12. Koskinen MT, Holopainen J, Pyörälä S, et al. Analytical specificity and sensitivity of a real-time polymerase chain reaction assay for identification of bovine mastitis pathogens. Dairy Sci 2009;92:952–9.

13. Koskinen MT, Wellenberg GJ, Sampimon OC, et al. Field comparison of real-time polymerase chain reaction and bacterial culture for identification of bovine mastitis bacteria. J Dairy Sci 2010;93:5707–15.

14. Katholm J. 2010. Available at: www.landbrugsinfo.dk/Kvaeg/Maelkekvalitet/Sider/ Streptococcus-agalactiae-an-increasing-problem.aspx. Accessed March 7, 2012.

15. Sears PM, Smith BS, English PB, et al. Shedding pattern of *Staphylococcus aureus* from bovine intramammary infections. J Dairy Sci 1990;73:2785–9.

16. Dohoo IR, Smith J, Andersen S, et al. Diagnosing intramammary infections: evaluation of definitions based on a single milk sample. J Dairy Sci 2011;94:250–61.

17. Walker JB, Rajala-Schultz PJ, DeGraves FJ. The effect of inoculum volume on the microbiologic detection of naturally occurring *Staphylococcus aureus* intramammary infections. J Vet Diagn Invest 2010;22:720–4.

18. Olde Riekerink RG, Barkema HW, Veenstra S, et al. Prevalence of contagious mastitis pathogens in bulk tank milk in Prince Edward Island. Can Vet J 2006;47:567–72.

19. Østerås O, Sølverød L, Reksen O. Milk culture results in a large Norwegian survey: effects of season, parity, days in milk, resistance, and clustering. J Dairy Sci 2006; 89:1010–23.

20. Bradley AJ, Leach KA, Breen JE, et al. Survey of the incidence and aetiology of mastitis on dairy farms in England and Wales. Vet Rec 2007;160:253–7.

21. Piepers S, De Meulemeester L, de Kruif A, et al. Prevalence and distribution of mastitis pathogens in subclinically infected dairy cows in Flanders, Belgium. J Dairy Res 2007;74:478–83.

22. USDA-APHIS. Prevalence of contagious mastitis pathogens on US dairy operations, 2007 APHIS Veterinary Services Info Sheet. #N533.1008. Washington, DC: APHIS, USDA; 2007.

23. Duarte RS, Miranda OP, Bellei BC, et al. Phenotypic and molecular characteristics of *Streptococcus agalactiae* isolates recovered from milk of dairy cows in Brazil. J Clin Microbiol 2004;42:4214–22.

24. Keefe G, Chaffer M, Ceballos A, et al. Effects of *Streptococcus agalactiae* on the Colombian dairy industry. Third International Symposium on Mastitis and Milk Quality, St. Louis (MO). National Mastitis Council Inc, Verona (WI); American Association of Bovine Practitioners, Auburn (AL); 2011;3:155.

25. Gianneechini R, Concha C, Rivero R, at al. Occurrence of clinical and sub-clinical mastitis in dairy herds in the West Littoral Region in Uruguay. Acta Vet Scand 2002;43:221–30.

26. Katholm J, Rattenborg E. The surveillance program of *Streptococcus agalactiae* in Danish dairy herds 1989–2008. Mastitis Research into Practice 5th IDF Mastitis Conference, Christchurch (NZ). Vetlearn*, Wellington (NZ); 2010. p. 241–6.

27. Olde Riekerink RG, Barkema HW, Scholl DT, et al. Management practices associated with the bulk-milk prevalence of *Staphylococcus aureus* in Canadian dairy farms. Prev Vet Med 2010;97:20–8.

28. Reyher KK, Dufour S, Barkema HW, et al. The National Cohort of Dairy Farms: a data collection platform for mastitis research in Canada. J Dairy Sci 2011;94:1616–26.

29. Moret-Stalder S, Fournier C, Miserez R, et al. Prevalence study of *Staphylococcus aureus* in quarter milk samples of dairy cows in the Canton of Bern, Switzerland. Prev Vet Med 2009;88:72–6.

30. Sampimon O, Barkema HW, Berends I, et al. Prevalence of intramammary infection in Dutch dairy herds. J Dairy Res 2009;76:129–36.

31. De Vliegher S, Fox LK, Piepers S, et al. Invited review: Mastitis in dairy heifers: nature of the disease, potential impact, prevention, and control. Dairy Sci 2012;95:1025–40.

32. Hillerton JE, Bramley AJ, Staker RT, et al. Patterns of intramammary infection and clinical mastitis over a 5 year period in a closely monitored herd applying mastitis control measures. J Dairy Res 1995;62:39–50.

33. Zadoks RN, Allore HG, Hagenaars TJ, et al. A mathematical model of *Staphylococcus aureus* control in dairy herds. Epidemiol Infect 2002;129:397–416.

34. Zadoks RN, Middleton JR, McDougall S, et al. Molecular epidemiology of mastitis pathogens of dairy cattle and comparative relevance to humans. J Mammary Gland Biol Neoplasia 2011;16:357–72.

35. Neave FK, Dodd FH, Kingwill RG, et al. Control of mastitis in the dairy herd by hygiene and management. J Dairy Sci 1969;52:696–707.

36. Schukken YH, Barkema HW, Lam TJGM, et al. Improving udder health on well managed farms: mitigating the "perfect storm." In Mastitis control: from science to practice. Wageningen (Netherlands): Wageningen Academic Publishers; 2008. p. 21–35.

37. Dufour S, Fréchette A, Barkema HW, et al. Invited review: effect of udder health management practices on herd somatic cell count. J Dairy Sci 2011;94:563–79.

38. Berry EA, Scrivens M, Hillerton JE. Milking machine test survey of UK herds. Vet Rec 2005;157:147–8.

39. Reneau J K, Chastain JP. Premilking cow prep: adapting to your system. Proceedings. Regional Meeting of the National Mastitis Council, Harrisburg (PA). National Mastitis Council, Inc, Verona (WI); 1995. p. 46.

40. Watters RD, Schuring N, Erb HN, et al. The effect of premilking udder preparation on Holstein cows milked 3 times daily. J Dairy Sci 2012;95:1170–6.

41. Wagner AM, Ruegg PL. The effect of manual forestripping on milking performance of Holstein dairy cows. J Dairy Sci 2002;85:804–9.

42. Elmoslemany AM, Keefe GP, Dohoo IR, et al. The association between bulk tank milk analysis for raw milk quality and on-farm management practices. Prev Vet Med 2010;95:32–40.

43. Dufour S, Dohoo IR, Barkema HW, et al. Manageable risk factors associated with the lactational incidence, elimination, and prevalence of *Staphylococcus aureus* intramammary infections in dairy cows. J Dairy Sci 2012;95:1283–300.

44. NMC. Summary of peer-reviewed publications on efficacy of premilking and postmilking teat disinfectant published since 1980. Available at: http://www.nmconline.org/docs/Teatbibl.pdf. Accessed March 5, 2012.

45. Borucki Castro SI, Berthiaume R, Laffey P, et al. Iodine concentration in milk sampled from Canadian farms. J Food Prot 2010;73:1658–63.

46. Rasmussen MD, Galton DM, Petersson LG. Effects of premilking teat preparation on spores of anaerobes, bacteria, and iodine residues in milk. J Dairy Sci 1991;74: 2472–8.

47. Wallace JA, Schukken YH, Welcome F. Measuring stimulation's effect with milk flow curves. Proceedings 42nd Annual Meeting of the National Mastitis Council, Fort Worth (TX). National Mastitis Council Inc, Verona (WI); 2003;42:86.

48. Maroney M, Ruegg P, Tayar F, et al. Use of Lactocorder® to measure milking performance. Proceedings 43rd Annual Meeting of the National Mastitis Council, Charlotte (NC). National Mastitis Council, Inc., Verona (WI); 2004;43:341.

49. Ruegg P. The seven habits of highly successful milking routines. Available at: www.wcds.ca/proc/2006/Manuscripts/Ruegg2.pdf. Accessed March 7, 2012.

50. Olde Riekerink RGM, Sampimon OC, Eerland VJ, et al. Comparing bacterial counts on bare hands with gloved hands during milking. In Mastitis control: from science to practice. Wageningen (Netherlands): Wageningen Academic Publishers; 2008. p. 77–82.

51. Hogeveen H, Huijps K, Lam TJ. Economic aspects of mastitis: new developments. NZ Vet J 2011;59:16–23.

52. O'Callaghan EJ. Measurement of liner slips, milking time, and milk yield. J Dairy Sci 1996;79:390–5.

53. Rasmussen MD, Frimer ES, Decker EL. Reverse pressure gradients across the teat canal related to machine milking. J Dairy Sci 1994;77:984–93.

54. Mein, G.A., and D. A. Reid. Milking-time test and guidelines for milking unit. Proceedings 35th Annual Meeting of the National Mastitis Council, Nashville (TN). National Mastitis Council Inc, Verona (WI); 1996;35:235.

55. National Mastitis Council. Recommended Mastitis Control Program. Available at: www.nmconline.org/docs/NMCchecklistNA.pdf. Accessed April 9, 2012.

56. Wilson DJ, Gonzalez RN, Sears PM. Segregation or use of separate milking units for cows infected with *Staphylococcus aureus*: effects on prevalence of infection and bulk tank somatic cell count. J Dairy Sci 1995;78:2083–5.

57. Zecconi A, Piccinini R, Fox LK. Epidemiologic study of intramammary infections with *Staphylococcus aureus* during a control program in nine commercial dairy herds. J Am Vet Med Assoc 2003;223:684–8.

58. Middleton JR, Fox LK, Smith TH. Management strategies to decrease the prevalence of mastitis caused by one strain of *Staphylococcus aureus* in a dairy herd. J Am Vet Med Assoc 2001;218:1615–8.

59. Fox LK, Hancock DD. Effect of segregation on prevention of intramammary infections by *Staphylococcus aureus*. J Dairy Sci 1989;72:540–4.

60. Hogan JS, Harmon RJ, Langlois BE, et al. Efficacy of an iodine backflush for preventing new intramammary infections. J Dairy Sci 1984;67:1850–9.

61. Smith TW, Eberhart RJ, Spencer SB, et al. Effect of automatic backflushing on number of new intramammary infections, bacteria on teatcup liners, and milk iodine. J Dairy Sci 1985;68:424–32.

62. Roy JP, Du Tremblay D, DesCôteaux L, et al. Effect of precalving intramammary treatment with pirlimycin in nulliparous Holstein heifers. Can J Vet Res 2007;71:283–91.

63. Makovec JA, Ruegg PL. Antimicrobial resistance of bacteria isolated from dairy cow milk samples submitted for bacterial culture: 8,905 samples (1994-2001). J Am Vet Med Assoc 2003;222:1582–9.

64. Erskine R J, Walker RD, Bolin CA, et al. Trends in antibacterial susceptibility of mastitis pathogens during a seven-year period. J Dairy Sci 2002;85:1111–8.

65. Farnsworth R, Stewart S, Reid D. Dealing with *Streptococcus agalactiae* mastitis 2011. Available at: www.ansci.umn.edu/dairy/Quality_Counts_2012/factsheets/F-MC-2_Dealing_with_strep_ag_mastitis.pdf. Accessed March 7, 2012.

66. Barkema HW, Schukken YH, Zadoks RN. Invited review: The role of cow, pathogen, and treatment regimen in the therapeutic success of bovine *Staphylococcus aureus* mastitis. J Dairy Sci 2006;89:1877–95.

67. van den Borne BH, Nielen M, van Schaik G, et al. Host adaptation of bovine *Staphylococcus aureus* seems associated with bacteriological cure after lactational antimicrobial treatment. J Dairy Sci 2010;93:2550–8.

68. Roy JP, Keefe GP. Systematic review: What is the best antibiotic treatment for *Staphylococcus aureus* intramammary infection of lactating cows in North America? Vet Clin Food Anim 2012;28:39–50.

69. Pinzón-Sánchez C, Cabrera VE, Ruegg PL. Decision tree analysis of treatment strategies for mild and moderate cases of clinical mastitis occurring in early lactation. J Dairy Sci 2011;94:1873–92.

70. Steeneveld W, van Werven T, Barkema HW, et al. Cow-specific treatment of clinical mastitis: an economic approach. J Dairy Sci 2011;94:174–88.

71. Middleton JR, Luby CD, Adams DS. Efficacy of vaccination against staphylococcal mastitis: a review and new data. Vet Microbiol 2009;134:192–8.

72. Pereira UP, Oliveira DG, Mesquita LR, et al. Efficacy of *Staphylococcus aureus* vaccines for bovine mastitis: a systematic review. Vet Microbiol 2011;148:117–24.

73. Robert A, Seegers H, Bareille N. Incidence of intramammary infections during the dry period without or with antibiotic treatment in dairy cows: a quantitative analysis of published data. Vet Res 2006;37:25–48.

74. Barkema HW, Green MJ, Bradley AJ, et al. Invited review: The role of contagious disease in udder health. J Dairy Sci 2009;92:4717–29.

75. Middleton JR, Fox LK, Gay JM, et al. Use of pulsed-field gel electrophoresis for detecting differences in *Staphylococcus aureus* strain populations between dairy herds with different cattle importation practices. Epidemiol Infect 2002;129:387–95.

Managing Environmental Mastitis

Joe Hogan, PhD*, K. Larry Smith, PhD

KEYWORDS

- Mastitis • Bedding • Dairy cows • Intramammary infections

KEY POINTS

- Coliform bacteria, streptococci, and enterococci are the most common etiologic agents of environmental mastitis.
- The primary agents of environmental mastitis are of fecal origin but can also heavily contaminate organic materials such as bedding, feed, and soil in the cows' surroundings.
- Washed sand contains 100-fold fewer mastitis pathogens per gram of bedding compared with common organic bedding materials.
- Management keys to reducing exposure of cows to environmental mastitis pathogens include frequent manure removal, eliminating standing water in the cow's walking lanes and loafing areas, and avoiding overcrowding of animals in barns and pastures.
- Populations of mastitis pathogens increase in the cow's environment as ambient temperature and moisture increases.
- Rates of environmental mastitis are greatest during the dry period and early lactation compared with other stages of lactation.

The most common environmental mastitis pathogens among herds of North America are those grouped as coliforms and environmental streptococci. The term *"coliform mastitis"* frequently is used incorrectly to identify mammary disease caused by all gram-negative bacteria.[1] Genera classified as coliforms are *Escherichia, Klebsiella,* and *Enterobacter.* Other gram-negative bacteria frequently isolated from intramammary infections include species of *Serratia, Pseudomonas,* and *Proteus.*[2] Coliform bacteria occupy many habitats in the cow's environment. *Escherichia coli* are normal inhabitants of the gastrointestinal tract of warm blooded animals. Both *Klebsiella* spp and *Enterobacter* spp populate soils, grains, water, and intestinal tracts of animals. *Serratia marcesens* share many environmental sources with *Klebsiella* spp and

Salaries and research support were provided by state and federal funds appropriated to the Ohio Agricultural Research and Development Center, The Ohio State University.
The authors have nothing to disclose.
Ohio Agricultural Research and Development Center, The Ohio State University, Wooster, OH 44691, USA
* Corresponding author.
E-mail address: hogan.4@osu.edu

Enterobacter spp. *Pseudomonas* spp and *Proteus* spp commonly contaminate drop hoses used to wash udders before milking.

The group of bacteria collectively labeled environmental streptococci includes *Streptococcus uberis*, *Streptococcus dysgalcatiae*, and *Enterococcus* spp.[3] The environmental streptococci, *S uberis* in particular, have been isolated from bedding materials, soil, rumen, feces, vulva, lips, nares, mammary gland, and teats.[4,5] Feed stuffs such as silages and green chop forages may also be a source of these pathogens and infections of the reproductive tract may contribute to environmental and teat end contamination.[6]

STALL BEDDING IS A KEY ENVIRONMENTAL SOURCE

The key to controlling environmental mastitis to an economically acceptable level within a herd is to reduce the exposure of cows to the pathogens. Although bacteria that cause environmental mastitis are among the etiologic agents commonly responsible for infectious respiratory and urogenital diseases in dairy cows,[7] the spread of these bacteria from other regions of the body to the mammary gland via the vascular or lymphatic systems appears minimal. Intramammary infections caused by environmental mastitis pathogens typically result from the bacteria traversing the teat canal and multiplying in the gland. These bacterial species are chemotropic organisms requiring organic material to use as food. Coliforms and streptococci cannot live on teat skin for long periods of time. If these bacteria are present in large numbers on teat skin, it is the result of recent contamination. Therefore, the number of these bacteria on teat skin is a reflection of the cow's exposure to the contaminating environment.[8,9]

Cows lay down 12 to 14 hours a day, and their teats are in direct contact with the bedding or other materials where they rest. Populations of the bacteria in bedding are related to the number of bacteria on teat ends and rates of clinical mastitis.[9,10] Therefore, reducing the number of bacteria in bedding generally results in a decrease in environmental mastitis. Coliforms cannot live on teat skin for long periods of time. If these bacteria are present in large numbers on teat skin, it is the result of recent contamination from a source such as bedding. Hygiene and proper management of stall, lots, and pastures are essential.

Sand Bedding

Ideally, bedding should be inorganic materials that are low in moisture content and contain few nutrients for bacteria to use. The bedding material that we recommend most for controlling environmental mastitis is washed sand. Compared to organic materials such as sawdust, recycled manure, straw, and dirt, washed sand consistently contains 100-fold fewer mastitis pathogens per gram of bedding.[10] The effectiveness of sand for reducing exposure of mastitis pathogens to mammary glands is due to the inorganic properties of sand. However, as organic content and moisture in sand bedding increase during the common practice of on-farm reclaiming sand from sand-laden manure, the mastitis pathogen populations also increase.[11] A realistic goal for dry matter of sand used for bedding is greater than 95%. Organic matter in sand bedding should be less than 5%.

Organic Bedding

Many farms are forced to use organic bedding materials that are compatible with liquid manure–handling systems. Little advantage exists in using one organic material over the use of another. For example, straw tends to have highest streptococcal counts, while sawdust has the highest coliform counts in comparisons among these bedding materials.[10] Any material to be used as bedding should be stored in a dry area to prevent saturation by rain and ground moisture. Composting organic materials is an effective way to reduce bacterial counts before use as bedding. However, although many organic bedding materials have relatively few mastitis pathogens prior to use, the pathogen populations often increase 10,000-fold within hours after use as bedding.[12] Fresh bedding tends to absorb moisture from the cows' environment for use by the great number of bacteria that are constantly present in manure and soiled bedding.

Organic materials used as bedding in North America have historically been affordable byproducts of the grain crops or the forestry and wood industry. Two trends have caused a shift from these organic bedding sources to the use of recycled manure solids on many dairies. First, the availability of sawdust, wood shavings, and straw has diminished with the increased of use of these products for home heating fuel and landscaping mulch. Second, the use of methane digesters on some dairies results in available solids and the profitability of digesters necessitates the use of solids for bedding. In general, bacterial counts in manure solids are similar to those in sawdust. The key to successful use of manure solids is to lower the moisture content, thus lowering the bacterial counts of mastitis pathogens. A realistic goal for manure solids when placed in stalls is 35% dry matter.

Regardless of the bedding used, removing wet and soiled material from the back third of stalls will significantly reduce the bacterial counts. Stalls should be raked a minimum of twice daily when animals are moved to be milked. A practice that is often successful in herds using manure solids is the daily complete replacement of bedding in back third of stalls. Spraying bedding with disinfectant and adding powdered lime to bedding have met with little practical success in reducing bacterial counts.[13] These practices cause an initial decline in bacterial populations, but pathogen numbers quickly recover. Twice-a-day application of powdered lime may be necessary to sustain an advantage in lowering bacterial numbers. Standing water and mud should be avoided in stalls, holding areas, and lots. Overcrowding of free-stall barns increases the manure contaminating the alleys and lanes. The accumulated manure in alleys will splatter on hooves and legs to contaminate bedding with organic matter and inoculate the bedding with fecal bacteria. Cows' access to dirt-manure lots also should be limited during rainy seasons. Outbreaks of coliform mastitis are common during rainy seasons when cows are exposed to dirt-manure lots and lanes leading to the milking parlors.

Seasonal Effects

Climatic factors that affect the risk to environmental mastitis are temperature and humidity. As the ambient temperature and moisture increase, populations of pathogens increase in the cow's environment and the mammary defense systems to combat infections become compromised. Growth rates of coliforms and environmental streptococci are greatest during warm, wet weather. The effects of season on bacterial populations in bedding are quite dramatic in regions that experience a wide variation of temperatures within a year. In general, the impact of bedding on exposure of cows in confinement housing decreases during cold weather and increases as temperatures and humidity increase.[10] Previous trials have shown a strong correlation between bacterial counts in bedding and both ambient temperature and relative humidity.[14] Overcrowding of barns with cows will exasperate the effects of heat and humidity. Therefore, adequate ventilation of barns and proper stocking rates are essential to moderate the effects of heat and humidity in housing areas.

Dry Lots and Corrals

Dirt and manure covered corrals are commonly used to house cows in semiarid and arid areas where temperatures are seldom below freezing for an extended time. Exposure to pathogens generally is low during the dry seasons as moisture content of the dirt-manure mixture is low. However, as density of cows increase under shade structures and around feeding areas and water troughs, excess wet organic matter should be removed or spread out to be dried.[15] Climatic factors affecting exposure in herds where cows are maintained on dry lots differ from those of in-stall barns. The rainy seasons of late fall through early spring are when bacterial populations are greatest. Manure in dry lots during the summer tends to be desiccated, thus limiting the moisture essential for bacterial growth.

Grazing Systems

The majority of research on the effects of grazing systems on mammary health has been conducted outside of North America. However, the overriding principle of reducing pathogen exposure by the use of grazing pastures appears universal. Grazing management systems often decrease pathogen loads in the cows' environment compared with total confinement systems. Turf-covered soil in grazing paddocks typically have minimal contamination with environmental mastitis pathogens when compared with organic bedding in stalls or loose housing. Bacterial exposure increases as forage is closely grazed and stocking rate increases.[16,17] Ample time between rotation of cows on paddocks is needed to allow forage regrowth over soil and manure load to dissipate.

Barren soil due to overgrazing and trampling can harbor elevated populations in the cows' environment.[18] Areas around feed troughs, exercise lots, and lanes often expose cows to bacterial concentrations comparable to that in organic bedded stalls. Removal of wet organic matter and replacement with dry, inorganic materials will reduce exposure. Similar to dry lots, solar radiation and drying during summer months reduce bacterial contamination in these areas compared with rainy winter months.[17]

Maternity and Dry Cow Lots

As evidenced later in the article, the rate of new intramammary infections caused by environmental mastitis pathogens is greater during the dry period than during lactation. Management and hygiene of dry cow housing and maternity areas should be priorities. Fortunately, the management practices for reducing mastitis pathogen exposure in dry cow and maternity facilities are similar to those for lactating cow housing. Dry cow areas should be well drained and free of excess manure. Dirt-covered areas can expose cows to pathogen levels comparable to those in free-stalls. Box stalls and loose housing areas should be cleaned to the foundation base regularly. Manure packs are to be avoided because they generally contain extremely high counts of pathogens that are dangerous to both dam and calf.

Milking Hygiene

Milking time hygiene is the basis for control of contagious mastitis but has less influence on environmental mastitis. The use of germicidal teat dips postmilking will have minimal effect on incidence of new intramammary infections caused by coliform or environmental streptococci. Teat dip efficacy is dependent on the time of application relative to milking and the pathogens causing mastitis. Most germicidal teat dips effectively and rapidly destroy microbes on teat skin by chemical or biological action. However, the persistency of germicidal activity is limited and neutralized by organic material such as milk and manure.[1] Therefore, although most germicidal products will kill coliforms on teat skin, exposure to these pathogens occurs primarily between milkings, long after the killing activity of the dips has diminished.

Predipping teats before milking in an effective disinfectant reduces new intramammary infections caused by coliforms during lactation. Field trials have shown predipping reduces the incidence of clinical mastitis by 50% in herds with low levels of contagious mastitis.[19] Current recommendations in North America for predipping include forestripping the first few streams of milk, removing excess manure and dirt from teats, dipping teats in the germicidal teat dip, allowing teat dip to contact teat skin at least 30 seconds, and manually drying teats with either individual paper towels or freshly laundered cloth towels.

Barrier dips form a physical obstruction between teat skin and the environment. Latex, acrylic, and polymer based products form a physical seal over the teat end to impede entrance into the udder between milkings. The use of some latex barrier teat dips may reduce the incidence of coliform mastitis, but the efficacy of physical barrier teat dips against other pathogens is minimal. Barrier teat dips containing germicides have not been shown to be more effective than conventional germicidal dips in reducing environmental mastitis in controlled studies.[20]

MONITORING CLINICAL MASTITIS

The ultimate measure of success in reducing exposure to environmental mastitis pathogens is improvement in mammary health. Bulk tank and monthly cow somatic cell counts (SCCs) are poor milk quality indicators of environmental mastitis. The prevalence of intramammary infections caused by environmental pathogens within a herd is seldom great enough to cause bulk tank SCCs of higher than 250,000/mL, but approximately 85% of coliform and 50% of environmental streptococcal infections will cause clinical mastitis. Surveys of herds with low bulk tank SCCs[21] have shown the average rate of clinical mastitis to be 46 cases per year in a 100-cow herd (3.8% of cows per month). The high frequency of clinical cases and relatively short duration of these intramammary infections render the use of individual cow SCC and bulk tank SCC as poor indicators of the prevalence of disease caused by these bacteria. For example, prevalence of intramammary infections caused by environmental mastitis pathogens seldom exceeds 5% of quarters in a herd; however, 20% and 15% of cows in well-managed herds are annually diagnosed with clinical mastitis caused by coliforms and environmental streptococci, respectfully. A realistic goal for rate of total clinical cases in a well-managed herd is 2% of cows per month.

The severity of clinical mastitis caused by environmental pathogens ranges from mild local signs to death. The vast majority of clinical coliform and environmental streptococcal clinical cases are characterized by only abnormal milk and a swollen gland. Only about 10% of clinical coliform cases result in systemic signs including fever, anorexia, and altered respiration.[22,23] Despite the relatively low percentage of clinical coliform cases yielding systemic signs, coliform bacteria have an exaggerated reputation for causing severe mastitis. The basis for this distinction originates from the point that the coliforms are the most common cause of systemic illness resulting from mastitis. Survey averages suggest that coliform bacteria are the culprits of 60% to 70% of severe clinical cases involving systemic signs.[22,23] Therefore, the general conclusions concerning severity of clinical coliform cases are that few coliform intramammary infections cause systemic clinical signs, but the majority of clinical cases resulting in systemic signs are caused by coliform bacteria.

Stage of lactation has a tremendous impact on cows' susceptibility to environmental mastitis. Recording the number of clinical cases and documenting the stage of lactation when they occur will aid in determining when cows are at greatest risk to clinical mastitis. Rates of new intramammary infections caused by coliforms are generally greater during the dry period than during lactation. Therefore, the thrust of herd management strategies for reducing environmental exposure should focus on dry period and early lactation. During the dry period, susceptibility to intramammary infections is greatest at the 2 weeks after drying off and the 2 weeks prior to calving. Many infections acquired during the dry period persist to lactation and become clinical cases. Research has shown that 65% of coliform clinical cases that occur in the first 2 months of lactation are intramammary infections that originated during the dry period.[22] Coliforms are adept at infecting the mammary gland during the transitional phase from lactating to fully involuted mammary gland. However, K pneumoniae, Serratia, and Pseudomonas are more capable than E coli at surviving in the mammary gland from the onset of involution until calving. Distribution of infections reveals that the greatest proportion of K pneumoniae infections present at calving originated in the first half of the dry period.[24] E coli infections present at calving and early lactation most often originate during the last 2 weeks of the dry period.

Rate of intramammary infections during lactation is highest at calving and decreases as days in milk advance. The prevalence coliform mastitis in a herd seldom exceeds 5% of lactating quarters because coliform infections tend to be short duration during lactation. The average duration of E coli intramammary infections during lactation is less than 10 days. Duration of intramammary infections caused by K pneumoniae average about 21 days. Chronic infections of greater than 90 days caused by E coli or K pneumoniae are relatively rare.[22] A major difference between intramammary infections caused by coliform bacteria and those caused by other gram-negative bacteria is the duration that bacteria persist in the mammary gland. Intramammary infections caused by Serratia spp and Pseudomonas spp often are less severe and more likely chronic infections, compared with E coli intramammary infections, and may persist multiple lactations.

The dynamics of environmental streptococcal mastitis across the stages of lactation are similar to those of coliform bacteria. The dry period is the time of greatest susceptibility to new environmental streptococcal intramammary infections. The rate of environmental streptococcal intramammary infections was 5.5-fold greater during the dry period than during lactation.[24] Environmental streptococcal intramammary infections tended to be short-duration infections with only a relatively few becoming chronic. Average duration of environmental streptococcal intramammary infections is less than 2 weeks.[22] During lactation, the incidence of clinical mastitis is greatest the first week after calving and decreased throughout the first 305 days in milk. Interestingly, rate of environmental streptococcal clinical cases increased in cows with extended lactations (>305 days) and is comparable to that of cows in peak lactation. Therefore, the use of management practices that encourage the use of extended calving intervals (thus a larger percentage of cows with extended days in milk) may impact the prevalence of environmental streptococcal intramammary infections in a herd.

SUMMARY

Many of the practices and principals of management for reducing the exposure of dairy cows to environmental mastitis pathogens were introduced a quarter of a century ago[22–25] and have been the subject of numerous reviews.[1,3,21] The common theme for reducing mastitis pathogens in the cows' environment is reducing moisture and organic contamination.[1] Frequent manure removal, avoiding overstocking of cows, taking precautions to eliminate stagnant water around cows, and providing clean, dry inorganic bedding for cows to lay on are important management considerations. These factors of environmental hygiene transcend stall barns, manure pack barns, open corrals, and pasture systems. The emphasis of control should center on protecting periparturient animals during wet, hot periods of the year when mastitis pathogen growth in the environment is greatest. As the dairy industry in North America changes and progresses to adapt to economic, social, and environmental demands, the old adage of keeping cows cool, dry, and comfortable remains paramount in managing environmental mastitis.

REFERENCES

1. Hogan J, Smith KL. Coliform mastitis. Vet Res 2003;34:507–19.
2. National Mastitis Council. Gram-negative bacteria. In: Laboratory handbook on bovine mastitis. Madison (WI): The National Mastitis Council, Inc; 1999. p. 85-115.
3. Hogan J, Smith KL. Environmental streptococcal mastitis: facts, fables, and fallacies. In: Proceedings of the 42nd Annual Meeting of the National Mastitis Council. Fort Worth (TX). Verona (WI): National Mastitis Council, Inc; 2003. p. 162–71.
4. Bramley AJ. Sources of *Streptococcus uberis* in the dairy herd. I. Isolation from bovine faeces and from straw bedding of cattle. J Dairy Res 1982;49:369–73.
5. Kruze J, Bramley AJ. Sources of *Streptococcus uberis* in the dairy herd. II. Evidence of colonization of the bovine intestine by *Str. uberis*. J Dairy Res 1982;49:375–9.
6. Petersson-Wolfe CS, Adams S, Wolf SL, et al. Genomic typing of enterococci isolated from bovine mammary glands and environmental sources. J Dairy Sci 2008;91: 615–9.
7. Epperson WB, Hoblet KH, Smith KL, et al. Association of abnormal uterine discharge with new intramammary infection in the early postpartum period in multiparous dairy cows. J Am Vet Med Assoc 1993;202:1461–4.
8. Rendos JJ, Eberhart RJ, Kesler EM. Microbial populations of teat ends of dairy cows, and bedding materials. J Dairy Sci 1975;58:1492–500.
9. Zdanowicz M, Shelford JA, Tucker CB, et al. Bacterial populations on teat ends of dairy cows housed in free stalls and bedded with either sand or sawdust. J Dairy Sci 2004;87;1694–701.
10. Hogan JS, Smith KL, Hoblet KH, et al. Bacterial counts in bedding materials used on nine commercial dairies. J Dairy Sci 1989;72:250–8.
11. Kristula MA, Rogers W, Hogan JS, et al. Comparison of bacteria populations in clean and recycled sand used for bedding in dairy facilities. J Dairy Sci 2005;88:4317–25.
12. Gooch CA, Hogan JS, Glazier N, et al. Use of post-digested separated manure solids as freestall bedding: case study. In: Proceeding of the 46th Annual Meeting of the National Mastitis Council. Tampa (FL). Verona (WI): National Mastitis Council, Inc; 2006. p. 151–60.
13. Hogan JH, Bogacz VL, Thompson LM, et al. Bacterial counts associated with sawdust and recycled manure bedding treated with commercial conditioners. J Dairy Sci 1999;82:1690–5.
14. Hogan JS, Smith KL, Todhunter DA, et al. Bacterial counts associated with recycled newspaper bedding. J Dairy Sci 1990;73:1756–61.
15. Spencer H. Free stall and corral management as related to mastitis control. In: Proceedings of the Regional Meeting of the National Mastitis Council. Madison (WI). Verona (WI): National Mastitis Council, Inc; 1996. p. 60–2.
16. Green MJ, Bradley AJ, Medley GF, et al. Cow, farm, and management factors during the dry period that determine the rate of clinical mastitis after calving. J Dairy Sci 2007;90:3764–76.

17. Lopez-Benavides MG, Williamson JH, Pullinger GD, et al. Field observations on the variation of *Streptococcus uberis* populations in a pasture-based dairy farm. J Dairy Sci 2007;90:5558–66.
18. Lacy-Hulbert J, Benavides ML, Williamson J, et al. Ecology of *Streptococcus uberis* within a pasture-based dairying system. Proceeding of the 46th Annual Meeting of the National Mastitis Council. Tampa (FL). Verona (WI): National Mastitis Council, Inc; 2006. p. 134–44.
19. Pankey JW. Hygiene at milking time in the prevention of bovine mastitis. Br Vet J 1989;145:401–9.
20. National Mastitis Council. Summary of peer-reviewed publications on efficacy of premilking and postmilking teat disinfectants published since 1980. In: Proceedings of the 51st Annual Meeting of the National Mastitis Council. St Petersburg (FL). Verona (WI): National Mastitis Council, Inc; 2012. p. 235–49.
21. Smith KL, Hogan JS. Environmental mastitis. Large Anim Vet 1992;47:16–20.
22. Smith KL, Todhunter DA, Schoenberger PS. Environmental mastitis: cause, prevalence, prevention. J Dairy Sci 1985;68:1531–53.
23. Hogan JS, Smith KL, Hoblet KH, et al. Field survey of mastitis in low somatic cell count herds. J Dairy Sci 1989;72:1547–56.
24. Smith KL, Todhunter DA, Schoenberger PS. Environmental pathogens and intramammary infection during the dry period. J Dairy Sci 1985;68:402–17.
25. Erskine RJ, Eberhart RJ, Hutchinson LH, et al. Incidence and types of clinical mastitis in dairy herds with high and low somatic cell counts. JAVMA 1988;192:761–5.

Mycoplasma Mastitis
Causes, Transmission, and Control

Lawrence K. Fox, MS, PhD

KEYWORDS

- *Mycoplasma* • Mastitis • Epidemiology • Control

KEY POINTS

- *Mycoplasma* sp are categorized as contagious mastitis pathogens, and it appears that *Mycoplasma* mastitis is a growing problem in the United States.
- The herd prevalence of mycoplasma mastitis pathogens has been estimated through culture and analysis of bulk tank milk samples.
- *Mycoplasma* sp that have been associated with mastitis have been considered contagious in nature, transmitted at milking time from a reservoir, the infected udder; via fomites, hands of a milker, milking unit liners, or udder wash cloths; to an uninfected cow. Additionally, evidence is presented that would suggest that *Mycoplasma* sp are spread on dairy herds by aerosols, nose to nose contact, and are spread hematogenously to the mammary gland to cause mastitis and arthritis.

INTRODUCTION

The first reported case of *Mycoplasma* mastitis was that of Hale and coworkers.[1] This Connecticut research group described the difficulties in isolating the pathogen that infected approximately 30% of a dairy herd. They had success when they allowed incubation of milk cultures to proceed for 5 days under 10% CO_2. They named the isolated organism *Mycoplasma agalactiae* var *bovis*, currently known as *M bovis*. This first described outbreak was remarkable in that it affected a large proportion of the herd, spread to multiple quarters of the same cow, and the agent was difficult to culture. Shortly after this report, Carmichael and coworkers of New York,[2] as reported by Jasper[3] and Stuart and coworkers of Great Britain,[4] reported *Mycoplasma* mastitis cases. One can imagine that following the report by Hale and coworkers,[1] researchers[1,4] and others applied the culture techniques described and were able to isolate *Mycoplasma* sp from cases of mastitis that might have previously been considered

The author has nothing to disclose.
Department of Veterinary Clinical Sciences, College of Veterinary Medicine, 100 Grimes Way, ADBF 2043, Washington State University, Pullman, WA 99164-7060, USA
E-mail address: fox@wsu.edu

Vet Clin Food Anim 28 (2012) 225–237
http://dx.doi.org/10.1016/j.cvfa.2012.03.007
0749-0720/12/$ – see front matter © 2012 Elsevier Inc. All rights reserved.

Table 1				
Percentage of cases of *Mycoplasma* mastitis by species				
Report	*M bovis*	*M californicum*	*M bovigenitalium*	*Other*
Jasper (1980)[15]	51	16	5	28
Kirk et al (1997)[16]	48	11	25	16
Boonyayatra et al (2011)[17]	85	5	1	9

idiopathic. Thus, 50 years ago it was apparent that *Mycoplasma* mastitis was a problem, perhaps an emerging problem.

Today it is recognized that *Mycoplasma* mastitis affects cattle around the world.[5,6] *Mycoplasma* sp are categorized as contagious mastitis pathogens[7] and it appears that *Mycoplasma* mastitis is a growing problem in the United States.[3,8–10] Moreover, given the difficulty in culturing the pathogen that was first noted 50 years ago, there is reason to suspect that cases of *Mycoplasma* mastitis are underreported.[11] In this review the epidemiology of *Mycoplasma* mastitis will be discussed, followed by a discussion of the host–pathogen interaction and elements associated with control of the disease. A focus of this article will be the presentation of recent findings that would explain why *Mycoplasma* may be an emerging mastitis pathogen.

EPIDEMIOLOGY

Mycoplasma sp are pathogens associated with several cattle diseases, primarily otitis media, inflammation of the urogenital tract, arthritis, pneumonia, and mastitis.[12,13] The most prevalent species causing these diseases is *M bovis*.[5,14] With respect to *Mycoplasma* mastitis, *M bovis* is the predominant causative agent and *M californicum* and *M bovigenitalium* appear to the next most common (**Table 1**).

Jasper[15] summarized the agents associated with cases of clinical *Mycoplasma* mastitis during a 14-year period and found that *M bovis* and *californicum* were the most common. The third most common was *M alkalescens,* which comprised approximately 12% of intramammary infections, followed by *M bovigenitalium* at 5% (see **Table 1**). Kirk and coworkers[16] surveyed bulk tank milk from a cooperative of 267 dairies in CA monthly for 6 years. The annual prevalence of tanks with *Mycoplasma* sp known to be mastitis agents ranged from 1.2% to 3.1% of tank samples. They reported that *M bovis, californicum,* and *bovigenitalium* were the most consistently the *Mycoplasma* mastitis agents isolated. Boonyayatra and colleagues[17] examined milk samples from 248 cases of clinical mastitis from a variety of sources over several years and reported 85% were *M bovis,* 5% were *M californicum,* and only 1% were *M bovigenitalium.* In the surveys reported in **Table 1**, it is clear that *M bovis* and *M californicum* appear to be the 2 most prevalent *Mycoplasma* mastitis pathogens. Other species that have been noted as causes of *Mycoplasma* mastitis include *M arginini, bovirhinis, canadense,* dispar, bovine group 7, and F-38.[18]

Prevalence

Prevalence of contagious mastitis pathogens estimates have been made through culture and analysis of bulk tank milk samples.[9,19] The major contagious mastitis pathogens identified this way in the United States are *Staphylococcus aureus, Streptococcus agalactiae,* and *Mycoplasma* sp, with herd level prevalence of 43.0%, 2.6%, and 3.2%.[9] In this survey,[9] the herd size affected the prevalence of only *Mycoplasma* mastitis, with the prevalence of other contagious mastitis pathogens unaltered by the number of cows per herd. In large herds (>500 cows), the prevalence of *Mycoplasma* mastitis was 14.4%. Results from a previous study were similar as it was reported that the percentages of *Mycoplasma* positive bulk tanks from herds with less than 100, 100 to 499, and more than 500 cows was 2.1%, 3.9%, and 21.7%.[8] In the later survey, regional differences were noted with 9.4% of the operations in the West having one positive *Mycoplasma* bulk tank culture, with operations in the Northeast and Midwest with less than 3% and the Southeast having 6.6%. Presumably, the regional differences are a function of herd size as herds in the West tend to have the most cows and herds in the Northeast and Midwest tend to have the fewest number of cows.[20]

Based on bulk tank surveys, the prevalence of *Mycoplasma* mastitis varies across the globe. In the European Union countries of Belgium, France, and Greece, the range in prevalence was less than 1% to 5.4% of herds.[21–23] Yet surveys done in Mexico,[24] Iran,[25] and Australia[26] indicate prevalence estimates as high as 55% to 100% of herds. In New Zealand, McDonald and coworkers[27] surveyed 244 herds and could not detect *Mycoplasma* sp in any bulk tank samples, suggesting a very low prevalence. The wide variation in global prevalence may be a function of exposure to these agents. Importation and mixing of cattle have been reported to lead to outbreaks of *Mycoplasma* diseases. For example, the first reported case of *Mycoplasma* cattle disease in Ireland occurred in 1993 and was attributed to the relaxation of import controls within the European Union.[28] Exposure of naïve cattle to this agent led to the appearance and then a significant increase in bovine *Mycoplasma* diseases.[28] Herd replacement cattle exposed to cattle outside the herd, either imported or reared off-site, increased with increasing herd size, a biosecurity risk factor.[29] It was found that herd size[10,30] and culling[30] were risk factors for increased herd prevalence of *Mycoplasma* mastitis. Presumably this is a result of herd expansion, the entrance of new cattle with symptomatic, or asymptomatic carriage of new strains of *Mycoplasma* sp into the herd. Thus, the elevated prevalence of *Mycoplasma* mastitis in herds, and herds of some countries, where cattle movement into and out of a herd is common, could explain the increased prevalence of this disease.

Cow-level prevalence is more difficult to estimate. It has been reported that in Great Britain, less than 1% of cows are affected by *Mycoplasma* mastitis.[31] *Mycoplasma* mastitis has most often been reported as a clinical disease. A survey of clinical mastitis in New York indicates that *Mycoplasma* sp are the cause of 1.5% of cases.[32]

Transmission

Mycoplasma sp that have been associated with mastitis have been considered contagious in nature, transmitted mostly at milking time from a reservoir, the infected udder; via fomites, hands of a milker, milking unit liners, or udder wash cloths; to an uninfected cow.[7] Strict milking time hygiene practices of disinfectant of udders before milking using single service towels, use of gloves by milkers, post-milking unit disinfection, and disinfection of teats post-milking were very effective in controlling the traditional contagious mastitis pathogens of *S aureus* and *S agalactiae*.[33] It has been assumed, but not tested, that such practices would be effective in the control of *Mycoplasma* mastitis.

Mycoplasma sp can spread from one bovine body site to another presumably via lymph or peripheral blood systems. *Mycoplasma* sp associated with mastitis have been isolated from the blood of cattle.[34–36] In outbreaks with *Mycoplasma* mastitis, it is not unusual to find cases of *Mycoplasma* arthritis.[37–41] Similarly, a field outbreak of *Mycoplasma*-associated bovine respiratory disease was associated with outbreaks of arthritis.[41] The link between arthritic *Mycoplasma* disease events and mastitis or pneumonia is indicative that internal somatic spread of this agent is not uncommon. Often multiple organ sites of cattle can be colonized and it is clear that the strain causing the disease is most often the same strain that is widely disseminated throughout the body.[35] This is also been shown by Jain and colleagues,[42] who experimentally induced intramammary infections with *Mycoplasma* sp in lactating cows and found that the apparent strain inoculated was shed at the mucosal surfaces of the eyes, nose, vagina, and rectum, within hours to days after inoculation. With this experiment, they also demonstrated vertical transfer of the agent as a calf, born during the trial from one experimentally infected cow, became colonized by the agent.[42] Moreover, in an outbreak of *Mycoplasma* mastitis, the agent was found colonizing the nares of cattle, both cows and/or calves.[43,44] The strain causing mastitis was found from nasal swab samples collected from cows and calves.[40] Thus, transmission of *Mycoplasma* sp associated with bovine mastitis may occur within the cow internally, from one infected organ site to the udder or reverse; and between cows from indirect udder to udder contact at milking time; or perhaps by shedding of the pathogen through external mucosal surfaces of an infected or colonized animal to a naïve animal.

Transmission of *Mycoplasma* sp from environmental sources to the udder has been discussed.[18] In this review, the authors report on 2 studies, 1 in Italy and 1 in Germany, where it was found that *M bovis* survived in and on multiple surfaces at various temperatures for up to 8 months. Materials studied were those that could be typically found on dairies including sponges, stainless steel, wood, rubber, glass, and water. Justice-Allen and coworkers[45] in Utah discovered that *Mycoplasma* could live for up to 8 months in a sand pile. The sand originated from a herd with an outbreak of *Mycoplasma* mastitis. *Mycoplasma* was also isolated in sand from 2 other dairies. The authors[45] suggested that sand could be a reservoir for *Mycoplasma* mastitis. However, in a separate investigation where there appeared to be a link between sand bedding and a clinical mastitis outbreak, it was found that the strains of *Mycoplasma* sp in the bedding had a completely different DNA fingerprint than those causing mastitis (Fox and Corbett, unpublished data, 2008). Utah researchers[46] investigated the possible transmission of *M bovis* from sand to naïve dairy calves during a 105-day trial. Although calves housed on sand bedding with *M bovis* carried this agent for periods of time during the trial, there was no evidence of carriage beyond transient colonization and no specific antibody titers formed against the agent. The authors concluded that there was no evidence that the contaminated bedding would serve as a source of *M bovis* disease transmission to naïve dairy calves. Thus, although it is clear that environmental sources could serve as a reservoir for *Mycoplasma* mastitis, there is no evidence to support that *M bovis* transmission from the environment to a cow is a likely mechanism involved in *Mycoplasma* mastitis.

Carriage

Most cases of mastitis are subclinical and the greatest loss to a dairy is a result of the subclinical nature of the disease.[47] Jasper[48] indicates that a significant number of cows might be shedding *Mycoplasma* pathogens in their milk without symptoms. Perhaps given the difficulty, expense, and the historically low prevalence of the *Mycoplasma* mastitis, a good estimate of the prevalence of subclinical *Mycoplasma* mastitis infections has not been reported.

It is well established that *Mycoplasma* sp can be isolated from mucosal surfaces of clinically normal calves and cows.[40,49] The prevalence of calves shedding *M bovis* at the nares was 34% in herds with noted *Mycoplasma* mastitis and only 6% in herds apparently free of disease.[49] The prevalence of mucosal surface shedding by asymptomatic carriers with the same clone of *M bovis* causing a *Mycoplasma*-associated disease outbreak may be as high as 21% to 47% of cattle in a dairy herd.[40] These findings indicate that *Mycoplasma* shedding by ostensibly healthy cattle is not uncommon but may be far more likely in herds experiencing a current outbreak.

The role of the asymptomatic *Mycoplasma* carrier animal in an outbreak of mastitis is not clear. It is known that *M bovis* carriage in the lungs of beef cattle calves is approximately that of dairy calves in situations without apparent *Mycoplasma* disease. Carriage increases when cattle are stressed, such as when they are moved from their place of rearing and then comingled in different locations as in feedlots.[12] Climatic stresses and *Mycoplasma* disease outbreaks have also been documented. Episodes of *Mycoplasma* pneumonia were observed in a closed beef herd where a number of calves became diseased after a spring storm.[50] Only 1 strain of *M bovis* was identified from pulmonary samples. Given the herd[50] was closed, it could be suspected that the strain identified was asymptomatically carried by cattle of this herd, and with climatic stresses and potentially associated compromised hosts, the *M bovis* strain was able to transform cattle from symptomless to diseased. Thus, a change in the environment of the calf, a move away from their accustomed setting, a change in climate, and/or the exposure to potential new strains of *Mycoplasma* sp can increase the prevalence of carriage of these agents and such carriage might be associated with subclinical or clinical disease.

A dairy herd will generally increase the exposure of its herd, to outside animals, through the purchase of replacements and via off-site rearing of calves. The University of Idaho dairy with approximately 90 to 100 lactating cows was historically free of *Mycoplasma* mastitis, and ostensibly other *Mycoplasma* diseases were rare or nonexistent. An outbreak of *Mycoplasma*-associated diseases at the University of Idaho dairy began shortly after a state institutional herd contracted with the dairy to raise their calves. The institutional herd also leased their primparae to the university dairy.[40] Within 2 months of initiating the contract, several cases of *Mycoplasma* diseases in calves and mastitis in cows developed. Diseased animals were culled from the herd, and during the third month of the initial outbreak, samples of mucosal surfaces of all animals were collected. Nearly 25% of all animals were shedding the same clone of *M bovis* from the mucosal surfaces as that causing disease. Yet, within 6 months only 1 cow and 1 calf were shedding the clone. During the course of the next year, the outbreak strain was infrequently detected. However, the outbreak clone was the only cause of *Mycoplasma* mastitis, with 4 cases occurring in total. One case spontaneously cured, and the other 3 cases were removed from the herd. New strains of *Mycoplasma* sp were detected, and these strains appeared to be very similar to the outbreak clone. None of these similar strains caused disease. These findings suggest an outbreak strain may be widely disseminated within a herd initially, with a few cases of disease, but concomitant with the dissolution of the outbreak is the reduction of shedding of the agent from mucosal surfaces. Additionally, the authors[40] concluded that the outbreak strain originated with the animals exposed to the institutional dairy herd and thus was imported into the herd. Punyapornwithaya and colleagues[41] also reported on an outbreak of *Mycoplasma* mastitis that appeared to originate with an imported heifer. The *M bovis* clone that caused mastitis in the original heifer at parturition also caused mastitis, pneumonia, and arthritis in the home herd of lactating cows. The strain then "ran its course" and disappeared after 4 months. A similar outbreak of *M bovis* disease was reported to start with mastitis.[44] Here an imported heifer developed mastitis at parturition, and within a few weeks several of the homebred cows developed *M bovis* mastitis, 1 cow developed arthritis, and several calves developed pneumonia. These reports[40,41,44] demonstrate that in an outbreak, there is the potential for multiple animals to become infected with several forms of *Mycoplasma* disease. In aggregate, these studies[40,41] indicate that a single clone of *M bovis* can readily transmit through the herd, but only a small proportion of cows become infected, and both asymptomatic carrier(s) or diseased animals can be the nidus of the outbreak. The nature of transmission might have been during milking time in one herd[41] but in the other[40] it was concluded by the authors that nose-to-nose contact was the most likely means of transmission. Pulmonary transmission would account for the rapid spread, the involvement of both lactating and nonlactating animals, and the involvement of both respiratory and joint diseases. Both Bicknell and colleagues[51] and Jasper[49] discuss the role of the asymptomatic carrier in *Mycoplasma* mastitis disease outbreaks. Both warn that asymptomatic carriers may be reservoirs of disease, although neither author presents evidence that such an outcome is likely or unlikely.

Jasper[49] indicates that some dairy managers will cull asymptomatic *Mycoplasma* carriers and some will isolate carriers until shedding subsides; successful control can be achieved with either method. The odds of an asymptomatic carrier causing an outbreak is unknown. Additionally, preferential culling or isolation of carrier animals was not apparently necessary to control *Mycoplasma* mastitis, and no animal appeared to be an asymptomatic carrier prior to the appearance of *Mycoplasma* mastitis.[40] Additionally, a cow or cows with *Mycoplasma* mastitis may not pose a risk to the development of an outbreak and may not need to be preferentially culled to control transmission.[52] It appears that asymptomatic carriage of *Mycoplasma* sp is involved in a *Mycoplasma* mastitis outbreaks. However, the definitive role carrier animals play in the outbreak and how they should be controlled are unclear. If culling asymptomatic carriers is chosen as a *Mycoplasma* mastitis control strategy, then it should be used judiciously while considering the number of potential culls and their proximity to susceptible animals. Isolation of affected animals and monitoring new carrier and infected animals might be effective tools of control of *Mycoplasma* mastitis.

CHARACTERISTICS OF PATHOGENIC *MYCOPLASMA* SP

Razin and Hayflick[52] have recently reviewed the research on *Mycoplasma* sp. They report that the *Mycoplasma* sp evolved from gram-positive bacteria in a degenerative evolution where these simple organisms lost the ability to produce a cell wall, one manifestation of the diminution of the genome. Razin and Hayflick[53] wrote that *Mycoplasma* cells have essentially 3 organelles: cell membrane, ribosomes, and densely packed circular DNA. The *Mycoplasma* cell is spherical about 0.3 to 0.8 μm in diameter. The species have a significant requirement for fatty acids and sterols and intermediate metabolic pathways are often truncated. *Mycoplasma* sp are perhaps the smallest and most simple self-replicating bacteria.[54] Given their simple nature and fastidious growth requirements, they find ecological niches within their host. In cases of intramammary infections, *Mycoplasma* sp do not appear to often cause a significant, if any, febrile response,[48,55,56] which may be consistent with their nature to colonize cows asymptomatically.

Mycoplasma sp lack a cell wall and thus are inherently resistant to beta-lactam antibiotics. The study of the pathogenicity of *Mycoplasma* organisms is diverse given that there are more than 100 *Mycoplasma* sp, with most of these pathogens specific for one or a few host species. Yet it appears that the pathogenic characteristics of *Mycoplasma* sp in general are (1) adherence to host cells, (2) internalization into host cells, (3) immunomodulatory characteristics, and (4) ability to colonize host tissue without causing fulminant disease.

Several *Mycoplasma* sp including *M bovis* possess adhesion molecules as part of their cell membranes, which allow them to bind to host tissue cells.[57] *M pneumonia*, for example, possesses a protein complex (P1, P30, P116, HMW1-3, A, B, and C) that provides for structural and functional adherence to cells and enables gliding mobility.[58] *M bovis* possesses variable surface lipoproteins (Vsps) that are involved in adherence to host cells.[59-61] These Vsps are part of a complex bacterial system that is notably most antigenically diverse and associated with much variation in gene expression.[60,62,63] Browning and colleagues[64] describe the high-frequency phase variation of the multigene families that encode surface proteins that are part of the *Mycoplasma* sp genome. They indicate that it has been generally accepted that the antigenic variation that results from the genetic phase variation is an immune evasion characteristic, although this hypothesis has not been tested.

Adherence to mammary epithelial surfaces is a characteristic of contagious mastitis pathogens, and this adherence characteristic appears to differentiate the contagious from the noncontagious mastitis pathogens.[65,66] It would be logical to assume that since *Mycoplasma* sp are considered contagious mastitis pathogens and as *Mycoplasma* mastitis pathogens are likely to produce cytadhesins, they would also have the ability to adhere to mammary epithelial cells, although this has been untested.

There may be other benefits to these adhesion proteins. The ability to adhere to host cell mucosal surfaces may enable the *Mycoplasma* sp to access nutrients including amino acids, nucleic acids, fatty acids, and sterols.[67] *Mycoplasma* sp tend to have truncated intermediate metabolic pathways[53] and thus have significant nutrient requirements, especially for sterols and fatty acids.

Pathogens that have the ability to invade and survive within the host cell have the advantage of the protection that the host cell affords against the host's own immune response and antimicrobial therapy. The mastitis pathogen *Staphylococcus aureus* has been described to possess this factor.[68] The ability to invade mammary epithelial cells may be a function of the virulence of the *S aureus* mastitis pathogen.[69] *Mycoplasma* sp have the ability to invade eukaryotic host cells.[70-72] There is evidence to indicate that *M bovis* can invade peripheral blood mononuclear cells and erythrocytes in vitro[73] and in both renal tubular epithelial cells and hepatocytes in clinically diseased bull calves determined at necropsy.[74] van de Merwe and colleagues[73] acknowledge that what might have seemed to be *M bovis*–induced invasion might have been a phagocytic response by specific immunocytes. However, *M bovis* appeared to be internalized by lymphocytes and erythrocytes. Not only would such internalization afford the pathogen protection from the immune response and antibiotic treatment, but this characteristic would enable it to reach multiple organ systems, consistent with the ability of *M bovis* to spread to multiple body sites of diseased cattle.[35,55]

M bovis has the ability to modulate the immune system. Findings by van der Merwe and colleagues[73] and Vanden Bush and Rosenbusch[75] indicate the pathogen secretes a peptide, a factor that can inhibit lymphocyte proliferation. This factor appears in the culture supernatant.[73] In addition, *M bovis* can cause immunomodulation of both the humoral and cell-mediated responses. Antibody titers may be reduced in *M bovis*–affected cattle,[76] and the ratio of IgG1 to IgG2 was reversed in some pneumonic calves.[77,78] An alteration in the T-helper cell response to *M bovis* lung infections was noted,[79] and there was evidence indicating that anti-inflammatory cytokine production was altered by an *M bovis* infection.

CONTROL

Historically, it has been thought that *Mycoplasma* mastitis might be best controlled by a test and slaughter program. Cows with *Mycoplasma* mastitis need to be identified and culled from the herd.[6,18,80] A critical component of this *Mycoplasma* mastitis control program is a monitoring system. First, a potential problem with *Mycoplasma* mastitis must be known and cows suspected of *Mycoplasma* mastitis must be identified and verified as diseased. Culture of bulk tank milk on a regular basis is a method to monitor a herd's *Mycoplasma* mastitis status,[10,16,81] and such regular sampling and culture of bulk tank milk as a monitor of *Mycoplasma* mastitis in a herd have been advocated.[52] It is generally believed that the culture of *Mycoplasma* sp from bulk tank milk is indicative of at least one herd cow having *Mycoplasma* mastitis, although a negative culture does not necessarily indicate that the herd is free of this disease.[82] If a herd has zero tolerance of *Mycoplasma* mastitis, then a positive bulk tank culture must be followed by the identification of cows with mastitis. Generally, cows with recent or chronic cases of clinical mastitis would be identified and milk from infected mammary quarters cultured and tested for *Mycoplasma* sp. Additionally, cows with elevated milk somatic cell counts would be identified and milk cultured. Cows once identified with *Mycoplasma* mastitis would be culled from the herd. However, the process of collection of a sample, transport to the laboratory, and culture and identification of the agent can take at least 4 to 7 days, an interim period. Cows may be penned with other infirm cows without *Mycoplasma* mastitis during this interim period. The transmission of *Mycoplasma* mastitis within these hospital pens might be as much as 100-fold more than in the cow's home pen.[41] Thus, hospital pen cows must be managed carefully to control this disease such that *Mycoplasma* mastitis is not transmitted to the home pens, when cows falsely believed to be free of this disease are returned.

The test and slaughter method of control might not be required. Some[53,83,84] reported that control could be achieved without culling, although another report indicated success with specific removal of cows with *Mycoplasma* mastitis.[85] *Mycoplasma* mastitis as a contagious mastitis pathogen should be controlled by full milking time hygiene practices that include disinfectant in the udder premilking wash, single service towels used to clean and dry udders premilking, use of clean gloved hands by milkers, milking unit backflush, and postmilking teat disinfection.[52] Biosecurity practices of isolation of all cattle before entry into a new herd, the testing of those cattle for carriage of *Mycoplasma* sp and elimination of those testing positive prior to entry into the herd, would in theory be an effective control strategy. Yet such a strategy does not appear to be a most common practice.[52] Quarantine of incoming animals requires considerable management as a practice. Quarantine as a control of a disease like *Mycoplasma* mastitis, that is emerging but affects a minority of cattle and herds, may not be cost effective. Yet *M bovis* was believed to be asymptomatically carried from imported cows into a herd believed to have been free of *Mycoplasma* mastitis.[40] Such carriage resulted into an outbreak of *Mycoplasma* diseases, mastitis, arthritis, and pneumonia, in cows and replacements in this herd.

Control of *Mycoplasma* mastitis via treatment is generally not viewed as a primary strategy. It is clear from previous discussion that the immune system will respond to *Mycoplasma* sp as a foreign agent. Yet it is also clear that *Mycoplasma* sp have the ability to evade the immune system by altering their surface proteins and inducing immunomodulatory effects. Perhaps the latter 2 characteristics would explain in part the heretofore lack of a successful development of mastitis vaccines against this agent.[6,18] An excellent review of *Mycoplasma* mastitis therapy can be found in

Jasper.[3] In that review, it is clear that although in vitro sensitivity of *Mycoplasma* mastitis agents exists for a broad range of non–beta-lactam antibiotics, success with antibiotic therapy in vivo has been unrewarding. Bushnell[80] indicated that based on his field experience, antibiotic therapy of *Mycoplasma* was not an economically viable control strategy.

SUMMARY

Mycoplasma mastitis is an emerging mastitis pathogen. Herd prevalence has increased over the past decade, and this increase parallels the increase in average dairy herd size. It has been documented that the importation of cattle into a herd can result in new cases of *Mycoplasma* disease in general and *Mycoplasma* mastitis specifically. Thus, expanding herds are likely to have a greater incidence of this disease. Transmission of the agent can result from either contact with diseased animals or with colonized or asymptomatically infected cattle. Initial transmission might occur via nose-to-nose contact and result in an outbreak of *Mycoplasma* mastitis, or it might occur during the milking time. This would suggest that new, incoming animals should be quarantined before being comingled with original herd animals. Quarantining does not seem to be a biosecurity strategy often practiced in control of *Mycoplasma* mastitis and may not be warranted in herds with excellent milking time hygiene practices. The ability to monitor for the incipient stages of an outbreak, often done through bulk tank milk culturing, is recommended.

ACKNOWLEDGMENTS

The author wishes to acknowledge the excellent editorial assistance of Dorothy Newkirk in preparation of this manuscript.

REFERENCES

1. Hale HH, Helmboldt CF, Plastridge WN, et al. Bovine mastitis caused by a Mycoplasma species. Cornell Vet 1962;52:582–91.
2. Carmichael LE, Guthrie RS, Fincher MG, et al. Bovine *Mycoplasma* mastitis. In: Proceedings of the 67th annual meeting of the U.S. Livestock Sanitary Association 1963;1964. p. 220–34.
3. Jasper DE. Bovine Mycoplasmal mastitis. In: Cornelius CE, Simpson, BF, editors. Advances in veterinary sciences and comparative medicine. New York: Academic Press; 1981. p. 121–57.
4. Stuart P, Davidson I, Slavin G, et al. Bovine mastitis caused by a Mycoplasma. Vet Rec 1963;75:59–64.
5. Nicholas RAJ, Ayling RD. Mycoplasma bovis: disease, diagnosis, and control. Res Vet Sci 2003;74:105–12.
6. Fox LK, Kirk JH, Britten A. Mycoplasma mastitis: a review of transmission and control. J Vet Med 2005;52:153–60.
7. Fox LK, Gay JM. Contagious mastitis. Vet Clin North Am Food Anim Pract 1993;9: 475–87.
8. APHIS-USDA. *Mycoplasma* in bulk tank milk in U.S. dairies. APHIS Info Sheet No. 395.053. Fort Collins (CO): APHIA-USDA; 2003.
9. APHIS-USDA. Prevalence of contagious mastitis pathogens on U.S. dairy operations, 2007. APHIS Info Sheet No. 533.1008. Fort Collins (CO): APHIA-USDA; 2008.
10. Fox LK, Hancock DD, Mickelson A, et al. Bulk tank milk analysis: Factors associated with appearance of *Mycoplasma* sp in milk. J Vet Med Ser B 2003;50:235–40.

11. Nicholas R, Ayling R, McAuliffe L. Mycoplasma mastitis. Vet Rec 2007;160:382–3.

12. Maunsell FP, Woolums AR, Francoz D, et al. Mycoplasma bovis infections in cattle. J Vet Intern Med 2011;25:772–83.

13. Gourlay RN, Howard CJ. Human and animal Mycoplasmas. In: Tully JG, Whitcombs RF, editors. The mycoplasmas. New York: Academic Press; 1979. p. 49–102.

14. Maunsell FP, Donovan GA. *Mycoplasma bovis* infection in young calves. Vet Clin North Am Food Anim Pract 2009;25:139–77.

15. Jasper DE. Prevalence of mycoplasmal mastitis in the western states. Calif Vet 1980;43:24–6.

16. Kirk JH, Glenn K, Ruiz L, et al. Epidemiologic analysis of Mycoplasma spp isolated from bulk-tank milk samples obtained from dairy herds that were members of milk cooperative. J Am Vet Med Assoc 1997;211:1036–8.

17. Boonyayatra S, Fox LK, Gay JM, et al. Discrimination between Mycoplasma and Acholeplasma species of bovine origin using digitonin disc diffusion assay, nisin disc diffusion assay, and conventional polymerase chain reaction. J Vet Diag Invest 2012;24(1):7–13.

18. Gonzalez RN, Wilson DJ. Mycoplasma mastitis in dairy herds. Vet Clin North Am Food Anim Pract 2003;19:199–221.

19. Farnsworth RJ. Microbiologic examination of bulk tank milk. Vet Clin North Am Food Anim Pract 1993;9:469–74.

20. USDA-ERS. Profits, costs, and the changing structure of dairy farming/ERR-47 Economic Research Service/USDA. 2006. Available at: www.ers.usda.gov/publications/err47/err47b.pdf. Accessed March 24, 2012.

21. Filioussis G, Christodoulopoulos G, Thatcher A, et al. Isolation of *Mycoplasma bovis* from bovine clinical mastitis cases in Northern Greece. Vet J 2007;173:215–8.

22. Arcangioli MA, Chazel M, Sellal E, et al. Prevalence of *Mycoplasma bovis* udder infection in dairy cattle: preliminary field investigation in southeast France. N Z Vet J 2011;59:75–8.

23. Passchyn P, Piepers S, De Meulemeester L, et al. Between-herd prevalence of *Mycoplasma bovis* in bulk milk in Flanders, Belgium. Res Vet Sci 2012;92(2):219–20.

24. Miranda-Morales RE, Rojas-Trejo V, Segura-Candelas R, et al. Prevalence of pathogens associated with bovine mastitis in bulk tank milk in Mexico. Ann N Y Acad Sci 2008;1149:300–2.

25. Ghazaei C. Mycoplasmal mastitis in dairy cows in the Moghan region of Ardabil State, Iran. J S Afr Vet Assoc 2006;77:222–3.

26. Ghadersohi A, Hirst RG, Forbes-Faulkener J, et al. Preliminary studies on the prevalence of *Mycoplasma bovis* mastitis in dairy cattle in Australia. Vet Microsc 1999;65:185–94.

27. McDonald WL, Rawdon TG, Fitzmaurice J, et al. Survey of bulk tank milk in New Zealand for *Mycoplasma bovis*, using species-specific nested PCR and culture. N Z Vet J 2009;57:44–9.

28. Blackburn P, Brooks C, McConnell W, et al. Isolation of *Mycoplasma bovis* from cattle in Northern Ireland from 1999 to 2005. Vet Rec 2007;161:452–3.

29. APHIS-USDA. Dairy 2007. Biosecurity practices on U.S. dairy operations, 1991–2007. APHIS Info Sheet No. 544.0510. Fort Collins (CO): APHIA-USDA; 2010.

30. Thomas CB, Willeberg P, Jasper DE. Case-control study of bovine mycoplasmal mastitis in California. Am J Vet Res 1981;42:511–5.

31. Bradley AJ, Leach KA, Breen JE, et al. Survey of the incidence and etiology of mastitis on dairy farms in England and Wales. Vet Rec 2007;160:253–7.

32. Hertl JA, Schukken YH, Bar D, et al. The effect of recurrent episodes of clinical mastitis caused by gram-positive and gram-negative bacteria and other organisms on mortality and culling in Holstein dairy cows. J Dairy Sci 2011;94:4863–77.
33. Neave FK, Dodd FH, Kingwill RG, et al. Control of mastitis in the dairy herd by hygiene and management. J Dairy Sci 1969;52:696–707.
34. Jain NC, Jasper DE Dellinger JD. Cultural characters and serological relationships of some Mycoplasmas isolated from bovine sources. J Gen Microbiol 1967;49:401–10.
35. Biddle MK, Fox LK, Evans MA, et al. Pulsed-field gel electrophoresis patterns of *Mycoplasma* isolates from various body sites in dairy cattle with *Mycoplasma* mastitis. J Am Vet Med Assoc 2005;227:445–59.
36. Fox LK, Muller FJ, Wedam ML, et al. Clinical *Mycoplasma bovis* mastitis in prepubertal heifers on 2 dairy herds. Can Vet J 2008;49:1110–2.
37. Byrne WJ, Ball HJ, McCormack R, et al. Elimination of *Mycoplasma bovis* mastitis from an Irish dairy herd. Vet Rec 1998;142:516–7.
38. Houlihan MG, Veenstra B, Christian MK, et al. Mastitis and arthritis in two dairy herds caused by *Mycoplasma bovis*. Vet Rec 2007;160:126–7.
39. Wilson DJ, Skirpstunas RT, Trujillo JD, et al. Unusual history and initial clinical signs of *Mycoplasma bovis* mastitis and arthritis in first-lactation cows in a closed commercial dairy herd. J Am Vet Med Assoc 2007;230:1519–23.
40. Punyapornwithaya V, Fox LK, Hancock DD, et al. Association between an outbreak strain causing *Mycoplasma bovis* mastitis and its asymptomatic carriage in the herd: a case study from Idaho, USA. Prev Vet Med 2010;93:66–70.
41. Punyapornwithaya V, Fox LK, Hancock DD, et al. Incidence and transmission of *Mycoplasma bovis* mastitis in Holstein dairy cows in a hospital pen: a case study. Prev Vet Med 2011;98:74–8.
42. Jain NC, Jasper DE, Dellinger JD. Experimental bovine mastitis due to Mycoplasma. Cornell Vet 1969;59:10–28.
43. Jasper DE, Al-Aubaidi JM, Fabricant J. Epidemiologic observations on Mycoplasma mastitis. Cornell Vet 1974;64:407–15.
44. Byrne WJ, Ball HJ, McCormack R, et al. Elimination of *Mycoplasma bovis* mastitis from an Irish dairy herd. Vet Rec 1998;142:516–7.
45. Justice-Allen A, Trujillo J, Corbett R, et al. Survival and replication of *Mycoplasma* species in recycled bedding sand and association with mastitis on dairy farms in Utah. J Dairy Sci 2010;93:192–202.
46. Wilson DJ, Justice-Allen A, Goodell G, et al. Risk of *Mycoplasma bovis* transmission from contaminated sand bedding to naive dairy calves. J Dairy Sci 2011;94:1318–24.
47. Blosser TH. Economic losses from and the national research program on mastitis in the United States. J Dairy Sci 1979;62:119–27.
48. Jasper DE. The role of Mycoplasma in bovine mastitis. J Am Vet Med Assoc 1982;181:158–62.
49. Bennett RH, Jasper DE. Nasal prevalence of *Mycoplasma bovis* and IHA titers in young dairy animals. Cornell Vet 1977;67:361–73.
50. Butler JA, Pinnow CC, Thomson JU, et al. Use of arbitrarily primed polymerase chain reaction to investigate *Mycoplasma bovis* outbreaks. Vet Microbiol 2001;78:175–81.
51. Bicknell SR, Gunning RF, Jackson G, et al. Eradication of *Mycoplasma bovis* infection from a dairy herd in Great Britain. Vet Rec 1983;112:294–7.
52. Punyapornwithaya V, Fox LK, Hancock DD, et al. Time to clearance of Mycoplasma mastitis: the effect of management factors including milking time hygiene and preferential culling. Can J Vet Res 2012, in press.
53. Razin S, Hayflick L. Highlights of Mycoplasma research: an historical perspective. Biologicals 2010;38:183–90.

54. Razin S, Yogev D, Naot Y. Molecular biology and pathogenicity of Mycoplasmas. Microbiol Mol Biol Rev 1998;62:1094–156.
55. Jain NC, Jasper DE, Dellinger JD. Serologic response of cows to *Mycoplasma* under experimental and field conditions. Am J Vet Res 1969;30:733–42.
56. Kauf AC, Rosenbusch RF, Paape MJ, et al. Innate immune response to intramammary *Mycoplasma bovis* infection. J Dairy Sci 2007;90:3336–48.
57. Szathmary S, Rajapakse N, Szekely I, et al. Binding of Mycoplasmas to solid phase adsorbents. Acta Vet Hung 2005;53:299–307.
58. Tabassum I, Chaudhry R, Chourasia BK, et al. Identification of an N-terminal 27 kDa fragment of *Mycoplasma pneumoniae* P116 protein as specific immunogen in *M pneumoniae* infections. BMC Infect Dis 2010;10:350.
59. Lysnyansky I, Rosengarten R, Yogev D. Phenotypic switching of variable surface lipoproteins in *Mycoplasma bovis* involves high-frequency chromosomal rearrangements. J Bacteriol 1996;178:5395–401.
60. Lysnyansky I, Sachse K, Rosenbusch R, et al. The vsp locus of *Mycoplasma bovis*: gene organization and structural features. J Bacteriol 1999;181:5734–41.
61. Thomas A, Leprince P, Dizier I, et al. Identification by two-dimensional electrophoresis of a new adhesin expressed by a low-passaged strain of *Mycoplasma bovis*. Res Microbiol 2005;156:713–8.
62. Lysnyansky I, Ron Y, Sachse K, et al. Intrachromosomal recombination within the vsp locus of *Mycoplasma bovis* generates a chimeric variable surface lipoprotein antigen. Infect Immun 2001;69:3703–12.
63. Nussbaum S, Lysnyansky I, Sachse K, et al. Extended repertoire of genes encoding variable surface lipoproteins in *Mycoplasma bovis* strains. Infect Immun 2002;70: 2220–5.
64. Browning GF, Marenda MS, Noormohammadi AH, et al. The central role of lipoproteins in the pathogenesis of mycoplasmoses. Vet Microbiol 2011;153:44–50.
65. Frost AJ, Wanasinghe DD, Woolcock JB. Some factors affecting selective adherence of microorganisms in the bovine mammary gland. Infect Immun 1977;15:245–53.
66. Wanasinghe DD. Adherence as a prerequisite for infection of the bovine mammary gland by bacteria. Acta Vet Scand 1981;22:109–17.
67. Caswell JL, Archambault M. *Mycoplasma bovis* pneumonia in cattle. Anim Health Res Rev 2007;8:161–86.
68. Craven N, Anderson JC. Phagocytosis of *Staphylococcus aureus* by bovine mammary gland macrophages and intracellular protection from antibiotic action in vitro and in vivo. J Dairy Res 1984;51:513–23.
69. Bayles KW, Wesson CA, Liou LE, et al. Intracellular *Staphylococcus aureus* escapes the endosome and induces apoptosis in epithelial cells. Infect Immun 1998;66:336–42.
70. Andreev J, Borovsky Z, Rosenshine I, et al. Invasion of HeLa cells by *Mycoplasma penetrans* and the induction of tyrosine phosphorylation of a 145-kDa host cell protein. FEMS Microbiol Lett 1996;132:189–94.
71. Yavlovich A, Katzenell A, Tarshis M, et al. *Mycoplasma fermentans* binds to and invades HeLa cells: involvement of plasminogen and urokinase. Infect Immun 2004; 72:5004–11.
72. Buim MR, Buzinhani M, Yamaguti M, et al. *Mycoplasma synoviae* cell invasion: elucidation of the Mycoplasma pathogenesis in chicken. Comp Immunol Microbiol Infect Dis 2011;34:41–7.
73. van der Merwe J, Prysliak T, Perez-Casal J. Invasion of bovine peripheral blood mononuclear cells and erythrocytes by *Mycoplasma bovis*. Infect Immun 2010;78: 4570–8.

74. Maeda T, Shibahara T, Kimura K, et al. *Mycoplasma bovis*-associated suppurative otitis media and pneumonia in bull calves. J Comp Pathol 2003;129:100–10.
75. Vanden Bush TJ, Rosenbusch RF. Characterization of a lympho-inhibitory peptide produced by *Mycoplasma bovis*. Biochem Biophys Res Commun 2004;315:336–41.
76. Boothby T, Jasper DE, Zinkl JG, et al. Prevalence of Mycoplasmas and immune responses to *Mycoplasma bovis* in feedlot calves. Am J Vet Res 1983;44:831–8.
77. Howard CJ, Parsons KR, Thomas LH. Systemic and local immune responses of gnotobiotic calves to respiratory infection with *Mycoplasma bovis*. Vet Immunol Immunopathol 1986;11:291–300.
78. Nicholas RA, Ayling RD, Stipkovits L. An experimental vaccine for calf pneumonia caused by *Mycoplasma bovis*. Vaccine 2002;20:3569–75.
79. Vanden Bush TJ, Rosenbusch RF. Characterization of the immune response to *Mycoplasma bovis* lung infection. Vet Immunol Immunopathol 2003;94:23–33.
80. Bushnell RB. Mycoplasma mastitis. Vet Clin North Am Large Anim Pract 1984;6:301–12.
81. Wilson DJ, Goodell G, Justice-Allen A, et al. Herd-level prevalence of *Mycoplasma* spp mastitis and characteristics of infected dairy herds in Utah as determined by a statewide survey. J Am Vet Med Assoc 2009;235:749–54.
82. Biddle MK, Fox LK, Hancock DD. Patterns of Mycoplasma shedding in the milk of dairy cows with intramammary Mycoplasma infection. J Am Vet Med Assoc 2003;223:1163–6.
83. Jackson G, Boynton E. A mild outbreak of bovine mastitis associated with *Mycoplasma bovigenitalium*. Vet Rec 1991;129:444–6.
84. Mackie DP, Finley D, Brice N, et al. Mixed Mycoplasma mastitis outbreak in a dairy herd. Vet Rec 2000;147:335–6.
85. Brown MB, Shearer JK, Elvinger F. Mycoplasma mastitis in a dairy herd. J Am Vet Med Assoc 1990;196:1097–101.

The "Other" Gram-Negative Bacteria in Mastitis
Klebsiella, Serratia, and More

Ynte Schukken, DVM, PhD[a],[*], Matt Chuff, DVM[a],
Paolo Moroni, DVM, PhD[a],[b], Abhijit Gurjar, DVM, PhD[a],
Carlos Santisteban, DVM[a], Frank Welcome, DVM, MBA[a],
Ruth Zadoks, DVM, PhD[a],[c]

KEYWORDS

• Mastitis • Klebsiella • Serratia • Raoultella • Treatment • Prevention

KEY POINTS

• Mastitis due to gram-negative bacteria is a common occurrence in dairy farms with a low bulk somatic cell count.

• All gram-negative bacteria have lipopolysaccharides (LPS) as a major part of their outer membrane. The biological activity of LPS resides predominantly within the lipid A fraction that anchors LPS in the bacterial outer membrane.

• Klebsiella spp intramammary infections cause a severe inflammatory response, while Serratia spp intramammary infections are usually associated with less severe clinical signs.

• Klebsiella spp and Serratia spp intramammary infections may occur in within farm clonal outbreaks.

• Severity of infections with gram-negative bacteria may be reduced by vaccination with a core antigen vaccine. Treatment of Klebsiella intramammary infections may result in an important increase in bacterial cure compared to untreated controls.

Gram-negative bacteria are an important cause of bovine mastitis throughout the world. With the advance of our understanding of the main risk factors for classic contagious bacteria such Streptococcus agalactiae and Staphylococcus aureus, we have observed a decrease in the prevalence of these 2 mastitis pathogens. However, this decrease has gone hand in hand with an increase in the incidence of intramammary

The authors have nothing to disclose.
[a] Quality Milk Production Services, Cornell University, 240 Farrier Road, Ithaca, NY 14853, USA;
[b] Department of Veterinary Pathology, Hygiene and Public Health, Università degli Studi di Milano, Via Celoria 10, Milan, Italy; [c] Moredun Research Institute, Pentlands Science Park, Bush Loan, Penicuik, Midlothian EH26 0PZ, Scotland
* Corresponding author.
E-mail address: yschukken@cornell.edu

Vet Clin Food Anim 28 (2012) 239–256
http://dx.doi.org/10.1016/j.cvfa.2012.04.001
0749-0720/12/$ – see front matter © 2012 Elsevier Inc. All rights reserved.

infections (IMIs) due to gram-negative bacteria.[1,2] Gram-negative bacteria, mostly coliforms (E coli, Klebsiella spp, and Enterobacter spp), cause 40% of all cases of clinical mastitis (CM),[2,3] and up to 25% of cows in well-managed herds are annually diagnosed with CM caused by coliforms.[3,4] The most common coliform species are Escherichia coli and Klebsiella spp.[5-8] The incidence of CM arising from gram-negative bacterial infection is inversely related to bulk milk somatic cell count (SCC)[1]; economic losses attributed to gram-negative IMI can be expected to increase as dairy farmers continue to strive for lower bulk milk SCC. Here, we will not focus on E coli but on the "other" gram-negative bacteria, which are predominantly Klebsiella spp and Serratia spp, while briefly discussing other gram-negative bacteria such as Raoultella spp and Enterobacter spp. First, a more general discussion on gram-negative bacteria and their bacterial characteristics and immune response patterns is provided. Then we will focus on the individual bacterial species and finally discuss the major new findings with regard to the "other" gram-negative mastitis causing bacteria.

GRAM-NEGATIVE BACTERIA
Enterobacteriaceae

Some of the more common clinically important genera of the family Enterobacteria-ceae are Salmonella, Shigella, Proteus, Escherichia, Citrobacter, Enterobacter, Serratia, Klebsiella, Morganella, Yersinia, Edwardsiella, and Providencia. These genera include recognized mastitis pathogens such as E coli, and Klebsiella spp but also the less well-known but known mastitis-causing organisms such as Raoutella spp, Pseudomonas spp, Enterobacter spp, Shigella spp, and Citrobacter spp. The Enter-obacteriaceae are rod shaped, are all gram-negative, and are typically diagnosed in the laboratory with the use of the MacConkey agar plates.[9] Lactose fermenters such as E coli, Enterobacter, and Klebsiella will produce acid, which lowers the pH of the MacConkey agar below 6.8 and results in the appearance of red/pink colonies. Some organisms ferment lactose slowly or weakly. These include Serratia spp and Citro-bacter spp. Non–lactose-fermenting bacteria such as Proteus spp and Shigella spp cannot utilize lactose and will use peptone instead. This forms ammonia, which raises the pH of the agar, and leads to the formation of white/colorless colonies on the MacConkey plate.[9]

One of the several unique characteristics of gram-negative bacteria is the structure of the outer membrane. The outer membrane consists of a complex lipopolysaccha-ride (LPS) whose lipid portion may act as an endotoxin. This LPS structure is present in all gram-negative bacteria but is structurally different between and within gram-negative bacterial species.[10,11]

Lipopolysacharides

Bacterial LPSs are the major component of the outer membrane of gram-negative bacteria. They have a structural role since they contribute to the cellular rigidity by increasing the strength of cell wall.[12] The LPS structure also mediates contacts with the external environment and will allow different species to live under different environmental conditions. The low permeability of the outer membrane acts as a barrier to protect bacteria from a number of environmental stressors, including antimicrobial compounds. The LPSs also have an important role in the activation of the host innate immunity.[12] For that reason, LPSs are considered pathogen-associ-ated molecular patterns.[13] The LPSs are macromolecules generally with 3 defined components: the lipid A fraction, the inner and out core oligosaccharide, and, finally, a polysaccharide portion, the O-chain.[11] In some gram-negative bacterial strains,

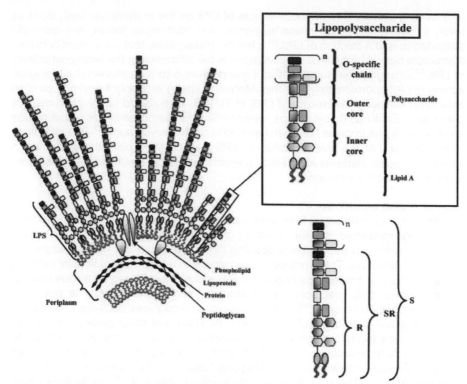

Fig. 1. Schematic representations of the enterobacterial Gram-negative cell wall (*left*), a lipopolysaccharide structure (*right*), R, SR, and S indicate the structures of rough-type, semi-rough type (with only one O-chain subunit) and smooth-type lipopolysaccharides, respectively. [*From* Caroff M, Karibian D. Structure of bacterial lipopolysaccharides. Carbohydr Res 2003;338(23):2431–47; with permission.]

there is no O-chain and these strains are identified as "rough types" as opposed to the "smooth types" when the O-chain is present. The O-chains are in direct contact with the host during infection and form the basis for serotype classification.[11] **Fig. 1** shows a schematic representation of the gram-negative cell wall.

Although LPS is not actively secreted by the bacterial cells, small amounts of the LPSs are released into the bacterial environment under circumstances such as cell division. Larger amounts are released when the bacteria are killed by antibiotics, phagocytosis, or the complement complex.

The role of LPS in the activation of the host immune response is dose dependent. Small amounts of LPSs can be used as a protective compound by stimulating the immune system.[14,15] Large amounts of LPSs, however, induce high fever, increase heart rate, and lead to septic shock and death by lung and kidney failure, intravascular coagulation, and systemic inflammatory response.[11] The biological activity of LPS resides predominantly within the lipid A fraction that anchors LPS in the bacterial outer membrane. Lipid A differs between species in acyl side chain number and length; however, the overall structure and synthetic pathway are conserved between gram-negative bacteria. The lipid A structure of *E coli* consisting of 6 acyl chains and 2 phosphate groups and is one of the most potent stimulators of the innate immune system through its binding to Toll-like receptor 4 (TLR4) in a tight connection to the

LPS binding protein.[13] Deleterious effects of LPS on the mammalian host, such as fever, inflammation, acute phase response, and multiorgan failure, are generally attributed to lipid A fraction of LPS.[10] It has been suggested that the variability in lipid A structure between bacterial species explains the difference in the biological activity of LPS.[10] Changing the number of acyl groups from 6 to 5 decreases the biological activity of LPS approximately 100-fold. Moreover, lipid A with only 4 acyl groups is an antagonist (blocking the binding of LPS) of TLR4.[16] With regard to the main mastitis pathogens, E coli has 6 acyl groups, whereas Serratia marcescens has 5 acyl groups and Klebsiella pneumoniae has been reported to have 7 acyl groups.[17] This difference in the structure of the lipid A portion of LPS may partly explain the difference in immune response patterns and clinical presentation that is observed between these 3 important mastitis pathogens.

Immune response patterns

The innate immune response is characterized by the rapid activation of antimicrobial host defense mechanisms in the mammary gland of the cow.[10] The ability to respond to a large number of pathogens is possible through evolutionary conserved pattern recognition receptors. These receptors are capable of recognizing molecular patterns that are shared by bacterial pathogens. TLR4, which is expressed on a wide array of cell types, including macrophages, neutrophils, and epithelial cells, is one such pattern recognition receptor.[10] The TLR4 receptor recognizes bacterial LPS, particularly the lipid A fraction of LPS. Activation of TLR4 and other pattern recognition receptors leads to the generation of an inflammatory response that is modulated, in part, by cytokine production.[10] Proinflammatory cytokines, such as tumore necrosis factor (TNF)-α and interleukin (IL)-1β, are potent inducers of the acute-phase immune response, fever, and neutrophil migration to the site of infection.[18] Cytokines, such as IL-10, contribute to the resolution of inflammation by inhibiting proinflammatory cytokine production and providing a negative feedback to the initial proinflammatory response.[18] In a series of experimental IMIs, Bannerman and coworkers provided a unique insight in the comparative activation of the innate immune response after a challenge with a number of gram-negative bacterial species.[19–21] Since these scientists were using similar methodologies throughout the challenge trials, it is now possible to compare the innate immune response of the host to IMIs with these gram-negative bacteria. **Fig. 2** shows the response of the challenged cows to an experimental IMI with E coli, K pneumoniae, and S marcescens. The results in this figure make it very clear that the innate response between these 3 pathogens differs sharply, with the most severe response observed after K pneumoniae IMI and the more modest response observed after an IMI with S marcescens. This difference in response was apparent in both the proinflammatory response as shown by the concentration of TNF-α (**Fig. 2**, top) and in the regulatory immune response as shown by the concentrations of the cytokine IL-10 (**Fig. 2**, bottom). As we will observe later, these innate immune responses are very predictive of the observed clinical response and the risk of death or culling after an IMI with any of these 3 pathogens under field conditions. Although the precise mechanism of the difference in innate immune response is not fully clear, the functional form of LPS in these 3 organisms is likely to play a role in the observed pathogenicity.

KLEBSIELLA MASTITIS

Differences in the pathogenicity of E coli, Klebsiella spp, and Serratia spp as mastitis pathogens have been noted.[18,22] These differences include a longer duration of infection for Klebsiella spp and Serratia spp compared to E coli.[23] Also, Klebsiella spp

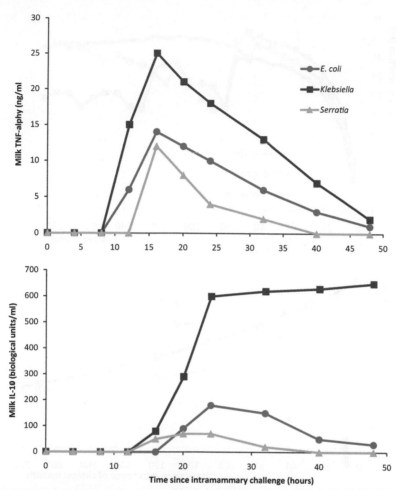

Fig. 2. Cytokine profiles after experimental challenge infections with 3 different gram-negative bacterial species. Milk TNF-α concentrations (in ng/mL) (*top*) and milk IL-10 concentrations (*bottom*) after intramammary challenge infection with *E coli, K pneumonia,* and *S marcescens. (Data from* Bannerman DD. Pathogen-dependent induction of cytokines and other soluble inflammatory mediators during intramammary infection of dairy cows. J Anim Sci (13 Suppl):10–25 2009;87).

IMIs appear to be more severe than *Serratia spp* IMIs, while *Serratia spp* IMIs appear to be less severe compared to *E coli* IMIs. *Klebsiella* mastitis occurs more frequently in herds that have a low bulk milk SCC than in herds with medium or high bulk milk SCC.[1] Severity of clinical episodes, poor response to vaccination, and the paucity of effective treatments make *Klebsiella* mastitis especially troublesome compared with *E coli*.[4,5,24] The severity of CM due to *Klebsiella* spp was highlighted in a series of reports from our research team. In a report on the effect of pathogen-specific CM on milk production of affected cows,[25] a difference in milk production loss between *E coli* and *Klebsiella* spp IMIs became clear (**Fig. 3**, top). The duration of milk production loss was substantially longer in cases of *Klebsiella* spp compared to clinical cases due to *E coli*. Similarly, the risk of culling[26] after a case of CM was substantially larger in cases of *Klebsiella* spp

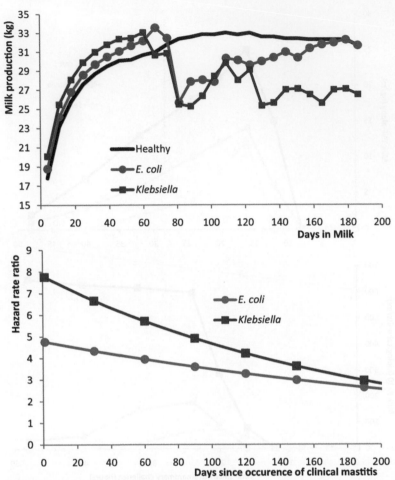

Fig. 3. Milk production effects (*top*) of an *E coli* and a *Klebsiella* spp case of clinical mastitis compared to milk production of healthy herd mates. The milk production loss pattern in *Klebsiella* spp indicates an earlier onset and a longer duration of milk production loss compared to *E coli*, whereas the severity of loss (indicated by the nadir) is approximately similar. Hazard rate ratio (bottom) of cows with a case of *E coli* or *Klebsiella spp* in early lactation. (*Data from* Gröhn YT, Wilson DJ, González RN, et al. Effect of pathogen-specific clinical mastitis on milk yield in dairy cows. J Dairy Sci 2004;87(10):3358–74; and Gröhn YT, González RN, Wilson DJ, et al. Effect of pathogen-specific clinical mastitis on herd life in two New York State dairy herds. Prev Vet Med 2005;71(1-2):105–25.).

mastitis compared to *E coli* CM (**Fig. 3**, bottom). These findings were in line with observations of others where *Klebsiella* CM turned out to be more severe compared to *E coli* mastitis.[5,24]

Klebsiella Outbreaks

Classically, *Klebsiella* spp IMIs are considered to be of environmental origin. The implication of this is that improving environmental hygiene and optimizing the cow's immune response would prevent these infections. Environmental infections are

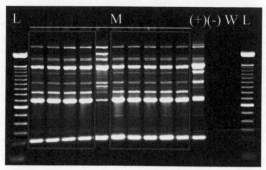

Fig. 4. An electrophoresis gel depicting the result of an RAPD analysis of the DNA of *K pneumoniae* isolates from 10 cases of clinical mastitis on a single dairy farm. The text above the gels indicate the cow number, quarter and date of the clinical case, (+) and (–) for positive and negative controls, W for a water control, and L for DNA ladder,. The 2 boxes show that 9 of 10 clinical cases were caused by the same clone of *K pneumoniae*.

considered to be not contagious, and the practical implication of that is that every IMI would be associated with its own bacterial strain of *Klebsiella*.[27] This is in stark contrast to contagious infections, where many IMIs share the same strain (or clone) of a bacterial species.[28] With the advance of molecular diagnostic techniques, the differentiation between clonal and nonclonal outbreaks of IMIs on dairy farms has become possible for routine outbreak evaluations. Munoz and colleagues[29] described the occurrence of two *Klebsiella* spp mastitis outbreaks on a single dairy farm. *Klebsiella* isolates from milk, feces, and environmental sources were compared using random amplified polymorphic DNA (RAPD). The first mastitis outbreak on the described farm was caused by a single strain of *Klebsiella pneumoniae*, which was detected in milk from 8 cows. In **Fig. 4**, an example of a clonal *K pneumoniae* outbreak on a New York dairy farm is shown. This RAPD type was also isolated from the rubber liners of milking machine units after milking of infected cows and from bedding in the outbreak pen. This observed predominance of a single strain would indicate contagious transmission of the organism or exposure of multiple cows to an environmental point source. When the authors implemented intervention methods that targeted the prevention of transmission via the milking machine as well as improvement of environmental hygiene, no new cases with the initial RAPD type were observed. A second outbreak of *Klebsiella* mastitis that occurred several months later on the same farm was caused by multiple RAPD types, which rules out contagious transmission and indicates infections originating from the environment.[29] Using the RAPD technique has shown to be useful in distinguishing clonal versus nonclonal outbreaks using several gram-negative mastitis pathogens.

Vaccination and Treatment

A mutant *E coli* O111:B4 known as J5 has been used for the development of a bacterin to reduce mastitis severity due to coliform organisms.[30] This mutant is deficient in the enzyme uridine 5′-diphosphate-galactose 4-epimerase so that it cannot attach the 0 side chains of LPS (**Fig. 1**). Without the O side chains, the core oligosaccharide with the bound lipid A becomes exposed and can stimulate antibody response by the host. The induced antibodies may react with the core region and lipid A of all LPSs, regardless of bacterial species. Commercial vaccines developed against the J5 core antigen of coliform bacteria have been in use for approximately 15 years,[31] Reduction of coliform CM in vaccinates compared with controls has been reported.[31,32] However, more often, J5 vaccination is associated with a reduction in severity and improved herd survival.[32,33] Wilson and colleagues[34] showed that the milk loss due to CM was substantially less among J5 vaccinates compared to controls; however, this protective effect of vaccination waned with increasing time since the last vaccination. It was recently reported that J5 vaccination was also associated with survival advantages after a case of clinical coliform mastitis.[34] Particularly, Wilson and colleagues[34] reported that vaccinates with Klebsiella CM were less likely to be culled for mastitis compared to unvaccinated controls. Together these data indicate that J5 vaccination is one of the tools available to reduce losses due to clinical Klebsiella spp mastitis.

Studies reporting on treatment efficacy of antibiotic treatment of Klebsiella mastitis have generally shown a very limited efficacy of antibiotic treatment.[24] In this study by Roberson and coworkers,[24] 37% of Klebsiella-infected quarters from cows with mild to moderate CM cured within 1 week, and 47% cured within 36 days. A field study of naturally occurring severe CM caused by coliform organisms showed that intramuscular treatment with ceftiofur reduced the risk of death or culling.[5] A proportion of approximately 50% cure was observed after intramuscular ceftiofur treatment of 8 animals with severe CM, while cure in controls animals was approximately 25%.[5] For systemically mild CM cases that were predominantly caused by E coli, however, intramuscular ceftiofur treatment did not have beneficial effects.[35] In a recent study on mild and moderate clinical coliform mastitis in 6 large dairy farms, it was reported that across farms and coliform species, 5-day treatment with intramammary ceftiofur resulted in a significantly higher probability of cure compared to no treatment.[12] Across herds and bacteriologic species, bacteriologic cure was 73% in the treated animals and 38% in control animals. For Klebsiella-infected quarters, this was 57% in treated animals versus 19% in control animals.[12] Although treatment of Klebsiella mastitis is not as successful as treatment of most gram-positive bacteria, the availability of third-generation cephalosporins for CM treatments appears to provide an important tool for the treatment of CM caused by this organism (Fig. 5).

Prevention

Identification of potential sources of Klebsiella is important for implementation of preventive measures that decrease exposure and limit the risk of udder infections (Fig. 6). Bedding materials from wood byproducts, such as sawdust and shavings, can be sources of Klebsiella organisms on dairy farms.[36,37] Furthermore, fecal shedding of Klebsiella by about 70% of healthy dairy cows has been documented recently.[38,39] Consequently, feces and manure also constitute sources of exposure to Klebsiella for dairy cows.[7,40] Direct contact of the teat ends with materials that contain Klebsiella, such as bedding, feces, manure splash, water, milk, mattresses, legs, or liners, may provide the bacteria with access to the udder,[41] which may ultimately result in IMI and subsequent CM.[42] Dirty udders were a significant risk factor for presence of Klebsiella after udder preparation. Poor udder cleanliness scores have been associated with an increased risk of IMI[43] and increased somatic cell score.[44] High prevalence of Klebsiella before udder preparation was associated with lower efficacy of cleaning Klebsiella from teat ends, with high Klebsiella loads not fully removed by udder preparation.[41] Cows with an udder cleanliness score of 1 (very clean) were positive for Klebsiella spp at their teat-ends after the preparation of the udder was completed in 10% of samples, this increased to 40% with a score of 2 (intermediate cleanliness) and to 55% in cows with an udder cleanliness score of 3 (dirty). Evaluation of cow cleanliness

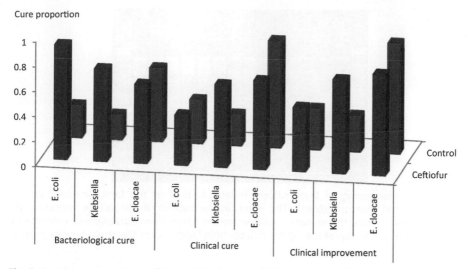

Cure proportion

Bacteriological cure | Clinical cure | Clinical improvement

Fig. 5. Least squares means of bacteriologic cure, clinical cure, and clinical improvement by bacterial species and treatment arm. Cows with nonsevere clinical coliform mastitis were randomized to obtain a 5-day ceftiofur treatment or remained untreated as a control group. (*Data from* Schukken YH, Bennett GJ, Zurakowski MJ, et al. Randomized clinical trial to evaluate the efficacy of a 5-day ceftiofur hydrochloride intramammary treatment on nonsevere gram-negative clinical mastitis. J Dairy Sci 2011;94:6203–15).

provides therefore an estimate of the degree of challenge to which dairy cows are exposed[41,45] and can be used as a tool to monitor and control bacterial exposure levels.[44,46,47] In summary, prevention of *Klebsiella* spp IMIs appears to be possible through careful monitoring and improving of hygiene in the environment of the cow. However, given the multiple ecological niches of *Klebsiella* spp in and around dairy cows, complete elimination of *Klebsiella spp* from dairy farms does not appear to be feasible.

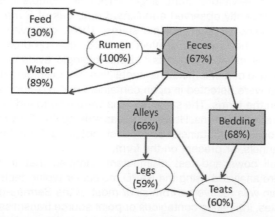

Fig. 6. *Klebsiella* prevalence in various sites in and around the dairy cow. (*From* Zadoks RN, Griffiths HM, Munoz MA, et al. Sources of Klebsiella and Raoultella species on dairy farms: be careful where you walk. J Dairy Sci 2011;94(2):1045–51; with permission.)

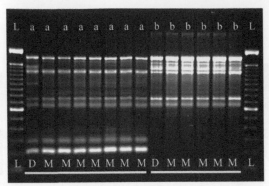

Fig. 7. Molecular typing of *S marcescens* isolates from 2 of the farms involved in the multistate *S marcensens* outbreak. The letters in the bottom of the picture indicate DNA ladder (L), isolate from the on-farm teat disinfectant (D) or from intramammary infections (M). The letters in the top of the figure indicate DNA ladder (L) or the strain type of isolate.

SERRATIA MASTITIS

The most common *Serratia* species in bovine mastitis are *S marcescens*[48–51] and *S liquefaciens*.[52,53] *Serratia* spp are ubiquitous in the environment and on dairy farms they have been isolated from bedding,[50,54] fecal materials, and in the parlor environment.[54] *Serratia* mastitis has been reported from North America,[23,55] Europe,[56,57] and Australia[54] and occurs under a wide variety of management conditions.

Infection with *Serratia* can result in clinical or subCM. Clinical episodes can alternate with subclinical episodes of infection.[52,55] Subclinical infections are more common than for other gram-negative bacteria.[48,50,58] The mean duration of *Serratia* IMI has been reported as 55 days to 4 months,[58,59] while individual infections can last as long as 10 months[48] or even 3 years.[59]

Serratia Outbreaks

Serratia mastitis is a rare occurrence on dairy farms and most reports on *Serratia* mastitis describe observations from single cases or multiple cases in a single herd.[23,48,55,60] We recently observed a multiherd outbreak of *S marcescencs* IMI in approximately 50 dairy herds in multiple states. These observations provided an opportunity to study the organism's effect on SCC, milk production, and survival across multiple cows in multiple herds.[51] Epidemiologic evidence associated the outbreaks with the use of a chlorhexidine-containing teat disinfectant on the affected herds. *Serratia* spp were detected in open containers and dip-cups with the product that were in use on the farms. The same bacteria were also found in milk samples of dairy cattle on the affected farms. However, it was striking that *S marcescens* was not cultured from unopened containers of product obtained from the manufacturer, through sales channels, or present on the farm.

Isolates from all cows and teat disinfectant samples that tested positive for *S marcescens* were analyzed using the RAPD molecular typing technique.[51] In each herd, a single strain was recovered from all or most of the *Serratia*-positive milk and disinfectant samples, indicating contagious or point source transmission of this strain on the farm of origin. As shown in **Fig. 7**, in each herd, the most common strain of *Serratia* was also isolated from a teat disinfectant containing chlorhexidine, implying that this product may have acted as point source or fomite. However, product samples originating from the affected herds and multiple batches of the chlorhexidine teat disinfected yielded a different RAPD pattern for each individual herd (see **Fig. 7**) and batch of product (ie, patterns were herd specific and not consistent within batches). It was concluded that the chlorhexidine-containing teat disinfectant allowed growth of *Serratia* spp in the product, but that there was no evidence for contamination of the product at the manufacturing plant. Product contamination appeared to occur on the farm and resulted in a within-herd outbreak of a farm-specific *S marcescens* strain. Resistance of *Serratia* spp and other gram-negative bacteria to biocides has been reported before[61] and in generally contributed to the presence of multidrug efflux pumps in the resistant strains.[62]

This multistate outbreak provided an unique opportunity to further study the clinical impact of *S marcescens* infections in dairy cows. In most herds where the outbreak was diagnosed, *Serratia* infections were clinically mild or even subclinical, as previously reported.[55,59,60] An increase in bulk milk SCC was often the only indication that a mastitis problem occurred. To study the impact of *S marcescens* IMIs on individual cows, further data collection in affected herds was initiated. Dairy herd improvement data were available for 20 of the herds involved in the outbreak. A comparison was made of cows known to be infected with *S marcesens* and cows known to be culture negative (controls). Approximately 100 cases of *S marcescens* and 400 frequently-matched noninfected control cows were available for further evaluation. Frequency matching was done based on age and days in milk at diagnosis. At cow level, detection of *Serratia* in a composite milk sample was associated with a significantly increased SCC compared to animals that were culture negative upon inclusion in the study (**Fig. 8A**). In this large multistate outbreak, detection of *Serratia* in a cow was not associated with a significant decrease in milk production compared to age and days in milk-matched herd mates (**Fig. 8B**). This is in strong contrast to milk production loss due to CM of *E coli* or *Klebsiella* spp, which were associated with a significant production losses of 13.10 kg/d and 9.94 kg/d, respectively (**Fig. 3**, Grohn and colleagues[25]). It was observed in the 20 dairy herds that *Serratia*-positive cows had a lower herd survival compared to negative control cows (**Fig. 8C**). Although there was no noticeable immediate loss to follow-up after diagnosis, culling for mastitis was the only culling reason that was significantly more common among *Serratia*-infected cows compared to control cows (see **Fig. 8B**). Culling of *Serratia*-infected cows because of recurrent CM has been reported,[52] and, as indicated previously, IMIs with *Serratia* are often chronic.[48,55] The scarcity of anecdotal reports on severe CM and death associated with *Serratia* cases in the large multistate outbreak, the delayed impact on culling, and the limited impact on production suggest that *Serratia* is much less pathogenic than other gram-negative bacteria such as *E coli* and *Klebsiella* spp. This is a very similar conclusion to the one that was reached based on experimental infections (see **Fig. 2**, Bannerman[18]),where a *S marcescens* challenge infection was associated with a shorter (eg, concentration of blood serum albumin in milk, an indicator of changes in vascular permeability) or lower (eg, concentrations of C5a, IL-8, IL-10, CD14, or interferon-γ in milk and LPS binding protein in milk and plasma) innate immune response.[19-21] It was suggested that a limited cytokine response contributes to the ability of bacteria to establish chronic IMIs.[19] Thus, observations from experimental infection studies match those of field studies in that *Serratia* infections tend to be less severe but more chronic than *E coli* and *Klebsiella* mastitis.

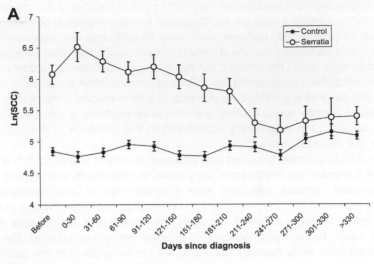

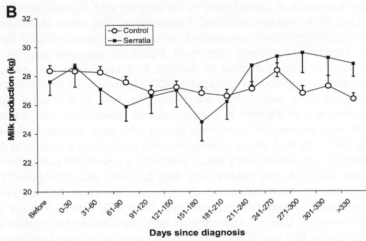

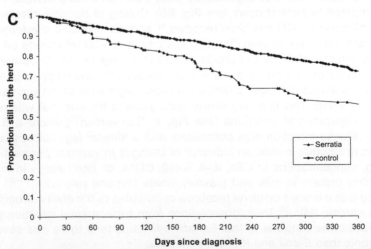

Treatment

Some authors report successful treatment of *Serratia* infections with an intramammary application of neomycin.[55,57] Other reports, however, suggest poor response of *Serratia* infections to antibiotic treatment.[23,52,63] The majority of *Serratia* infections appear to cure spontaneously.[23] In the multistate outbreak, we observed that *Serratia* was repeatedly isolated from 45% of animals for which multiple samples were available. In the remaining animals with multiple samples over time, a likely spontaneous cure was observed.

Prevention

Although the same preventative practices that would prevent gram-negative infection in general are expected to apply to *Serratia* infections, a single risk factor for *Serratia* IMIs stands out. Many outbreaks of *Serratia* mastitis in dairy herds are associated with chlorhexidine-containing teat disinfectants. Certainly not all chlorhexidine-containing teat disinfectants result in *Serratia* outbreaks, but some of these products are clearly associated with outbreaks of *Serratia* infections.[64] *S marcescens* strains have been reported to be resistant to biocides.[63] Outbreaks of *Serratia* spp in hospitals and other health care settings are frequently reported and often associated with the use of chlorhexidine.[65]

OTHER GRAM-NEGATIVE INFECTIONS

Several other gram-negative bacterial species have been associated with mastitis in dairy cows. These include *Shigella, Proteus, Citrobacter, Enterobacter, Yersinia,* and *Raoultella.* Among these species the ones that are more frequently associated with bovine mastitis are probably *Raoultella* and *Enterobacter.* Given the limited knowledge on *Raoultella* and *Enterobacter* mastitis cases, it is advisable that routine use of more advanced diagnostic procedures is used in mastitis research. It is expected that these species will show a higher incidence once proper diagnostics are in place.

Raoultella

Raoultella spp are a relatively new group of bacterial species. This new genus has been recently introduced after a reclassification of the genus *Klebsiella,* during a phylogenetic study based on the 16S rDNA and *rpoB* gene sequence. In most routine mastitis diagnostic laboratories, *Raoultella* spp will not be identified separately and will typically be reported as *Klebsiella* spp However, when more detailed diagnostics is performed, such as 16S sequencing, then an important number of the isolates previously identified as *Klebsiella* spp may be reported as *Raoultella* spp. In a recent field study on risk factors for *Klebsiella* spp mastitis, it was observed that several isolates from bedding material that had the phenotypic appearance of *Klebsiella* spp

---

Fig. 8. (*A*) Natural log of test day somatic cell counts in cows diagnosed with a *Serratia* spp IMI and frequency-matched noninfected controls. Data are presented relative to the first diagnosis of the *Serratia* spp IMI (day 0). (*B*) Milk production in kilograms per day in cows diagnosed with a *Serratia* spp IMI and frequency-matched noninfected controls. Data are presented relative to the first diagnosis of the *Serratia* spp IMI (day 0). (*C*) Within herd survival probability in cows diagnosed with a *Serratia* spp IMI and frequency matched not infected controls. Data are presented relative to the first diagnosis of the *Serratia* spp IMI (day 0).

were identified as being *Raoultella planticola* and *Raoultella terrigena*. This identification was based on rpoB sequencing.[66] In a large ecological study on New York dairy farms, Zadoks and colleagues[41] reported that genotypic identification of species using *rpoB* sequence data showed that *K pneumoniae* was the most common species in rumen content, feces, and alleyways, whereas *R planticola* was among the most frequent species among isolates from soil and feed crops.

Enterobacter spp

Enterobacter spp are routinely reported among the causes of CM on dairy farms.[1,2] In general, no further speciation of the *Enterabacter* spp is performed. In a number of recent studies, however, *rpoB* sequencing was performed and the dominant *Enterobacter* spp was reported to be *E cloacae*.[13,67,68] In the 2011 study of Schukken and colleagues,[13] *E cloacae* was the dominant cause of mild and moderate gram-negative CM on a farm. Clinical signs associated with *E cloacae* were generally mild compared to other coliform mastitis cases and spontaneous cure of infection and clinical signs was generally high (Schukken and colleagues,[13] **Fig. 5**). It was noteworthy that no different was observed in bacteriologic cure and clinical cure between ceftiofur-treated and nontreated control animals (Schukken and colleagues,[13] **Fig. 5**).

SUMMARY

Mastitis caused by gram-negative infections is of increasing importance on modern and well-managed dairy farms. Without a doubt, *E coli* tends to be the most important cause of these gram-negative infections when the data are tallied across farms.[1] However, more precise investigation of individual farms often reveals a farm-specific infection pattern where a single gram-negative bacterial species predominates. Several farms with a predominance of "other" gram-negative IMIs may be observed. We have shown the presence of outbreaks on individual dairy farms with *K pneumoniae*, *S marcescens,* and *Enterobacter cloacae*. On farms with a predominance of these "other" gram-negative infections, a detailed epidemiologic investigation may reveal the source of these infections.

It is quite surprising to identify the difference in host immune response pattern and the associated clinical and subclinical presentations of IMIs due to the different gram-negative organisms. Experimental and field observations would suggest that among the gram-negative bacterial causes of mastitis, *Klebsiella* spp are causing the most severe cases, closely followed by *E coli* and then much less clinical severity is observed in *Serratia* spp and *Enterobacter* spp cases. The precise mechanisms that would explain the difference in clinical severity are not known, but the most likely explanation appears to be the structure of the lipid A fraction of the LPS of the bacterial species. Important differences in the lipid A fraction of LPS between and within bacterial species are observed.

The prevention of IMIs with gram-negative bacteria has components that are generic across species and components that are species specific. Generic prevention may be obtained by improving hygiene and reducing exposure of teat ends to environmental contamination. Also the use of a J5 bacterin is expected to provide some reduction in severity of gram-negative IMIs across bacterial species. Specific prevention programs will depend on the actual transmission behavior of the dominant species causing IMIs in the herd. Several clonal outbreaks of gram-negative bacterial species have been described. In such situations, optimal milking procedures, segregation and culling of infected animals, and targeted treatment would be advisable. Even more specific are the prevention procedures associated with *S marcescens* outbreaks, where resistance against specific biocides will lead to transmission of infection through teat disinfectants. Removal of these biocides from the cow environment is than essential. Antimicrobial treatment of gram-negative bacteria has often considered to be of limited value and treatment should be more targeted toward cow survival and reduction of clinical symptoms. More recently, extended treatment with a third-generation cephalosporin was reported to be efficacious in the treatment of *E coli* and *Klebsiella* spp but not of *E cloacae*. Further investigations in effective treatment protocols for gram-negative IMIs are warranted.

REFERENCES

1. Barkema HW, Schukken YH, Lam TJGM, et al. Incidence of clinical mastitis in dairy herds grouped in three categories by bulk milk somatic cell counts. J Dairy Sci 1998;81:411–9.
2. Olde Riekerink RG, Barkema HW, Kelton DF, et al. Incidence rate of clinical mastitis on Canadian dairy farms. J Dairy Sci 2008;91:1366–77.
3. Erskine RJ, Eberhart RJ, Hutchinson LJ, et al. Campbell. Incidence and types of clinical mastitis in dairy herds with high and low somatic cell counts. J Am Vet Med Assoc 1988;192:761–5.
4. Smith KL, Hogan JS. Environmental Mastitis. Vet Clin North Am Food Anim Pract 1993;9:489–98.
5. Erskine RJ, Bartlett PC, VanLente JL, et al. Efficacy of systemic ceftiofur as a therapy for severe clinical mastitis in dairy cattle. J Dairy Sci 2002;85:2571–5.
6. Erskine RJ, Walker RD, Bolin CA, et al. Trends in antibacterial susceptibility of mastitis pathogens during a seven-year period. J Dairy Sci 2002;85:1111–8.
7. Munoz MA, Welcome FL, Schukken YH, et al. Molecular epidemiology of two Klebsiella pneumoniae outbreaks on a dairy farm in New York State. J Clin Microbiol 2007;45:3964–71.
8. Todhunter DA, Smith KL, Hogan JS, et al. Gram-negative bacterial infections of the mammary gland in cows. Am J Vet Res 1991;52:184–8.
9. National Mastitis Council. Laboratory handbook on bovine mastitis. Madison (WI): National Mastitis Council; 1999.
10. Schukken YH, Günther J, Fitzpatrick J, et al. Members of the Pfizer Mastitis Research Consortium. Host-response patterns of intramammary infections in dairy cows. Vet Immunol Immunopathol 2011;144(3/4):270–89.
11. Caroff M, Karibian D. Structure of bacterial lipopolysaccharides. Carbohydr Res 2003;338(23):2431–47.
12. De Castro C, Parrilli M, Holst O, et al. Microbe-associated molecular patterns in innate immunity: extraction and chemical analysis of gram-negative bacterial lipopolysaccharides. Methods Enzymol 2010;480:89–115.
13. Schukken YH, Bennett GJ, Zurakowski MJ, et al. Randomized clinical trial to evaluate the efficacy of a 5-day ceftiofur hydrochloride intramammary treatment on nonsevere gram-negative clinical mastitis. J Dairy Sci 2011;94:6203–15.
14. Petzl W, Günther J, Pfister T, et al. Lipopolysaccharide pretreatment of the udder protects against experimental Escherichia coli mastitis. Innate Immun 2011. [Epub ahead of print].
15. Gunther J, Petzl W, Zerbe H, et al. Lipopolysaccharide priming enhances expression of effectors of immune defence while decreasing expression of pro-inflammatory cytokines in mammary epithelia cells from cows. BMC Genom 2012;13(1):17–28.
16. Bardoel BW, van Strijp JA. Molecular battle between host and bacterium: recognition in innate immunity. J Mol Recognit 2011;24(6):1077–86.

17. Llobet E, Campos MA, Giménez P, et al. Analysis of the networks controlling the antimicrobial-peptide-dependent induction of Klebsiella pneumoniae virulence factors. Infect Immun 2011;79(9):3718–32.
18. Bannerman DD. Pathogen-dependent induction of cytokines and other soluble inflammatory mediators during intramammary infection of dairy cows. J Anim Sci 2009;87(13 Suppl):10–25.
19. Bannerman DD, Paape MJ, Goff JP, et al. Innate immune response to intramammary infection with Serratia marcescens and Streptococcus uberis. Vet Res 2004;35:681–700.
20. Bannerman DD, Paape MJ, Hare WR, et al. Characterization of the bovine innate immune response to intramammary infection with Klebsiella pneumoniae. J Dairy Sci 2004;87:2420–32.
21. Bannerman DD, Paape MJ, Lee JW, et al. Escherichia coli and Staphylococcus aureus elicit differential innate immune responses following intramammary infection. Clin Diagn Lab Immunol 2004;11:463–72.
22. Rajala-Schultz PJ, Gröhn YT. Comparison of economically optimized culling recommendations and actual culling decisions of Finnish Ayrshire cows. Prev Vet Med 2001;49:29–39.
23. Todhunter DA, Smith KL, Hogan JS, et al. Gram-negative bacterial infections of the mammary gland in cows. Am J Vet Res 1991;52(2):184–8.
24. Roberson JR, Warnick LD, Moore G. Mild to moderate clinical mastitis: efficacy of intramammary amoxicillin, frequent milk-out, a combined intramammary amoxicillin, and frequent milk-out treatment versus no treatment. J Dairy Sci 2004;87(3):583–92.
25. Gröhn YT, Wilson DJ, González RN, et al. Effect of pathogen-specific clinical mastitis on milk yield in dairy cows. J Dairy Sci 2004;87(10):3358–74.
26. Gröhn YT, González RN, Wilson DJ, et al. Effect of pathogen-specific clinical mastitis on herd life in two New York State dairy herds. Prev Vet Med 2005;71(1–2):105–25.
27. Paulin-Curlee GG, Singer RS, Sreevatsan S, et al. Genetic diversity of mastitis-associated Klebsiella pneumoniae in dairy cows. J Dairy Sci 2007;90:3681–9.
28. Zadoks RN, Schukken YH. Use of molecular epidemiology in veterinary practice. Vet Clin North Am Food Anim Pract 2006;22:229–61.
29. Munoz MA, Bennett GJ, Ahlström C, et al. Cleanliness scores as indicator of Klebsiella exposure in dairy cows. J Dairy Sci 2008;91(10):3908–16.
30. Teng NN, Kaplan HS, Hebert JM, et al. Protection against gram-negative bacteremia and endotoxemia with human monoclonal IgM antibodies. Proc Natl Acad Sci U S A 1985;82(6):1790–4.
31. Tyler JW, Cullor JS, Osburn BI, et al. Relationship between serologic recognition of Escherichia coli 0111:B4 (J5) and clinical coliform mastitis in cattle. Tyler JW, Cullor JS, Osburn BI, Bushnell RB, Fenwick BW. Am J Vet Res 1988;49:1950–4.
32. González RN, Cullor JS, Jasper DE, et al. Prevention of clinical coliform mastitis in dairy cows by a mutant Escherichia coli vaccine. Can J Vet Res 1989;53(3):301–5.
33. Wilson DJ, Grohn YT, Bennett GJ, et al. Milk production change following clinical mastitis and reproductive performance compared among J5 vaccinated and control dairy cattle. J Dairy Sci 2008;91(10):3869–79.
34. Wilson DJ, Grohn YT, Bennett GJ, et al. Comparison of J5 vaccinates and controls for incidence, etiologic agent, clinical severity, and survival in the herd following naturally occurring cases of clinical mastitis. J Dairy Sci 2007;90(9):4282–8.
35. Wenz JR, Garry FB, Lombard JE, et al. Short communication: efficacy of parenteral ceftiofur for treatment of systemically mild clinical mastitis in dairy cattle. J Dairy Sci 2005;88:3496–9.

36. Hogan JS, Smith KL, Hoblet KH, et al. Bacterial counts in bedding materials used on nine commercial dairies. J Dairy Sci 1989;72:250–8.
37. Zdanowicz M, Shelford JA, Tucker CB, et al. Bacterial populations on teat ends of dairy cows housed in free stalls and bedded with either sand or sawdust. J Dairy Sci 2004;87:1694–701.
38. Zadoks RN, Griffiths HM, Munoz MA, et al. Sources of Klebsiella and Raoultella species on dairy farms: be careful where you walk. J Dairy Sci 2011;94(2):1045–51.
39. Munoz MA, Ahlström C, Rauch BJ, et al. Fecal shedding of Klebsiella pneumoniae by dairy cows. J Dairy Sci 2006;89:3425–30.
40. Verbist B, Piessens V, Van Nuffel A, et al. Sources other than unused sawdust can introduce Klebsiella pneumoniae into dairy herds. J Dairy Sci 2011;94(6):2832–9.
41. Zadoks RN, Middleton JR, McDougall S, et al. Molecular epidemiology of mastitis pathogens of dairy cattle and comparative relevance to humans. J Mammary Gland Biol Neoplasia 2011;16(4):357–72.
42. Bramley AJ, Neave FK. Studies on the control of coliform mastitis in dairy cows. Br Vet J 1975;131:160–9.
43. Schreiner DA, Ruegg PL. Relationship between udder and leg hygiene scores and subclinical mastitis. J Dairy Sci 2003;86:3460–5.
44. Reneau JK, Seykora AJ, Heins BJ, et al. Association between hygiene scores and somatic cell scores in dairy cattle. J Am Vet Med Assoc 2005;227:1297–301.
45. Green MJ, Leach KA, Breen JE, et al. National intervention study of mastitis control in dairy herds in England and Wales. Vet Rec 2007;160:287–93.
46. Bartlett PC, Miller GY, Lance SE, et al. Managerial determinants of intramammary coliform and environmental streptococci infections in Ohio dairy herds. J Dairy Sci 1992;75:1241–52.
47. Ward WR, Hughes JW, Faull WB, et al. Observational study of temperature, moisture, pH and bacteria in straw bedding, and faecal consistency, cleanliness and mastitis in cows in four dairy herds. Vet Rec 2002;151:199–206.
48. Wilson DJ, Kirk JH, Walker RD, et al. Serratia marcescens mastitis in a dairy herd. J Am Vet Med Assoc 1990;196:1102–5.
49. Todhunter DA, Smith KL, Hogan JS. Serratia species isolated from bovine intramammary infections. J Dairy Sci 1991;74:1860–5.
50. Ruegg PL, Guterbock WM, Holmberg CA, et al. Microbiologic investigation of an epizootic of mastitis caused by Serratia marcescens in a dairy herd. J Am Vet Med Assoc 1992;200:184–9.
51. Muellner P, Zadoks R, Perez A, et al. The integration of molecular tools into veterinary and spatial epidemiology. Spatial Spatio-temporal Epidemiol 2011; 2(3):159–71.
52. Bowman GL, WD Hueston, Boner GJ, et al. Serratia liquefaciens mastitis in a dairy herd. J Am Vet Med Assoc 1986;189:913–5.
53. Nicholls TJ, Barton MG, Anderson BP. Serratia liquefaciens as a cause of mastitis in dairy cows. Vet Rec 1981;109:288–91.
54. Kamarudin MI, Fox LK, Gaskins CT, et al. Environmental reservoirs for Serratia marcescens intramammary infections in dairy cows. J Am Vet Med Assoc 1996;208: 555–8.
55. Barnum DA, Thackeray EL, Fish NA. An outbreak of mastitis caused by Serratia marcescens. Can J Comp Med Vet Sci 1958;22:392–5.
56. Di Guardo G, Battisti A, Agrimi U, et al. Pathology of Serratia marcescens mastitis in cattle. Zentralbl Veterinarmed B 1997;44:537–46.
57. Bradley AJ, Green MJ. A study of the incidence and significance of intramammary enterobacterial infections acquired during the dry period. J Dairy Sci 2000;83: 1957–65.

58. Todhunter DA, Smith KL, Hogan JS. Serratia species isolated from bovine intramammary infections. J Dairy Sci 1991;74:1860–5.
59. Hogan JS, Smith KL. Importance of dry period in Serratia mastitis outbreaks. Large Anim Pract 1997;May/June:20–5.
60. Ruegg PL, Guterbock WM, Holmberg CA, et al. Microbiologic investigation of an epizootic of mastitis caused by Serratia marcescens in a dairy herd. J Am Vet Med Assoc 1992;200:184–9.
61. Fox JG, Beaucage CM, Folta CA, et al. Nosocomial transmission of Serratia marcescens in a veterinary hospital due to contamination by benzalkonium chloride. J Clin Microbiol 1981;14:157–60.
62. Maseda H, Hashida Y, Konaka R, et al. Mutational upregulation of a resistance-nodulation-cell division-type multidrug efflux pump, SdeAB, upon exposure to a biocide, cetylpyridinium chloride, and antibiotic resistance in Serratia marcescens. Antimicrob Agents Chemother 2009;53(12):5230–5.
63. Isaksson A, Holmberg O. Serratia-mastitis in cows as a herd problem. Nord Vet Med 1984;36:354–60.
64. Hogan JS, Smith KL, Todhunter DA, et al. Efficacy of a barrier teat dip containing .55% chlorhexidine for prevention of bovine mastitis. J Dairy Sci 1995;78(11):2502–6.
65. Vigeant P, Loo VG, Bertrand C, et al. An outbreak of Serratia marcescens infections related to contaminated chlorhexidine. Infect Control Hosp Epidemiol 1998;19(10):791–4.
66. Munoz MA, Welcome FL, Schukken YH, et al. Molecular epidemiology of two Klebsiella pneumoniae mastitis outbreaks on a dairy farm in New York State. J Clin Microbiol 2007;45(12):3964–71.
67. Malinowski E, Lassa H, Kłossowska A, et al. Etiological agents of dairy cows' mastitis in western part of Poland. Pol J Vet Sci 2006;9(3):191–4.
68. Nam HM, Lim SK, Kang HM, et al. Prevalence and antimicrobial susceptibility of gram-negative bacteria isolated from bovine mastitis between 2003 and 2008 in Korea. J Dairy Sci 2009;92(5):2020–6.

Vaccination Strategies for Mastitis

R.J. Erskine, DVM, PhD

KEYWORDS

- Dairy • Mastitis • Vaccination

KEY POINTS

- Prevention of mastitis primarily relies on consistent application of proper milking practices and providing a clean dry environment for the cow.
- Use of core-antigen Gram-negative bacterins to reduce the severity of clinical coliform mastitis has been demonstrated to be successful, although limitations of this technology exist.
- Use of bacterins and other products to immunize dairy cattle against mastitis must be integrated with a total herd health management program.

Prevention of exposure is the foundation of infectious disease control programs, including mastitis. The tenets of mastitis prevention are maintaining cows in a clean, dry, comfortable environment and ensuring that recommended milking practices are consistently followed. Under the proper circumstances, vaccination can augment a herd mastitis control program. However, vaccination is essentially an insurance policy to mitigate losses that result from exposure, and subsequent infection, from mastitis pathogens. Similar to an insurance policy, the purchaser of the plan has to weigh expected benefits against costs and select a policy that best serves their individual needs. Thus, veterinarians who counsel dairy producers on mastitis vaccination programs should be able to assess the need, evaluate the available vaccines that could help resolve the problem, and establish a program that balances applied immunology with logistical reality of the dairy operation. Vaccination protocols should be designed to meet individual herd needs, and *only* applied as part of a comprehensive mastitis prevention program, and *not* as a proxy for inadequate management. This article will (1) briefly review immunologic principles of immunization, (2) consider the principles of evaluating the efficacy of mastitis vaccines, (3) cite the potential benefits and limitations of available commercial products and the most promising research, and (4) propose guidelines for immunization protocols.

The author has nothing to disclose.
Department of Large Animal Clinical Sciences, College of Veterinary Medicine, Michigan State University, D-202 Veterinary Teaching Hospital, East Lansing, MI 48824, USA
E-mail address: erskine@cvm.msu.edu

Vet Clin Food Anim 28 (2012) 257–270
http://dx.doi.org/10.1016/j.cvfa.2012.03.002
0749-0720/12/$ – see front matter © 2012 Elsevier Inc. All rights reserved.

VACCINE IMMUNOLOGY AND EFFICACY

Vaccination is a controlled exposure of the host defense system to a pathogen, or toxin, that ideally is robust enough to impart the immune system with increased surveillance and intensity of response, should that particular antigen be encountered again, but without the pathology of an actual infection. For better understanding of immunologic principles, and specifically mammary immunology, the reader is advised to seek in-depth reviews.[1–3]

Microbes are the primary cause of bovine mastitis, with the predominance of infections caused by bacteria. If invading pathogens are able to overcome the teat canal barrier, and gain entry into the gland, a series of innate host defenses help to limit bacterial growth. These include soluble factors such as complement, lactoferrin, and immunoglobulin and a cellular response that (1) functions to identify foreign agents, (2) changes local vasculature and recruits immune effectors (inflammation), and (3) enhances pathogen destruction though ingestion and killing by phagocytes. Innate host defenses differentiate host tissue from pathogens by recognition of molecules with regular patterns that are universal to many microbes but not on the body's own cells.[4] These pathogen-associated molecular patterns (PAMPs) are recognized and selectively bound by serum proteins and receptors in host cells, which are termed pathogen recognition receptors (PRRs).[4]

Toll-like receptors (TLRs) are an important class of PRRs that reside both on the cell surface and within host cells. These receptors act as the critical link between recognition of foreign agents and initiation of the host response by invoking gene expression and release of inflammatory cytokines (eg, interleukins, tumor necrosis factor-α) from the host cells.[4,5] Examples of specific pathogen targets bound by TLRs include peptidoglycan and lipoteichoic acid of gram-positive bacteria (TLR-2), gram-negative lipopolysaccharide (LPS; TLR-4), bacterial flagellin (TLR-5), and bacterial DNA, as CpG oligonucleotides (TLR-9).[1] Thus, much of both local inflammation and, if the infection is severe enough, systemic signs associated with mastitis are attributable to this response. Numerous cell types, including epithelial and endothelial cells, have been identified as possessing TLRs, which can contribute to an inflammatory response.[2] In addition to release of proinflammatory cytokines, phagocytic cells, such as macrophages, neutrophils, and natural killer cells, actively eliminate pathogens.[1]

If a pathogen survives innate host defenses, the adaptive, or acquired, immune system is triggered. This branch of the immune system recognizes specific antigens of pathogens, and if repeated exposure occurs, an immunologic "memory" initiates a faster and more intense response, of longer duration. It is antigen specificity, and the subsequent amnestic response, of the acquired immune response that serves as the basis for vaccination. The primary cells of acquired immunity are the lymphocytes. To date, the roles of the CD4+ (helper), CD8+ (cytotoxic and suppressor), and CD17 (phagocyte agonist) subsets in bovine mammary immunity are best understood.[2,6,7] B-lymphocytes, both as potential antigen processors and as precursors to immunoglobulin-producing plasma cells, also play a critical role.

Lymphocytes will respond to a specific microbial antigen only if the antigen (protein) is combined with a major histocompatibility complex (MHC) molecule on the surface of host cells, a process referred to as antigen presentation.[2] Cells such as macrophages and dendritic cells are particularly efficient in antigen processing, by phagocytzing, digesting, and presenting antigens on their membrane surface in conjunction with and MHC molecule. In response to antigen presentation, naïve lymphocytes then undergo clonal expansion and differentiation. A specific antigen can only be presented to a lymphocyte that solely recognizes that antigen.[4] Thus, successful immunization against a pathogen must link the invasion of the pathogen with recruitment of innate phagocytic cells, that recognize and digest the microbe, and subsequently present one of potentially hundreds of different protein antigens from the pathogen on the cell surface, in order attract and activate a matching lymphocyte that specifically recognizes the antigen. T-helper cells play a central role by (1) enhancing B-lymphocyte clonal expansion and differentiation to antibody-producing plasma cells and (2) completing the inflammatory response loop by releasing cytokines such as interleukin (IL)-17 and interferon-γ that stimulate phagocytes to more efficiently phagocytize and kill ingested microbes. Antigen-specific antibodies that arise from the acquired immune response also enhance phagocyte function by opsonizing microbes, thus assisting in target recognition and ingestion.

In ruminants, the lactating mammary gland must overcome numerous deficits relative to other tissues, in order to effectively respond to pathogen invasion. SCC, which in lactating dairy cattle are primarily leukocytes, are typically less than 10^5 cells/mL in uninfected glands, which is approximately 100-fold lower than in blood. Concentrations of factors such as immunoglobulin, lactoferrin, and complement are also lower in milk relative to plasma.[8] Additionally, the ability of circulating macrophages in milk to reenter tissue for antigen presentation remains speculative. Both macrophages and neutrophils in milk have decreased phagocytic ability, relative to blood.[3,9] Furthermore, phagocyte diapedesis and killing and lymphocyte mitogenic responses are markedly decreased during the periparturient period, and this may help contribute to increased incidence of mastitis at this stage of lactation.[7,10–13] Cows infected with *Staphylococcus aureus* have a subpopulation of CD8$^+$ lymphocytes within the mammary gland that suppress proliferation of CD4$^+$ lymphocytes, and this class of CD8$^+$ cells is preferentially trafficked into the gland during the postpartum period.[6]

Host-adapted pathogens, such as *S aureus*, with numerous virulence factors to help evade recognition and phagocytosis, further compromise the ability of host defenses to eliminate the infection. Thus, vaccination to prevent intramammary infection (IMI) following entry of pathogens into the gland has numerous barriers to overcome relative to other tissues.

Considerable variation in response to immunization between animals will exist even under ideal conditions. However, immunizing under such conditions as periods of extreme heat, which is especially pertinent for lactating cows, immediately after transportation, and concurrent outbreaks of other pathogens, such as *Salmonella* sp or *Mycoplasma* sp, should be avoided. Recent reports have suggested that cows with marked negative energy balance may also have profound alterations in immune cell function and expression of fatty acid precursors to inflammation.[14] Avoiding vaccination against severe coliform mastitis during stages of lactation when negative energy balance is typical may be problematic; this stage of lactation is also associated with increased risk of clinical mastitis.

The management–labor culture is also important to optimize vaccine response. *With present day marketing of vaccines through a variety of farm supply outlets, ensuring compliance with adequate immunization protocols is a critical need for veterinary oversight on many dairies.* In a Pennsylvania study, although 82% of dairy producers indicated that they routinely vaccinated their herds for bovine viral diarrhea, only 27% of the herds were found to be adequately vaccinated.[15]

The decision to employ a vaccine as part of a mastitis control program should be founded on the practitioner's ability to access peer-reviewed studies and to compare incidence and severity of natural infections between vaccinated animals and unvaccinated controls. Such studies should encompass a diversity of herd management practices and geographic regions. Unfortunately, such trials require large number of animals and long duration. Alternatively, challenge-exposure trials are often performed to assess vaccine efficacy. This type of trial requires fewer animals and less time, and many variables such as different strains of bacteria, challenge dose, and physiologic and lactation status of the animal can be uniformly standardized. Additionally, more comprehensive outcomes, including shedding of bacteria in milk, physical examination of the cow, and changes in biochemical parameters of serum and milk, can be reliably measured. However, these studies may have limited application in relation to the diversity of dairy farm management and environment, as well as among pathogens.

Changes in antibody levels, or titers, often serve as the gold standard to assess the response for an individual animal, or a population, to a vaccine. Failure of a vaccine to elevate titers is often regarded as a vaccination failure. However, predicting direct correlations between antibody titers and clinical outcome in the face of natural exposure is tenuous. A cow with half the serum titer for anti-J5 *Escherichia coli* antibodies compared to another cow is not twice as likely to succumb to severe coliform mastitis. Likewise, available research often does not report differences in cell mediated responses between vaccinated and unvaccinated cattle, which may be a better indicator of the duration of the amnestic response.

Appraisal of vaccine efficacy, as with therapeutics, should *not* be made on testimonials, especially herd-level impressions of "before-and-after" responses. Assertions of are often made on perceptions that initiating a vaccine program decreased the incidence and severity of mastitis cases, lowered somatic cell counts (SCC), increased milk production, etc, without employing a concurrent nonvaccinated control group for comparison. This is a frequent flaw in the evaluation of autogenous bacterins, in addition to a lack of quality control standards that are rigorously followed in commercial production. Mastitis incidence and SCC within a herd can rise and fall from many factors, including weather, changes in proportion of younger to older animals in the herd, history of herd additions, correction of milking techniques or deficiencies in equipment, and culling decisions.

Practitioners should realistically ask if the goal of immunization is to prevent new IMI or mitigate the severity of infections. The later goal would be prudent in the case of J5 *E coli* bacterins. Ultimately, a vaccine should be cost effective, present a minimal risk for anaphylaxis and injection lesions, and not affect milk production of lactating cattle. Finally, a vaccine should be administered as part of a herd mastitis control program only after ensuring that the targeted pathogen is a legitimate endemic concern for the udder health of the herd.

CORE-ANTIGEN GRAM-NEGATIVE BACTERINS

Gram-negative "core-antigen" bacterins (GNCABs) are commonly used on many dairy herds. The most extensively studied variants are formulated with a mutant strain of *E coli* O111:B4 (Rc mutant, commonly termed J5) lacking the "O" antigen capsule of the cell wall but with the core LPS, membrane proteins, and lipid A antigens intact. These core antigens are highly conserved among Gram-negative bacteria[16–18] and elicit cross-reactive anti–Gram-negative antibodies in J5 vaccinated cows.[18–20] Thus, dairy cattle immunized that with these bacterins develop immune resistance against a wide variety of gram-negative bacteria, including mastitis-causing coliforms.

Initial studies in California determined that higher serum anti-J5 *E coli* immunoglobulin G (IgG) was correlated with a lower incidence of clinical coliform mastitis.[21] A subsequent field trial demonstrated that cows administered 3 immunizations at drying off, 30 days after drying off, and in the postpartum period had a 5-fold decrease in the rate of clinical coliform mastitis in the first 100 days of lactation, compared to unvaccinated cows.[22] A field trial in Ohio using a similar dose regimen reported that J5 immunization did not reduce the prevalence of gram-negative IMIs at calving; however, 67% of the infections present at calving in unvaccinated cows developed clinical mastitis, compared to only 20% of the J-5 vaccinated cows.[23] Additionally, vaccination with J5 bacterin increased anti-J5 E coli IgG in serum and milk compared to unvaccinated controls,[23–25] although anti-J5 E coli antibody titers in milk are orders of magnitude lower than in serum. Following intramammary challenge of E coli, J-5 immunization reduced the severity of infection, but infections were not prevented.[23]

The pathogenesis of severe coliform mastitis is dependent on LPS-induced immune mediator responses, and a high proportion of severe coliform mastitis cases become bacteremic.[26] Thus, J5 bacterins may likely have a greater impact on the systemic effects of coliform mastitis, rather than local mammary inflammation. This concept is supported by a field trial from New York that determined 2 doses of J5 bacterin decreased the proportion of clinical mastitis cases that resulted in culling or death by 3-fold but did not reduce the overall incidence of clinical mastitis cases.[27] However, coliform mastitis cases contracted during the first 50 days of lactation resulted in less milk production loss among J5 vaccinated cattle.[28]

Gram-negative bacterins are regarded as weakly immunogenic in dairy cattle because they elicit poor amnestic IgG1 and IgG2 responses.[3] An Ontario study found that a substantial population of cows that were administered 2 J-5 bacterin doses during the dry period had poor antibody responses and a higher incidence of mastitis in the subsequent lactation.[29] This relatively short duration of immune protection is supported by several trials.[30–32] A New York study determined that cows vaccinated with 2 doses of J5 bacterin had less milk production loss following clinical mastitis and better survival in the herd compared to unvaccinated cows. However, this protection, as well as anti-J5 antibody titers, declined as lactation (and time since vaccination) progressed and was not existent by 75 days in milk.[30] In a Michigan study, hyperimmunization of cows with 6 doses of J5 bacterin resulted in a 3-fold decrease in severe clinical coliform mastitis from 42 to 126 days in milk, compared to cows that received 3 doses. This suggested that supplemental immunizations extended protection beyond that offered by traditional vaccination regimens.[31] A subsequent Michigan study determined that cows immunized with 5 doses of J5 bacterin had elevated anti-J5 E coli antibody IgG1 and IgG2 titers, relative to unvaccinated cows, for up to 60 to 90 days longer than cows administered 3 doses of J5 bacterin only.[32] Additionally, the best response to immunization, in terms of intensity and duration of antibody response, was gained when multiple immunizations were given as a series in different anatomical locations on the cow.[32]

In addition to the J5 E coli bacterin, an Re-17 mutant of Salmonella typhimurium bacterin toxoid is also available commercially. Peer reviewed literature in support of this product is limited. However, in an Arizona study, 2 immunizations in late pregnancy of this product was reported to reduce the incidence of clinical coliform mastitis cases and subsequent culling from coliform mastitis cases, during the first 150 days of lactation.[33] A recent product has been introduced in Europe that combines J5 E coli bacterin with S aureus SP 140 strain. At the time of this writing, evidence of the efficacy of this product to mitigate severe coliform mastitis, in peer reviewed literature, is lacking.

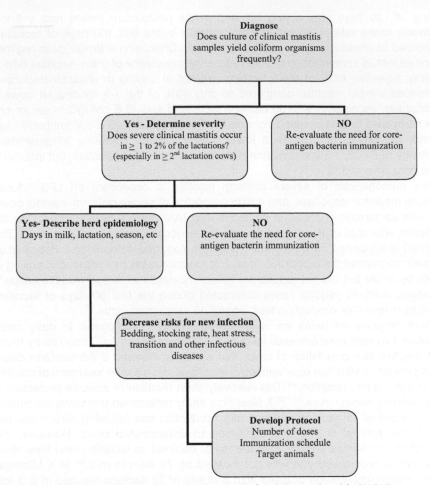

Fig. 1. Flow chart to design immunization protocols for dairy cattle with GNCABs.

STRATEGIES FOR IMMUNIZATION PROTOCOLS: GRAM-NEGATIVE CORE ANTIGEN BACTERINS

Use of GNCABs relies on 5 fundamental principles: (1) diagnose if coliform organisms cause a substantial portion of clinical mastitis within a herd, (2) determine the severity and incidence of clinical coliform mastitis cases, (3) describe the epidemiology of the problem in the herd, (4) decrease other herd risk factors that may contribute to clinical coliform mastitis, and (5) develop a vaccination protocol that best integrates immunology with herd needs and practical limitations. A flow chart to summarize this approach is presented in **Fig. 1**.

1. *Diagnose if coliform organisms cause a substantial portion of clinical mastitis.*

The most practical method to diagnose causative agents of clinical mastitis on dairy farms is milk bacteriology. Although culture of milk samples from individual clinical mastitis cases may often yield negative results, if a representative number of cases are sampled and cultured, the role of coliform organisms as causative agents will be better understood. Diagnosis of causative pathogens for mastitis cases cannot be based on clinical signs, appearance of milk from the affected quarter, or response to antimicrobial therapy. Failure to appreciate the demographics of causative agents in a herd leads to false expectations for a variety of mastitis control measures, including GNCAB use. This disappointment will especially be predictable in herds that experience a majority of clinical mastitis cases caused by water borne organisms such as *Pseudomonas* sp and *Prototheca*, mycotic organisms, *Mycoplasma bovis*, and gram-positive cocci. Typically, in low SCC herds (<200,000 cells/mL), 30% to 40% of cultured samples will yield coliform organisms, and if samples where no organism was isolated are excluded, the proportion of coliform cases can be 50% to 70%. Nonetheless, this should be confirmed in the laboratory.

2. *Determine the severity and incidence of clinical coliform mastitis cases.*

DeGraves and Fetrow[34] predicted J5 *E coli* bacterin use to be profitable if clinical coliform mastitis occurs in greater than 1% of lactations and would be profitable at all production levels. However, this estimate may have been conservative. Costs of therapy have increased, and the role of coliform cases in chronic, recurring mastitis has been better elucidated, and in some cases, host-adapted strains may act as a reservoir of infection to other cows.[35] Nonetheless, the primary benefit gained from GNCAB use is the mitigation of the severity, not the prevention of IMI. Ultimately, the frequency of severe clinical mastitis, caused by gram-negative organisms, is the primary motivator to immunize with these bacterins.

3. *Describe the epidemiology of the problem in the herd.*

The consensus of clinical trials and on farm use of GNCABs decreases the incidence of severe clinical mastitis and culling losses among vaccinated cows, in approximately the first 2 to 3 months of lactation. However, a careful review of the distribution of clinical mastitis cases, by stage of lactation, season, and lactation number, should be assessed on an individual herd basis. In some herds, a preponderance of severe mastitis cases may occur after peak milk (3–5 months after calving) and continue well into lactation.[31] Additionally, in many herds, cases are relatively rare in first lactation cows, have seasonal cycles, and may even be associated with routine changes in bedding. It is important to know the *when, where,* and *who* of severe mastitis cases in each herd, as this will alter the strategy of immunization regimens.

4. *Decrease other herd risk factors that may contribute to clinical coliform mastitis.*

It is not in the scope of this chapter to outline the complete epidemiology of coliform mastitis. However, primary risk factors, such as clean bedding, udder hygiene, and teat end condition, all play a role. Immunization with GNCABs should only be a part of a herd mastitis prevention program if fundamental mastitis control practices are part of herd routine management.

5. *Develop a vaccination protocol that best integrates immunology with herd needs and practical limitations.*

Ideally, immunization regimens offer a long duration of protection, preferably on an approximately annual cycle relative to calving. Many gram-negative bacterins, not just GNCABs, are limited in terms of duration of protection. Thus, *if* the response to labeled dosing of a GNCAB is falling short of herd mastitis goals, *then* additional doses may be considered to better target the occurrence of severe mastitis cases. Although hyperimmunization may be a useful tool, serum anti-J5 antibodies in cows administered 6 doses of J5 bacterin did not differ from cows administered 3 doses, when assayed at the start of the next lactation.[31] Newer vaccines, formulated with adjuvants that activate TLRs of innate immune cells, are under development in human and veterinary medicine. These may offer longer duration of protection and have been investigated for use in J 5 *E coli* bacterins.[36]

Care should be exercised in administering multiple gram-negative bacterins (leptospirosis, k-99 *E coli, Histophilus somni,* etc). LPS contamination is pervasive, although highly variable among gram-negative bacterins. One report determined a transient, 7% decline in milk production following immunization of lactating cows with a J5 bacterin.[37] Veterinarians should inquire of vaccine suppliers, on behalf of their clients, as to the LPS levels in vaccines.

If herd records support the strategy, many herds forego the use of GNCABs in first lactation cows or reserve immunization for seasons identified as high risk for severe coliform mastitis. Additionally, there is nothing sacred in dosing GNCABs during the standard dry period/post-calving regimens. Most cows will respond with increased antibody titers at about 10 to 14 days following immunization. If a need is identified to protect cows from severe coliform mastitis during the first 3 weeks after calving, an advantage may be gained by immunizing cows before drying off, at dry off, and 2 weeks before expected calving to maximize antibody titers at the time of calving. Rotation of serial injections to different anatomical injection sites improved the intensity and duration of the antibody response in periparturient dairy cows.[32] However, immunization protocols that are unnecessarily complicated and lead to poor compliance are best avoided.

Staphylococcus Aureus

S aureus mastitis occurs in many dairy herds. Because of the predominantly contagious nature of this organism, many herds have been able to maintain a low prevalence of IMI caused by this organism. Heifers have been demonstrated to be infected with this pathogen at calving, although this varies greatly between herds and geographic regions.[38] This pathogen generally causes only a small percentage of clinical mastitis cases, and subclinical infections often become chronic and unresponsive to therapy. The ability of this pathogen to establish long-term IMI varies between strains. However numerous virulence factors increase survival of the microbe in host tissues. As the duration of infection increases, fibrin deposition and microabscess formation further reduce the effectiveness of the immune response. The ability to survive intracellularly within phagocytes impairs both humoral immunity and drug therapy. Additionally, *S aureus* infections rarely elicit marked innate immune responses, compared to *E coli,* for example.[39] This allows the organism to avoid an acute phase immune response that may endanger existence in infected tissue.[39,40]

An effective vaccine against this pathogen needs to overcome several major obstacles: (1) marked variation in strains, thus the need for a conserved, universal antigen, (2) "immune stealth" virulence factors, especially the ability to survive intracellularly and unexposed to antibodies, and (3) difficulty in assessing impact of a vaccine on reducing deleterious clinical effects of infection and actual IMI status. The last point reflects the nature of *S aureus* IMI to shed bacteria in milk from infected glands in a cyclic fashion. Recurrence of *S aureus* in milk may occur up to 28 days after therapy in as much as 80% of quarters because of L-form transformation (an induced variant that lacks cell walls), and rigorous serial sampling should be part of a protocol to determine IMI because of low sensitivity for 1, or even 2 samples, to correctly identify negative quarters.[41,42]

Considerable effort, encompassing numerous antigens, virulence factors, and bacterial strains, has been made to develop an efficacious and practical *S aureus* vaccine. Much of the interest has focused on primiparous heifers. A bacterin containing a lysed culture of polyvalent phage types, including a variety of capsular serotypes, is commercially available in the United States (Lysigin; Boehringer Ingelheim, Ridgefield, CT, USA). This product originated from work in Louisiana that determined 2 initial doses 2 weeks apart, followed by doses at 6-month intervals, reduced IMI at calving caused by both coagulase-negative staphylococci (CNS) and S aureus.[43] However, a subsequent challenge-infection study determined that this bacterin did not prevent IMI, accentuate clearance of IMI, affect SCC, or milk yield post-challenge.[44] The Lysigin-vaccinated heifers did have improved clinical scores and shorter duration of clinical mastitis.[44] Although immunization with Lysigin increased serum anti–S aureus IgG1 in heifers, milk concentrations of IgG1, IgG2, or IgM were not affected.[45] In a subsequent report in lactating cows, representing multiple parities, 2 doses of Lysigin administered 14 days apart did not reduce the number of mammary quarters that developed new S aureus or CNS IMI, the time after vaccination to develop new IMI, or SCC.[46] The authors speculated that the bacterin may have induced insufficient opsonizing antibodies in milk to promote phagocytosis.[46]

A different formulation of a whole cell killed bacterin was found to reduce the number of quarters infected and SCC following an experimental challenge, although this effect was only reported for up to 13 days after the challenge.[47] A subsequent field study reported that 2 simultaneous doses administered to heifers, followed by an additional dose, resulted in higher anti–S aureus–specific antibodies throughout the subsequent lactation. The investigators also reported that vaccinated animals had an average increase of 0.5 kg of milk/d and lower SCC.[48] In this study, incomplete Freund's adjuvant was used as part of the initial biphasic dose. This adjuvant is known to cause significant injection site reactions and is not generally used in commercial products. One of the more intriguing developments by the same research group has identified a Target of RNAIII Activating Protein (TRAP), a highly conserved membrane protein among many species of staphylococci, including S aureus. This antigen may have the potential to become a specific and universal anti-staphylococcal vaccine.[49]

S aureus produces adhesins, virulence factors that promote attachment to host tissues and subsequent adhesion among bacterial cells, producing a biofilm that can resist phagocytosis. Surface polysaccharides are a key element of staphylococcal biofilm, and strains that express exopolysaccharide (slime associated antigenic complex [SAAC]) in high levels have been isolated.[50] A preliminary study demonstrated the immunization with a high-producing SAAC S aureus strain reduced the concentration of bacteria in infected quarters, compared to a bacterin composed of a low-producing SAAC strain or unvaccinated controls.[50] However, there was no effect on new IMI, and effects of vaccination were followed for only 14 days after challenge.

A commercial formulation of the SAAC S aureus bacterin, combined with E coli, has been approved in the European Union. Clinical reports suggest that this product improves udder health by reducing new infection rates and lowering SCC in vaccinated animals.[51,52] However, data presented thus far have not appeared in peer-reviewed publications, and details as to evaluation of new infection rates and cures have been based on tenuous definitions of IMI. Little data have been reported regarding the efficacy of the E coli component of this bacterin.

Use of S aureus vaccines would likely have limited use in many dairies, especially in herds with low prevalences of IMI, as is typical for herds with SCC less than 200,000 cells/mL. Thus, it is unlikely that S aureus bacterins will have a significant impact in herds that successfully control contagious mastitis by practicing excellent milking techniques and maintaining milking equipment. Conversely, herds that immunize in lieu of good management practices are likely to have disappointing results. Heifers may provide a viable opportunity for use of an effective staphylococcal bacterin, especially in herds where IMI in post-partum heifers are endemic. As previously mentioned, this varies greatly between herds and geographic regions. If a herd has a staphylococcal mastitis problem, bacterins may also reduce shedding of bacteria from milk of infected animals. Investigators have administered *S aureus* bacterins in an attempt to augment antimicrobial therapy, with conflicting results.[53,54]

Streptococcus sp

With the exception of *Streptococcus uberis*, little progress has been made in the development of vaccines against streptococcal mastitis. Arguably, with the ability to nearly eradicate *Streptococcus agalactiae* and, to some extent, *Streptococcus dysgalactia*, with effective control programs, the need for research to develop a vaccine against this group of pathogens is limited. However, control of *S uberis* has proved more difficult and is an important cause of both clinical and, more typically, subclinical mastitis. IMIs from this pathogen may occur throughout lactation and become chronic, and the pathogen has been demonstrated to internalize and persist in bovine mammary epithelial cells.[55,56] Thus, internalization may aid *S uberis* to avoid opsonization by antibodies and other innate serum factors, as well as phagocyte recognition. Within herds, multiple strains can be isolated from clinical mastitis cases, although the isolation of dominant strains have a tendency to be responsible for chronic cases.[57] This suggests that the environment of the cow is an important reservoir of infection, as well as a limited number of host-adapted strains that can be transmitted both within-cow and between-cows, possibly at milking.[57]

Early attempts by researchers in the United Kingdom to develop a vaccine for control of *S uberis* attempted the use of live vaccines in combination with an intramammary administration of a soluble cell extract.[58] A decrease in the development of clinical signs following experimental infection was realized, but the protection appeared to be strain specific.[58] Further research by the same research group determined that *S uberis* plasminogen activator, PauA, is an important virulence factor for acquiring nutrients in host tissue, and used this antigen for immunization in experimental infections.[59] Unfortunately, consistent clinical efficacy in large field trials and subsequent commercial application did not follow.

More recently, reports have identified a *S uberis* adhesion molecule (SUAM), a virulence factor that enhances adhesion to mammary epithelial cells, and subsequent internalization.[60] SUAM appears to be highly conserved among strains from diverse geographical locations, and thus could serve as a potential universal antigen.[61] Vaccination of dairy cows with 3 doses of recombinant SUAM (rSUAM), administered during the dry and peripartutient period, induced anti-rSUAM antibodies in serum and colostrum at calving.[62] Furthermore, the antibodies were found to reduce adherence and internalization of *S uberis* into bovine mammary epithelial cells in vitro.[62] Although this technology offers promise, results demonstrating the impact of this vaccine on live challenge models and, more important, wide-scale field trials have yet to be published. Particularly because of the ability of *S uberis* to internalize in host cells, a successful vaccine against this pathogen will likely need to stimulate cytotoxic CD8[+] lymphocytes that can recognize and destroy bacteria-infected host cells, in addition to antibody responses.

SUMMARY

Presently, the most successful use of vaccination strategies as part of a dairy herd mastitis control program involves GNCABs, of which the J-5 bacterins are best understood. Immunization protocols employing this technology should be adapted to individual herd needs. Ironically, the success of these bacterins may rely, in part, on the systemic pathogensis of severe coliform mastitis. Because immune function is impaired in the mammary gland of a lactating dairy cow, and the difficulty in maintaining effective concentrations of antibodies in milk following vaccination, vaccines developed against pathogens that cause more chronic IMI, while promising, have significant obstacles to overcome.

REFERENCES

1. Rainard P, Riollet C. Innate immunity of the bovine mammary gland. Vet Res 2006; 37:369–400.
2. Sordillo LM, Streicher KL. Mammary gland immunity and mastitis susceptibility. J Mamm Gland Biol Neoplasia 2002;7:135–46.
3. Kehrli, ME, Harp JA. Immunity in the mammary gland. Vet Clin North Am Food Anim Pract 2001;17:495–516.
4. Innate immunity. In: Murphy K, Travers P, Walport M, editors. Janeway's immunobiology. 7th edition. New York: Garland Science; 2008. p. 53–60.
5. Netea MG, Van Der Graaf C, Van Der Meer JW, et al. Toll-like receptors and the host defense against microbial pathogens: bringing specificity to the innate-immune system. J Leukoc Biol 2004;75:749–55.
6. Park YH, Fox LK, Hamilton MJ, et al. Suppression of proliferative responses of BoCD4C T lymphocytes by activated BoCD8C T lymphocytes in the mammary gland of cows with Staphylococcus aureus mastitis. Vet Immunol Immunopathol 2003;36: 137–51.
7. Shafer-Weaver KA, Sordillo LM. Bovine CD8C suppressor lymphocytes alter immune responsiveness during the postpartum period. Vet Immunol Immunopathol 1997;56: 53–64.
8. Smith KL, Schanbacher FL. Lactoferrin as a factor of resistance to infection of the bovine mammary gland. J Am Vet Med Assoc 1977;170:1224–7.
9. Mullan NA, Carter EA, Nguyen KA. Phagocytic and bactericidal properties of bovine macrophages from non-lactating mammary glands. Res Vet Sci 1985;38:160–6.
10. Preisler MT, Weber PS, Tempelman RJ, et al. Glucocorticoid receptor down-regulation in neutrophils of periparturient cows. Am J Vet Res 2000;61:14–9.
11. Kehrli ME Jr, Nonnecke BJ, Roth JA. Alterations in bovine neutrophil function during the periparturient period. Am J Vet Res 1989;50:207–14.
12. Waller KP. Mammary gland immunology around parturition. Influence of stress, nutrition and genetics. Adv Exp Med Biol 2000;480:231–45.
13. Cai TQ, Weston PG, Lund LA, et al. Association between neutrophil functions and periparturient disorders in cows. Am J Vet Res 1994;55:934–43.
14. Contreras GA, Sordillo LM. Lipid mobilization and inflammatory responses during the transition period of dairy cows. Comp Immunol Microbiol Infect Dis 2011;34:281–9.
15. Rauff Y, Moore DA, Sischo WM. Evaluation of the results of a survey of dairy producers on dairy herd biosecurity and vaccination against bovine viral diarrhea. J Am Vet Med Assoc 1996;209:1618–22.
16. Cullor JS. The Escherichia coli J5 vaccine: investigating a new tool to combat coliform mastitis. Vet Med 1991;86:836–44.
17. Tyler JW, Cullor JS, Spier SJ. Immunity targeting common core antigens of gram-negative bacteria. J Intern Med 1990;4:17–25.
18. Tyler JW, Cullor JS, Dellinger JD. Cross reactive affinity purification of immunoglobulin recognizing common gram-negative bacterial core antigens. J Immunol Methods 1990;129:221–6.

19. Tomita GM, Todhunter DA, Hogan JS, et al. Antigenic crossreactivity and lipopoly-saccharide neutralization properties of bovine immunoglobulin G. J Dairy Sci 1995; 78:2745–52.

20. Chaiyotwittayakun A, Burton JL, Weber PSD, et al. Hyperimmunization of steers with J5 Escherichia coli bacterin: effects on isotype-specific serum antibody responses and cross reactivity with heterogeneous gram-negative bacteria. J Dairy Sci 2004;87: 3375–85.

21. Tyler JW, Cullor JS, Osburn BI, et al. Relationship between serologic recognition of Escherichia coli O111: B4 (J5) and clinical coliform mastitis in cattle. Am J Vet Res 1988;49:1950–4.

22. Gonzalez RN, Cullor JS, Jasper DE, et al. Prevention of clinical coliform mastitis in dairy cows by a mutant Escherichia coli vaccine. Can J Vet Res 1989;53:301–5.

23. Hogan JS, Smith KL, Todhunter DA, et al. Field trial to determine efficacy of an Escherichia coli J5 mastitis vaccine. J Dairy Sci 1992;75:78–84.

24. Hogan JS, Weiss WP, Todhunter DA, et al. Efficacy of an Escherichia coli J5 mastitis vaccine in an experimental challenge trial. J Dairy Sci 1992;75:415–22.

25. Tomita GM, Ray CH, Nickerson SC, et al. A comparison of two commercially available Escherichia coli J5 vaccines against E. coli intramammary challenge. J Dairy Sci 2000;83:2276–81.

26. Wenz JR, Barrington GM, Garry FB, et al. Bacteremia associated with naturally occurring acute coliform mastitis in dairy cows. J Am Vet Med Assoc 2001;219: 976–81.

27. Wilson DJ, Grohn YT, Bennett GJ, et al. Comparison of J5 vaccinates and controls for incidence, etiologic agent, clinical severity, and survival in the herd following naturally occurring cases of clinical mastitis. J Dairy Sci 2007;90:4282–8.

28. Wilson DJ, Grohn YT, Bennett GJ, et al. Milk production change following clinical mastitis and reproductive performance compared among J5 vaccinated and control dairy cattle. J Dairy Sci 2008;91:3869–79.

29. Mallard BA, Wagter LC, Ireland MJ, et al. Effects of growth hormone, insulin-like growth factor I, and cortisol on periparturient antibody response profiles of dairy cattle. Vet Immunol Immunopathol 1997;60:61–76.

30. Wilson DJ, Mallard BA, Burton JL, et al. Association of Escherichia coli J5-specific serum antibody responses with clinical mastitis outcome for J5 vaccinate and control dairy cattle. Clin Vaccine Immun 2009;16:209–17.

31. Erskine RJ, VanDyk EJ, Bartlett PC, et al. Effect of hyperimmunization with an Escherichia coli J5 bacterin in adult lactating dairy cows. J Am Vet Med Assoc 2007;231:1092–7.

32. Erskine RJ, Brockett AR, Beeching ND, et al. Effect of changes in number of doses and anatomic location for administration of an Escherichia coli bacterin on serum IgG1 and IgG2 concentrations in dairy cows. Am J Vet Res 2010;71:120–4.

33. McClure AM, Christopher EE, Wolff WA, et al. Effect of Re-17 mutant Salmonella typhimurium bacterin toxoid on clinical coliform mastitis. J Dairy Sci 1994;77: 2272–80.

34. DeGraves FJ, Fetrow J. Partial budget analysis of vaccinating dairy cattle against coliform mastitis with an Escherichia coli J5 vaccine. J Am Vet Med Assoc 1991;199: 451–5.

35. Almeida RA, Dogan B, Klaessing S, et al. Intracellular fate of strains of Escherichia coli isolated from dairy cows with acute or chronic mastitis. Vet Res Commun 2011;35: 89–101.

36. Yancey RJ, Dominowski PJ, Erskine RJ, et al. Evaluations of J5 bacterins in cows with novel immunomodulating formulations (abstract). Fifth International Dairy Federation Mastitis Conference; Christchurch (New Zealand); 2010.
37. Musser JM, Anderson KL. Effect of vaccination with an *Escherichia coli* bacterin-toxoid on milk production in dairy cattle. J Am Vet Med Assoc 1996 209:1291–3.
38. Borm AA, Fox LK, Leslie KE, et al. Effects of prepartum intramammary antibiotic therapy on udder health, milk production, and reproductive performance in dairy heifers. J Dairy Sci 2006;89:2090–8.
39. Petzl W, Zerbe H, Günther J, et al. *Escherichia coli*, but not *Staphylococcus aureus* triggers an early increased expression of factors contributing to the innate immune defense in the udder of the cow. Vet Res 2008;39:18–26.
40. Middleton JR, Luby CD, Viera L, et al. Influence of *Staphylococcus aureus* intramammary infection on serum copper, zinc, and iron concentrations. J Dairy Sci 2004;87: 976–9.
41. Sears PM. Fettinger M, Marsh-Salin J. Isolation of L-form variants after antibiotic treatment in *Staphylococcus aureus* bovine mastitis. J Am Vet Med Assoc 1987;191: 681–4.
42. Sears PM, Smith BS, English PB, et al. Shedding pattern of Staphylococcus aureus from bovine intramammary infections. J Dairy Sci 1990;73:2785–9.
43. Nickerson SC, Owens WE, Tomita GM, et al. Vaccinating dairy heifers with a *Staphylococcus aureus* bacterin reduces mastitis at calving. Large Anim Pract 1999;20:16–28.
44. Middleton JR, Ma J, Rinehart CL, et al. Efficacy of different Lysigin formulations in the prevention of *Staphylococcus aureus* intramammary infection in dairy heifers. J Dairy Res 2006;73:10–9.
45. Luby CD, Middleton JR, Ma J, et al. Characterization of the antibody isotype response in serum and milk of heifers vaccinated with a *Staphylococcus aureus* bacterin (Lysigin). J Dairy Res 2007;74:239–46.
46. Middleton JR, Luby CD, Adams DS. Efficacy of vaccination against staphylococcal mastitis: a review and new data. Vet Microsc 2009;134:192–8.
47. Leitner G, Lubashevsky E, Glickman A, et al. Development of a *Staphylococcus aureus* vaccine against mastitis in dairy cows. I. Challenge trials. Vet Immun Immunopathol 2003;93:31–8.
48. Leitner G, Yadlin N, Lubashevsky E, et al. Development of a *Staphylococcus aureus* vaccine against mastitis in dairy cows. II. Field trials. Vet Immun Immunopathol 2003;93:153–8.
49. Leitner G, Krifucks O, Madanahally DK, et al. Vaccine development for the prevention of staphylococcal mastitis in dairy cows. Vet Immun Immunopathol 2011;142:25–35.
50. Prenafeta A, March R, Foix A, et al. Study of the humoral immunological response after vaccination with a *Staphylococcus aureus* biofilm-imbedded bacterin in dairy cows: possible role of the exopolysaccharide specific antibody production in the protection from *Staphylococcus aureus* induced mastitis. Vet Immun Immunopathol 2010;134:208–17.
51. Jiminez LM, Romero C. Efficacy of vaccination on mastitis epidemiology: field study. Proceedings of the 50th Annual National Mastitis Council Meeting. Verona (WI): National Mastitis Council; 2011. p. 171–2.
52. Noguera M, March R, Guix R, et al. Evaluation of the efficacy of a new vaccine against bovine mastitis caused by CNS field trial results. Proceedings of the 50th Annual National Mastitis Council Meeting. Verona (WI): National Mastitis Council; 2011. p. 187–8.

53. Luby CD, Middleton JR. Efficacy of vaccination and antibiotic therapy against *Staphylococcus aureus* mastitis in dairy cattle. Vet Rec 2005;157:89–90.
54. Smith GW, Lyman RL, Anderson KL. Efficacy of vaccination and antimicrobial treatment to eliminate chronic intramammary *Staphylococcus aureus* infections in dairy cattle. J Am Vet Med Assoc 2006;228:422–5.
55. Jayarao BM, Gillispie BE, Lewis MJ, et al. Epidemiology of *Streptococcus uberis* intramammary infections in a dairy herd. J Vet Med 1999;46:442.
56. Tamilselvam B, Almeida RA, Dunlap JR, et al. *Streptococcus uberis* internalizes and persists in bovine mammary epithelial cells. Microb Pathol 2006;40:279–85.
57. Zadoks RN, Gillespie BE, Barkema HW, et al. Clinical, epidemiological and molecular characteristics of *Streptococcus uberis* infections in dairy herds. Epidemiol Infect 2003;130:335–49.
58. Finch JM, Winter A, Walton AW, et al. Further studies on the efficacy of a live vaccine against mastitis caused by *Streptococcus uberis*. Vaccine 1997;15:1138–43.
59. Leigh JA. Vaccines against bovine mastitis due to Streptococcus uberis current status and future prospects. Adv Exp Med Biol 2000;480:307–11.
60. Almeida RA, Luther DA, Park HM, et al. Identification, isolation, and partial characterization of a novel Streptococcus uberis adhesion molecule (SUAM). Vet Microsc 2006;115:183–91.
61. Luther DA, Almeida RA, Oliver SP. Elucidation of the DNA sequence of *Streptococcus uberis* adhesion molecule (SUA) and detection of SUA in strains of *Streptococcus uberis* isolated from geographically diverse locations. Vet Microsc 2008;128:304–12.
62. Prado ME, Almeida RA, Ozen C, et al. Vaccination of dairy cows with recombinant *Streptococcus uberis* adhesion molecule induces antibodies that reduce adherence to and internalization of *S. uberis* into bovine mammary epithelial cells. Vet Immun Immunopathol 2011;35:145–56.

Treatment of Clinical Mastitis

Jerry R. Roberson, DVM, PhD

KEYWORDS

• Mastitis • Clinical signs • Culture • Treatment • Diagnosis

KEY POINTS

• Decision making in clinical mastitis management requires determining the severity level of each case.
• Treatment decisions should be based on culture results and culture results can be obtained within 1 day.
• Making treatment decisions based on culture results allows the practitioner the most justified and judicious use of animal medications.
• Nearly 50% of all clinical mastitis cases are treated inappropriately or unnecessarily.
• Although there are many treatments for clinical mastitis, good scientific studies demonstrating the efficacy of most treatments are lacking.

Clinical mastitis cases should be managed rather than simply treated. Many cases of clinical mastitis do not require any treatment. In this day and age of possible excessive antibiotic use, antibiotic resistance, and increased testing for drug residues, veterinarians should be especially judicial in their use of drug therapy for clinical mastitis cases. Knowledge of clinical mastitis severity levels, culture-based therapy (pathogen-directed therapy) and treatment efficacy are essential in effectively and efficiently managing clinical mastitis cases.

SEVERITY CLASSIFICATION SYSTEM

A first step in managing a case of clinical mastitis is to determine the severity level. A classification system introduced and preferred by clinical mastitis researchers in the last 15 years is the severity classification system of mild, moderate, and severe.[1] This system does not indicate the speed of clinical mastitis development—just the severity. However, the precise definition of each level is not completely agreed upon.[2]

Although not necessarily written, most dairy farms have established clinical mastitis treatment protocols usually based on severity level. Although only a few Kansas dairy farmers reported having a written mastitis severity scoring system, the majority of

The author has nothing to disclose.
Department of Large Animal Clinical Sciences, College of Veterinary Medicine, University of Tennessee, 2407 River Drive, Knoxville, TN 37996, USA
E-mail address: jrobers8@utk.edu

Vet Clin Food Anim 28 (2012) 271–288
http://dx.doi.org/10.1016/j.cvfa.2012.03.011

these farmers used increased treatments and greater duration of treatment with increasing mastitis severity.[3] The most common indicators of the severity of the cow with clinical mastitis among Kansas dairy producers were being off-feed and the cow's appearance.[3]

Using more objective parameters should lead to a more consistent and judicious treatment protocol. The parameters used should be objective, quick, easy to perform, and repeatable among different people. In the author's opinion, the parameters that appear to be most helpful for assessment purposes are rectal temperature (for objectivity), hydration status (as an indication for fluid therapy), and rumen strength and secretion color (as excellent indications of severe mastitis). Assessing these 4 parameters should take no more than a couple of minutes. Although the author is very comfortable relying on this system, it has not been rigorously tested against other systems.

Wenz and others evaluated 4 classification schemes for acute coliform mastitis.[1] The first system used systemic parameters of rectal temperature, hydration status based on degree of exophthalmoses, rumen contraction rate, and attitude based on signs of depression. The other 3 systems were slight variations from each other based on local inflammatory signs of the udder and used quarter firmness, quarter swelling, quarter pain, and secretion characteristics with or without systemic signs of illness. The system using systemic parameters scored 47% of cases studied as mild and 21% as severe, whereas the systems using local inflammatory signs averaged less than 10% as mild and 38% to 63% as severe. The first system was considered the most discerning and helpful in making management and treatment decisions. However, this system was not considered to allow cases to be treated aggressively enough in a subsequent Colorado study.[4] In the author's experience of evaluating cows with clinical mastitis, the presence of a hard swollen quarter does not appear to be especially important in regard to treatment but does signify greater severity. Clearly, a single severity scoring system is not likely to work well for all herds. In addition, ill-defined subjective parameters may lead to an excellent system being considered poor when used by a different herd or individual.

Once the severity level is determined, milk culture should follow to allow for optimum treatment/management. Simply put, treatment for mild and moderate cases can normally await culture results, although moderate cases should be reevaluated for increasing severity. Severe cases should be treated immediately.

Severity: The Mild Case

Mild cases are those that consist solely of abnormal milk. The cow is not affected systemically and the udder is not noticeably swollen or hard. Between 60% and 90% of clinical mastitis cases are mild.[5,6] The importance of classifying a case of clinical mastitis as mild is that there should be ample time to obtain culture results prior to determining the most appropriate means of managing the case.

Severity: The Moderate Case

While most researchers agree on what classifies a clinical mastitis case as mild, there are differences in opinion on what constitutes a moderate case. Some have used abnormal milk with an abnormal quarter (heat, swelling, pain) as moderate, and if there were any systemic signs, the case was classified as severe.[7] The author prefers a system that uses 6 different relatively objective parameters to determine the severity level.[8] Under this system, cows with abnormal milk and no more than 1 of the following signs (serum-colored secretion, decreased ruminal strength, dehydration, elevated temperature, increased heart rate, or increased respiratory rate) would be classified as moderate. In addition, cows with a hard swollen quarter would be considered at least moderate cases. Cows with moderate clinical mastitis are not emergencies but should be rechecked if there is any question as to severity. Moderate cases seldom require immediate treatment and can often wait for treatment until culture results are known. Moderate cases represent around 10% to 30% of cases.

Severity: The Severe Case

Cows with severe clinical mastitis have abnormal milk, may or may not have signs of mammary swelling, and have 2 or more of signs of systemic illness such as fever, tachycardia, tachypnea, dehydration, and/or decreased rumen function. Affected cows may be toxic and may be downers. These cows need immediate attention and cannot wait on culture results prior to treatment, although a culture should be taken. It is generally thought that the majority of severe clinical mastitis cases are due to coliform organisms. However, data from 2 separate studies suggest that about 50% of severe clinical mastitis cases are due to coliform organisms. Thus, it is important to recognize that gram-positive organisms may also result in severe clinical mastitis. A Virginia Tech study revealed that of 21 cows with severe clinical mastitis, only 10 were due to gram-negative organisms (*Escherichia coli, Klebsiella* sp, or *Pasteurella multocida*). The remaining 11 were due to environmental streptococcus (ES), *Arcanobacterium pyogenes,* or yeast.[9] A study by Erskine and others reported that 53.8% of severe clinical mastitis cases were due to coliform organisms.[10] If a case of clinical mastitis is truly severe, there will be microbial growth; no growth or negative cultures are extremely unlikely in the severe case. Thus, culture is still essential even for the severe clinical mastitis case.

CULTURE-BASED THERAPY (PATHOGEN-DIRECTED THERAPY)

The primary reason for antibiotic use on the dairy farm is mastitis. It is not surprising that the major reason for residue violations in milk is due to mastitis therapy. The majority of cows with clinical mastitis are treated with antibiotics. But this widespread use of antibiotics may be lessened as found in a study regarding on-farm culture that indicated that withholding treatment pending culture helps reduce antibiotic use.[11] A single method (blanket therapy) of managing clinical mastitis results in inappropriate and needless antimicrobial use. A 2008 study of 165 clinical mastitis cases in which 32% were no growth, 51% were *E coli*, 8% were ES, and 9% were "other" found that nearly 50% were treated unnecessarily or inappropriately.[12] Nearly all cases received oxytetracycline even though about 48% of isolates were resistant in vitro. Inappropriate or unjustified treatment was largely due to treatment of no growth cases, mild *E coli* cases, and in vitro antibiotic resistance. In only 17% of cases (all severe) was all antibiotic use considered justifiable. These findings should reinforce the need for culture-based therapy, which should increase bacterial cures, decrease unjustified drug use, and decrease the risk of bulk tank residues.

Culture-based therapy is simply a method of using the culture result of a milk sample to determine the most appropriate means of managing a case of clinical mastitis. Although many may argue the logistics, few would argue the value of this concept. Culture-based therapy, along with severity level, helps determine if antibiotic use is warranted. Ancillary treatment such as fluids and anti-inflammatory drugs should be used as necessary. A 1986 study confirmed difficulty in predicting the etiologic agent of a case of subclinical or clinical mastitis.[13] More recently, a study was conducted to determine if a decision-tree induction was able to predict the Gram-status of clinical mastitis using in-line sensor measurements from automatic milking systems. The researchers concluded that this method provided insufficient discriminative power to predict the Gram-status or the clinical mastitis pathogen itself.[14]

The logistics of using culture-based therapy has been challenging. Many dairies did not have a mechanism to get milk culture results back in a timely manner. When a diagnostic laboratory is not available and the herd veterinarian does not offer culturing services, culturing can be performed on the farm. Two Virginia herds tried culture-based therapy beginning in the year 2000 (J.R. Roberson, unpublished information). In one herd, the procedure was a failure due to frustration and lack of readily available help in reading the cultures and ultimately lack of interest in its use. In the other herd, the program was highly successful. When the successful herd began culture-based therapy, their rolling herd average somatic cell count (SCC) was between 300,000 and 400,000 cells/mL. For the following 2 years, the rolling herd average decreased to 107,000 cells/mL. The herd is cultured at dry-off, at freshening, if there is a drop in production, if the individual SCC is greater than 200,000 cells/mL and if there are any clinical cases. Clinical cases were not treated until culture results were available which was usually the next day (except for severe cases). Treatment was postponed until culture results were known in about 98% of clinical cases. Streptococcal infections were treated with cephapirin by label with a follow-up culture within 30 days. Mild to moderate E coli, Klebsiella, and no growth cases receive no treatment; these also had follow-up cultures. Antibiotic therapy for clinical mastitis had been cut roughly in half since the program was put in place, which agrees with a recent study by Lago and others.[7] Several more recent studies have demonstrated the benefits and feasibility of on-farm culture-based therapy.[7,11,15,16]

When culture results are known, treatment can be adjusted for the causative agent(s). Culture results will also help identify management correction areas for control if an outbreak develops. Culture follow-up is a seldom used but extremely beneficial method to document the efficacy of treatments used for severe clinical mastitis.[5]

TREATMENT OF MILD, MODERATE, AND SEVERE CLINICAL MASTITIS

In general, mild and moderate cases of clinical mastitis should only be treated when the culture result reveals a streptococcal, staphylococcal (an argument could be made against the treatment of Staphylococcus aureus), or a corynebacterial specie. Severe cases should be treated symptomatically followed by adjusting antibiotic use based on culture. Some cows with severe clinical mastitis will die within the first 24 hours regardless of heroic efforts taken (~10%–20% of severe cases). In a 2002 report, 13.5% of cows classified as having severe clinical mastitis died.[10] In an earlier study, 6 (14%) of 42 cows with coliform mastitis died despite intensive antibiotic and electrolyte therapy.[17] In the author's experience, cows that survive the first 24 hours are not likely to die. Initial efforts should be made to support the cow through the critical first 24 hours; afterward, equal efforts should be made to save the affected quarter(s). The objectives of treatment are to cure the infection, speed recovery to a clinical cure, save the affected quarter, and save the cow. The priority of these objectives changes somewhat based on the severity of the infection. When treating clinical mastitis the following acronym may be useful: FANO, where "F" = fluids, "A" = antibiotics, "N" = nonsteroidal anti-inflammatory drugs, and "O" = other medications that might help. The approach to treatment of clinical mastitis should vary according to the severity and culture result of clinical mastitis.

Fluids and Electrolytes

Cows with mild clinical mastitis and the majority of cows with moderate clinical mastitis do not require fluids. However, fluids are probably the most essential treatment consideration for saving the severe clinical cow. Fluids and electrolytes are necessary to help protect the kidney and other systems from the toxic effects of some antibiotics (eg, tetracycline) and anti-inflammatory drugs (eg, flunixin meglumine), as well as to offset hypovolemia and endotoxemia. Assessing hydration status by evaluating the degree of exophthalmoses is subjective. The author prefers the more objective skin pinch on the neck in a horizontal plane using both hands. If the neck skin remains pinched longer than 2 seconds, the cow is at least 5% dehydrated and fluid therapy is advised. If the rumen is still motile with enough strength to push the fist or stethoscope out of the paralumbar fossa 1 inch or more, oral fluids should be adequate. Cows with severe clinical mastitis due to streptococcal species or yeast usually have good rumen motility despite having fever and hard swollen quarters. If the rumen is extremely weak or inactive, intravenous (IV) fluids should be strongly considered.

For most adult Holstein cows, 10 to 12 gallons of oral fluids should suffice. Electrolytes should always be added to the oral fluids (~160 g NaCl and 60 g KCl). Alfalfa meal, nutrient/energy supplements, and oral calcium products can also be added and may be of benefit when oral fluids are given.

A 1997 study indicated that cows with severe clinical mastitis tend to have metabolic alkalosis.[18] Thus, unless a blood gas analysis can be performed to determine the metabolic pH status, isotonic fluids should be used if administering IV fluids. Greater than 40 L of isotonic fluids should be considered with up to 20 L given rapidly in the typical Holstein cow. Calcium, dextrose, and B vitamins can be added to IV fluids.

Additional fluids should then be considered on a daily basis as needed. Most severe clinical mastitis cases will require 2 or 3 fluid therapy treatments. Hypertonic saline (7.2%) may be used at 1 to 2 L IV. Although some cows will drink adequate quantities of water after hypertonic treatment, many will not and oral fluids should be administered. To reemphasize, if fluids are not adequately provided to the severe clinical mastitis case, the prognosis will suffer.

Antibiotics: Systemic

Systemic antibiotic therapy for mild and moderate clinical mastitis cases is not usually necessary. Wenz and others found no benefit of intramuscular (IM) ceftiofur in the treatment outcomes of systemically mild clinical mastitis.[6] However, systemic antibiotics are highly recommended for cows with severe clinical mastitis and should be directed against gram-negative organisms because they are most commonly isolated from blood of severely ill mastitic cows.[19] Wenz and coworkers isolated bacteria from the blood of 46 of 144 cows with acute coliform mastitis.[19] Greater than 40% of cows with severe clinical mastitis developed a bacteremia, usually due to a coliform (primarily E coli or Klebsiella pneumoniae; others included P multocida, Mannheimia hemolytica, Enterobacter agglomerans, Salmonella typhimurium, and Bacillus spp). Erskine and others reported that IM ceftiofur did not affect the outcome of severe clinical mastitis when all isolates were analyzed together.[10] However, when coliforms were evaluated separately, cows receiving IM ceftiofur had a significantly lower rate of death and culling (13.8%) versus cows with coliform mastitis that were not treated with systemic ceftiofur (37%). Erskine and others[10] also reported that none of the 48 cows with gram-positive cultures died regardless of treatment group, suggesting that systemic antibiotic therapy for gram-positive cases may be unnecessary. Fluid therapy in the dehydrated cow is essential if a drug with potential renal toxicity, such as tetracycline, is to be used. If slaughter as an option, a ceftiofur product should be used because of the short withdrawal time. Cows with severe clinical mastitis should be treated systemically for 3 to 5 days. The Wenz data suggest that bacteremia is reduced by half at 48 hours.[19] The use of gentamicin should be avoided, not only because of the prolonged withdrawal time but also because it has not proved to be effective.[20,21] Although there are some European studies demonstrating the efficacy of fluoroquinolones against coliform mastitis, extralabel use of fluoroquinolones and sulfonamides for mastitis treatment is illegal in the United States.

Antibiotics: Intramammary

Intramammary (IMM) antibiotic therapy for mild to moderate clinical mastitis cases should be based on culture result. Streptococcal clinical mastitis should be treated with an appropriate IMM antibiotic as the streptococci can be susceptible and, if not treated, may result in a chronic intramammary infection (IMI). However, mild to moderate coliform mastitis, especially if due to E coli, usually do not require IMM antibiotic therapy because most cases achieve a bacterial cure within a few days with no treatment.[8] Interestingly, Wenz and coworkers found that culture negative results at 7 days post-mastitis event were no higher than 50% for gram-negative mild clinical mastitis.[6] IMM antibiotics evaluated were pirlimycin and cephapirin with or without intramuscular ceftiofur. This study provides some evidence as to the lack of efficacy of commonly available IMM infusion products against gram-negative pathogens.[6]

Approved IMM antibiotic therapy for cases of severe clinical mastitis has been and is still sometimes ineffective. Until the introduction of IMM ceftiofur (Spectramast, Pfizer Animal Health, A Division of Pfizer, Inc, New York, NY, USA), approved IMM products were consistently ineffective against coliform mastitis. As with any case of clinical mastitis, IMM therapy should be based on culture. Most common mastitis pathogens can be identified sufficiently within 18 to 24 hours of plating. In fact, coliform organisms grow so quickly on standard blood agar that they can be presumptively identified by 6 to 8 hours after plating by performing a KOH string test on the visible growth.[22]

Intramammary antibiotic therapy is not absolutely necessary on the first day, if culture can be performed. Prior to the time that IMM ceftiofur (Spectamast) became available, I had used IMM ceftiofur (Excenel) successfully in cows with severe coliform clinical mastitis.[9] I used 6 mL (undiluted) every 12 hours for 3 days (total of 6 treatments). The time to a negative SNAP Beta-lactam test (IDEXX Laboratories, Westbrook, ME, USA) has ranged from 48 hours to 12 days. This is extra-label therapy; thus it is very important to test the milk for antibiotic residues prior to returning milk to the bulk tank. Most beta-lactam tests are capable of detecting ceftiofur. However, this extralabel usage of IMM ceftiofur will likely become illegal in the United States in 2012. In a dose titration trial of IMM ceftiofur (Spectramast), the 125 mg dose resulted in a bacterial cure of 70.4% compared to 41.3% in non-treated controls.[23] Although cure rates by organism were not listed, IMM ceftiofur at 125 mg was reported to be effective in treating clinical mastitis due to S aureus, coagulase-negative Staphylococcus (CNS), Streptococcus species and E coli. Other studies that specifically evaluated the efficacy of IMM ceftiofur (Spectramast) by label for severe coliform mastitis could not be found. One important consequence of using an effective IMM antibiotic is that coliform bacteria will die and release additional endotoxin. Thus, anti-inflammatory drugs must be onboard, especially if effective IMM drugs are being used. Approved IMM antibiotics should be used against

Streptococcus spp, whereas IMM antibiotics have no effect and therefore should not be used when yeast are cultured.

Anti-Inflammatory Drugs

Several studies have been conducted on the efficacy of anti-inflammatory therapy for cases of clinical mastitis without an overall consensus as to a consistent positive effect. Many of these studies were conducted on experimentally infected cattle; thus, the relevance of the study results should be viewed with caution for the naturally occurring severe clinical mastitis case. Dascanio and others could find no significant benefit of either phenylbutazone or flunixin melamine when compared to a negative control for cows with acute toxic mastitis.[24] A relatively recent study was conducted with meloxicam for mild clinical mastitis.[25] While the authors reported no difference in treatment failures or milk yield, the SCC was significantly lower in the meloxicam-treated group. Whether this lowered SCC is actually worthwhile is a matter for debate. A similar study conducted on moderate and or severe clinical mastitis cases is needed.

Although data are limited, it appears unlikely that the use of anti-inflammatory drugs will alter the outcome of the mild to moderate clinical IMI. Studies involving experimentally induced mastitis of cows that received either dexamethasone or isoflupredone prior to the onset of clinical signs have demonstrated a decreased severity of clinical signs.[26,27] Yet, clinical signs of mastitis are not apparent until about 12 hours post-infection. The efficacy of the glucocorticoids in naturally occurring severe clinical mastitis has not been published. However, as long as appropriate fluids and systemic antibiotics are administered, anti-inflammatory drugs may be beneficial and probably do no harm. Abortion is a possibility when dexamethasone is administered.

Other: Ancillary Treatments

Other pharmaceuticals and procedures can be used in cases of clinical mastitis as long as they do no harm. There are no published studies documenting the efficacy of these treatments. Supplemental calcium may be one the most beneficial treatments in that many cows, especially those in early lactation, will be at least subclinically hypocalcemic. Wenz and others reported that cows with moderate to severe coliform mastitis were significantly more likely to be hypocalcemic than were cows classified as mild.[28] Care must be taken in choosing the most appropriate method of administration. IV administration could be especially hazardous if the heart is already adversely affected by endotoxins. Likewise, oral calcium gels can be especially caustic to the dehydrated cow's mucous membranes. B vitamins may be given but their benefit has never been evaluated. Frequent milk-out (FMO) does not appear to be beneficial or harmful for coliform mastitis but may prolong the clinical phase in gram-positive clinical mastitis.[8,29] Although the majority of studies that mention FMO out do not report positive clinical efficacy, a recent study of acute *E coli* mastitis reported that FMO improved clinical cure.[30]

CLINICAL MASTITIS TREATMENT: SPECIFIC MASTITIS PATHOGENS

Prior to 1994, there were very few studies of mastitis treatment efficacy that used nontreated control cases. Although it is well known that the efficacy of a given treatment depends largely on the agent of mastitis,[31] few studies evaluated the effect of treatment on specific mastitis agents. Pirlimycin (Pirsue, Pfizer Animal Health, A Division of Pfizer, Inc, New York, NY, USA) is highly effective against *Streptococcus*

Box 1
Some items to consider when evaluating clinical mastitis treatment efficacy studies

1. Utilization of naturally occurring clinical mastitis cases.
2. Uses a nontreated control group.
3. Defines severity levels studied and treatment outcome parameters and parameters are objective as possible.
4. Investigators had full control of the cows.
5. Culturing is conducted prior to treatment, preferably once during treatment, once immediately after milk withdrawal time and once 3-4 weeks after the first treatment. For studies with chronic pathogens (eg, *Staphylococcus aureus*), cultures should be continued for at least 2 months.
6. Treatments were assigned randomly (systematically or truly random) and the method of randomization is specifically declared.
7. Treatment outcomes are assessed by severity level (mild, moderate, and severe).
8. Treatment outcomes are assessed by etiologic agent.

---

agalactiae but has no effect against *E coli*. Approximately 80% of clinical mastitis due to *E coli* are mild to moderate cases and most of these cases undergo spontaneous cure within a few days. Thus, an efficacy study, which did not use a nontreated control, of pirlimycin for clinical mastitis in a herd that had a high percentage of *E coli* mastitis might suggest that pirlimycin is an "effective" antibiotic for *E coli*. The severity level is also associated with the efficacy of a given product.[31] There are various other factors that might alter the interpretation of the results of a clinical trial. A 2004 study identified severity of mastitis, lactation number, previous mastitis this lactation and bacteriological findings as factors that influence outcome of treatment and these factors appear relevant as stratification factors in mastitis trials.[32] More properly conducted mastitis treatment efficacy studies are needed but progress is being made. Items to consider when evaluating mastitis treatment efficacy studies are presented in **Box 1**.

Clinical Mastitis Treatment: Environmental Streptococci

Simply put, streptococcal clinical mastitis should be treated with IMM antibiotics regardless of severity level. There is no antibiotic of choice. Typically, between 12% and 35% of clinical mastitis cases are due to ES.[33,34] Environmental streptococci clinical mastitis tends to present as mild to moderate but can present as severe clinical mastitis. Severity levels for 48 cows with clinical ES in a Virginia Tech study were 8.3% severe, 27% moderate, and 64.6% mild.[35] Severe cases usually present with elevated temperatures and heart rates, hard swollen quarter(s), and sometimes dehydration, but the rumen usually remains strong with the cow eating and lactating well. Five of the 48 cows with ES clinical mastitis had multiple quarters affected. The Virginia Tech findings are similar to those reported by Hogan and Smith in which 43% of clinical cases had signs limited to abnormal milk (mild), 49% involved abnormal milk and swollen gland (moderate), and 8% involved systemic signs of fever and anorexia (severe).[36]

The primary objective in managing a case of clinical mastitis due to ES should be a bacterial cure. Bacterial cure rates for clinical ES mastitis that do not receive antibiotic therapy are usually between 20% and 30%. The lack of antibiotic use for clinical mastitis due to ES could lead to a herd outbreak as documented in a Colorado case study.[37] The ES are usually susceptible to most approved IMM antibiotics, although the ES in the outbreak reported by Cattell[37] were resistant to cloxicillin.

Thus, antibiotic sensitivity testing would be prudent on occasion. Despite in vitro susceptibility to most approved IMM antibiotics, reported bacterial cures range from 20 to 90% with the average reported bacterial cure among 11 studies being around 60% (expect around 40% failures).[38-40]

Clinical efficacy studies using experimentally induced mastitis can be suggestive of treatment efficacy but true efficacy requires well-designed studies of naturally occurring clinical mastitis cases. A 2001 study of experimentally induced *Streptococcus uberis* clinical mastitis compared the treatment efficacy of no treatment to IMM and or parenteral antibiotics. The no treatment group (11 quarters) did not achieve clinical or bacterial cures by 6 days, whereas all other treatment groups had greater than 90% clinical cures by 6 days and greater than 70% bacterial cures by 6 days. The authors concluded that 100% clinical and bacteriological cure is achievable with 3 days of combined treatment.[41] The authors of the previous study followed up with a similar study of experimentally induced *S uberis* clinical mastitis and concluded that aggressive IMM treatment with a product containing penethemate, dihydrostreptomycin, framycetin, and prednisolone (Leo Yellow [Leo Animal Health, Princes Risborough, UK]) (administered twice a day for 3 days) was the most effective treatment for the fastest cure clinically and bacteriologically using the least antibiotic.[42] Although the results of studies of experimentally induced streptococcal clinical mastitis might differ from naturally occurring cases, all results indicate that antibiotics offer the best opportunity for achieving bacterial cures and subsequent complete resolution of the mastitis. These findings are echoed by a study in which IMM pirlimycin (Pirsue) was found to result in gram-positive mastitis resolution 1.8 times more frequently than nontreated quarters.[43] In a treatment efficacy study of naturally occurring clinical streptococcal mastitis, IMM amoxicillin (Amoximast [SmithKline-Beecham Animal Health, Exton, PA, USA]) appeared superior to the other treatments, not necessarily because of the 75% bacterial cure but more so because of the low cure rates for the other treatments: no treatment (29%), FMO (22%), and FMO with IMM amoxicillin (Amoxicillin) at night (18%).[8]

Several studies have evaluated the effect of extended antibiotic therapy for cases of streptococcal mastitis and the majority has found extended therapy to increase bacterial cure rates over conventional therapy.[44,45] Milne and others[45] reported that 55% of *S uberis* clinical mastitis cases that did not respond with a bacterial cure, when treated with conventional therapy, obtained a bacterial cure with extended IMM antibiotic therapy. They also found that some cases of *S uberis* mastitis would have falsely been identified as bacterial cures if not sampled at 21 days after the end of treatment. A 2004 treatment study of IMM ceftiofur (Spectramast) conducted on experimentally induced *S uberis* clinical mastitis showed a significantly higher percentage of bacterial cures by extended therapy (5 or 8 infusions at 24-hour intervals) when compared to label therapy (2 infusions at 24-hour intervals).[46] An unpublished Virginia Tech study (J.R. Roberson and F. Elvinger, unpublished information, 2010) compared IMM amoxicillin (Amoximast) by label (3 total treatments every 12 hours) to extended IMM amoxicillin (9 total treatments every 12 hours). Although results were not significantly different between the 2 groups, a higher percentage of the extended group obtained a clinical cure by 7 (37% vs 57%) and 30 (59% vs 76%) days, whereas the extended group actually had a lower bacterial cure by 10 (59% vs 48%) and 30 (67% vs 60%) days, respectfully. Anecdotally, I have had some success with treatment failures by using a different class of IMM antibiotic by label. The duration of the infection does not appear to greatly hamper the ability to achieve a bacterial cure. It is important to note that bacterial cure may and usually does precede clinical cure. Thus, the use of antibiotics until the milk is back to normal is probably unwarranted. Follow-up cultures to determine bacterial cures would be a useful procedure. When follow-up culture is not feasible, a low California Mastitis Test at 21 to 28 days would be suggestive of a bacterial cure. Frequent milk-out with or without IMM antibiotic therapy appears to be detrimental, extending time to clinical and bacterial recovery.[8]

Clinical Mastitis Treatment: S aureus

Management and treatment of S aureus are presented elsewhere, but a few comments may be worthy. The determination of a bacterial cure for most mastitis pathogens can reasonably be done with a couple of culture periods after the antibiotic withdrawal period (eg, 14 and 28 days). This same sampling schedule will not suffice for S aureus. Thus, studies that report high bacterial cures rates for S aureus should be viewed skeptically if long-term sampling has not been performed (long-term = at least 2–3 months post-treatment). In a study of extended IMM pirlimycin (Pirsue) with or without vaccination for S aureus, Timms reported 30-day bacterial cure rates of 18%, 38%, and 56%, but at 60 days, bacterial cures were only 14%, 17%, and 14%.[47]

However, some factors regarding which cows have the best chance of truly obtaining a bacterial cure are becoming evident. In a 2003 study of S aureus clinical mastitis treatment efficacy using parenteral penicillin alone or in combination with an IMM product, nearly 92% of first lactation cows affected by β-lactamase–negative strains obtained bacterial cures, compared to 67% of older cows.[48] However, the bacterial cure was based on only 1 or 2 follow-up cultures at 2 and 4 weeks or only at 4 weeks. Thus, it may be worthwhile to treat first lactation cows, but reported bacterial cure rates of older cows are likely misleading as long-term culturing is seldom performed.

Clinical Mastitis Treatment: Gram-Negative Pathogens

There is a movement among producers and veterinarians to treat gram-positive clinical mastitis and avoid antibiotic use for gram-negative clinical mastitis. Diagnostic tools are available for on-farm or clinic use to differentiate between these 2 major microbial groups. For most practical purposes, this is appropriate, but there are instances in which antibiotic treatment may be useful in managing a case of gram-negative coliform clinical mastitis. Although the coliforms are often managed as a group, it is important to realize that there are distinct differences in treatment necessity and success. As mentioned earlier, mild to moderate E coli clinical mastitis does not necessarily require any therapy. The majority of clinical mastitis due to E coli tends to be mild, as reported in a 2003 study: 62%, 27%, and 11% of E coli clinical mastitis cases were mild, moderate, and severe, respectively, and none of more than 50 cows with E coli had more than 1 quarter involved.[49] In work conducted at Virginia Tech, cephapirin (Cefa-Lak [Fort Dodge Animal Health, Syracuse, NY, USA]) and amoxicillin (Amoximast) were compared to no treatment on cases of mild to moderate E coli mastitis.[49] Neither product proved to be better than no treatment. Fourteen of 19 cows with mild-moderate E coli clinical mastitis that received no treatment obtained a bacterial cure by day 5, and all cows obtained a bacterial cure by day 1.[5] The data support the premise that mild to moderate cases of E coli mastitis do not require treatment.

Although mild-moderate E coli clinical mastitis cases may cure satisfactorily without treatment, cases of severe E coli mastitis usually require the ancillary treatments listed earlier as well as parenteral and IMM antibiotics. There is no definitive preference for the parenteral antibiotic other than being broad spectrum and perhaps it having a short withdrawal period. The IMM antibiotic choice is a little more problematic. Until IMM ceftiofur (Spectramast) became available, there was only 1 approved IMM therapy for *E coli*: ampicillin (Hetacin-K). However, experience has taught us that ampicillin is usually not effective against clinical *E coli* mastitis. Studies published in peer-reviewed journals that reported on the efficacy of IMM ampicillin (as the sole treatment) for clinical mastitis could not be found. In an Israeli study of experimentally induced *E coli*, an ampicillin and cloxacillin IMM preparation was significantly inferior to parenteral cefquinome therapy with or without IMM cefquinome.[50]

Because IMM ceftiofur (Spectramast) is approved for use in lactating cows with *E coli* clinical mastitis, it should the first choice IMM antibiotic when *E coli* mastitis treatment is warranted. In the author's opinion, IMM ceftiofur is warranted for severe cases of clinical mastitis and for the relatively rare cases of chronic *E coli* mastitis. However, a Michigan study found that IMM ceftiofur (200 mg) was no more successful in achieving a bacterial cure of chronic *E coli* mastitis than was no treatment.[51] The author has had success treating severe *E coli* clinical mastitis with 300 mg IMM ceftiofur (Excenel) twice a day for 6 total treatments.[52] The author could not find any reported research on the efficacy of per-label IMM ceftiofur (Spectramast) on severe *E coli* clinical mastitis.

A European study documented the efficacy of parenteral enrofloxacin against at least moderately severe *E coli* mastitis over nontreated controls.[53] However, in a 2010 European study, systemic enrofloxacin treatment did not result in greater bacteriological or clinical cure of acute clinical mastitis caused by *E coli* compared to supportive treatment alone when assessed 21 days post-treatment.[30] Because moderate and severe *E coli* mastitis cases were analyzed as a group, any efficacy among the severe cases might have been diluted by the moderate cases. A single IV dose of danofloxacin given to cows experimentally infected with *E coli* showed statistically significant lower local clinical scores and a more rapid return to preinoculation values over saline-treated controls.[54] Although enrofloxacin and danofloxacin are illegal to use in an extralabel manner in the United States, the study does suggests that cows with severe *E coli* mastitis may benefit from systemic antibiotics.

Whereas antibiotic therapy is either not necessary or not worthwhile for most coliform mastitis because many self-cure, clinical *Klebsiella* mastitis may be an exception as more than 50% may become chronic infections.[8] A similar observation was noted in an earlier study in which IMIs caused by *Klebsiella* were of significantly greater duration than *E coli* mastitis.[55] For *Klebsiella* clinical mastitis, 44%, 25%, and 31% of cases were mild, moderate, and severe, respectively.[49] Approximately 10% of *Klebsiella* cases involved more than 1 clinical quarter. Essentially, *E coli* IMIs tend to be of short duration, whereas *Klebsiella* IMIs have a greater tendency to become chronic, and of those that do self-cure, the clinical course is longer. Unfortunately, there are essentially no studies providing evidence of an effective treatment against *Klebsiella* clinical mastitis. **Fig. 1** shows data collected in a Virginia Tech study (both published and unpublished data) that indicate the ineffectiveness of various treatments for clinical *Klebsiella* mastitis.[8] Anecdotally, the more severe cases have resulted in a higher rate of cure than the mild cases. The optimum treatment for *Klebsiella* mastitis remains unknown.

P multocida tends to present as a moderate to severe clinical mastitis that may be successfully treated with IMM ceftiofur (Excenel, Pfizer Animal Health, A Division of Pfizer, Inc NY, NY, USA).[5] Based on the author's research data, *Citrobacter* may be managed in a similar manner to the mild-moderate *E coli*.[5] The author is unaware of any claimed successful treatments for *Serratia* or *Pseudomonas* spp.

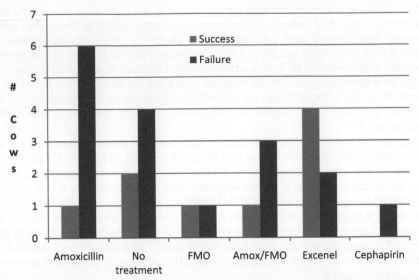

Fig. 1. Treatment success for cases of clinical mastitis due to *Klebsiella* sp. Amoxicillin (Amoximast) was administered per label. Amox/FMO, amoxicillin administered at night milking for 3 days with FMO occurring during the day; ceftiofur (Excenel), 300 mg administered via intramammary route every 12 hours for 3 days (6 treatments); cephapirin (Cefa-Lak) administered per label; FMO, frequent milk-out at 3 extra milkings per affected quarter per day for 3 days.

Clinical Mastitis Treatment: Coagulase-Negative Staphylococci and Other Coagulase-Positive Staphylococci

Typically, CNS and other coagulase-positive *Staphylococci* (CPS), other than S *aureus,* are considered minor mastitis pathogens, rarely causing moderate or severe clinical mastitis. The CNS and other CPS seem to be susceptible to approved IMM antibiotics in vitro, and again the goal should be a bacterial cure. For example, in one case monitored by the author, a CNS was recovered from clinical mastitis of both rear quarters and the cow received no treatment. The milk of this cow returned to normal by 4 days. However, a bacterial cure did not occur and the SCC in both rear quarters continued to be greater than 1 million for the duration of her lactation.[5]

Clinical Mastitis Treatment: Yeast/Prototheca

Both yeast and prototheca may produce clinical mastitis ranging from mild to severe. However, like ES, the severe cases tend to present as hard swollen quarters, some dehydration, and greatly elevated temperatures. The rumen usually continues to function well; affected cows continue to eat, drink, and milk. IMM antibiotics are completely ineffective against these organisms; in fact, yeast can utilize the nitrogen in the antibiotic for growth. Although it has been suggested that these cows need to be culled due to the contagious nature and chronicity, I have found that most of these cases clear spontaneously within 2 to 4 weeks. Symptomatic treatment for 1 to 2 days should be sufficient, and even that may not be necessary. IMM miconazole was attempted in 2 cows with naturally occurring *Candida* mastitis, but little, if any, effect was seen on subsequent culture results.[56] IMM therapy for fungal mastitis is not advised.

Clinical Mastitis Treatment: Arcanobacterium pyogenes

This gram-positive bacterial pathogen is very susceptible to IMM antibiotics in vitro; however, successful treatment in vivo tends to be rare. By the time clinical cases are identified, the chance of curing the infection and/or saving the quarter is unlikely. However, if cases are identified early, success has been recorded.[5] Because of the abscessation and necrosis involved, the infection should be attacked from both parenteral and IMM routes. Penicillin is the drug of choice, but a recent report indicated greater success with florfenicol and ceftiofur than penicillin.[57] Symptomatic treatment should also be considered as some cows will become systemically ill.

Clinical Mastitis Treatment: Bacillus

Bacillus cereus causes rare but severe clinical mastitis. I have seen at least 2 cases of gangrene of the udder due to *B cereus*. In one case the cow was severely ill. In the other case, the cow was not as severely affected but the teat of the affected quarter was dead. In both cases, the secretion was port wine in color. Occasionally, *Bacillus* spp are isolated from clinical mastitis cases. *Bacillus* spp are gram-positive organisms and should therefore be susceptible to approved IMM products.

MISCELLANEOUS MASTITIS TREATMENTS
Polymyxin B

Polymyxin B is reported to be a lipopolysaccharide-neutralizing agent. In a study by Ziv and others, IMM infusion of polymyxin B at 30 or 60 minutes after LPS IMM infusion failed to alter the clinicopathologic course of endotoxin-induced acute mastitis.[58] Specific data regarding the antiendotoxic or antibacterial benefit of polymyxin B in naturally occurring severe coliform mastitis cases could not be found. Ziv and others suggest the following dosage for polymyxin B sulfate: 100 mg in 10 to -20 mL sterile water for injection administered IMM once daily for 2 or 3 days; 5 mg/kg IM twice daily for 2 days.[59] The milk and meat withdrawal is not precisely known, but Ziv and others report that polymyxin B was well absorbed from a mammary gland infusion in a severe quarter and that the drug could be detected in the milk for up to 9 milkings.

Homeopathy

Although more clinical trials of homeopathic mastitis treatment have been published in recent years, to date, there are no published well-designed studies that clearly indicate efficacy. A study published in 2004 investigated the use of a homeopathic complex to treat cases of clinical mastitis in buffaloes.[60] The authors reported cures of 80% to 97% for fibrosed and nonfibrosed quarters, respectively. Yet, there were no controls, cure was not specifically defined, and bacteriologic studies were not performed. These same authors performed a similar study and reported that homeopathic combination medicine resulted in cures (defined as normal milk and udder and normal California Mastitis Test [CMT]) of 86.6% for acute nonfibrosed mastitis compared to 59.2% cures for a historical antibiotic group.[61] Some of the concerns with this study are the lack of nontreated controls, the lack of milk cultures, the use of a historical antibiotic group, and the fact that cows receiving the homeopathic combination that did not respond within the first few days were excluded from the study. In a small study comparing homeopathy, placebo, and antibiotic treatment of clinical mastitis in dairy cows, evidence of efficacy of homeopathic treatment beyond placebo was not found.[62]

Oxytocin

Although the use of oxytocin to treat cases of clinical mastitis is a commonly recommended adjunct therapy, there is little evidence to suggest that it is actually effective. When used as the sole treatment for experimentally induced S uberis clinical mastitis, clinical cures were minimal and mastitis severity increased.[42] A 1993 study by Guterbock and others indicated that oxytocin alone was at least equally effective (or ineffective) as IMM antibiotics.[63] This study was historic in that it was one of the first to use, or practically so, a nontreated control in that oxytocin has no effect on mastitis agents nor does it decrease inflammation. Although oxytocin can assist with milk let-down in many mastitis cases, and thereby assist in removal of mastitis related components, it has not proved very helpful for milk removal in severe swollen quarters as the milk ducts are likely blocked by inflammatory products and debris (pus).

Frequent Milk-Out

There are few peer-reviewed articles that indicate that FMO is beneficial in the treatment of clinical mastitis. A 2004 study found no benefit and suggested that FMO may be detrimental in obtaining clinical cures for ES.[8] A more recent study reported that milking 4 times as a supportive therapy for mild, moderate, and severe antimicrobially treated mastitis cases cannot be recommended.[64] A review of the history and studies regarding the efficacy of FMO for clinical mastitis is available.[65] The only study, to date, that reported improved efficacy with FMO indicated that use of frequent milking significantly improved clinical cure for naturally occurring acute E coli mastitis on day 2.[30] Based on the study's data, it appears that only 26 of 90 cows were milked out frequently (at least 2 additional milkings per day), and of the 26, 17 were treated with enrofloxacin, leaving only 9 control cows that received FMO alone.

SUMMARY

In summary, culture-based therapy and severity levels are key to management of clinical mastitis. Antibiotic therapy should be strongly considered for gram-positive clinical mastitis. Antibiotic therapy is not necessary for mild-to-moderate gram-negative clinical mastitis. Antibiotic therapy is warranted for practically all severe clinical mastitis as well as fluids and anti-inflammatory drugs. Clinical mastitis cases due to yeast and fungal pathogens or no growth isolates do not warrant antibiotic therapy.

REFERENCES

1. Wenz JR, Garry FB, Barrington GM. Comparison of disease severity scoring systems for dairy cattle with acute coliform mastitis. J Am Vet Med Assoc 2006;229:259–62.
2. Smith KL, Hillerton JE. What do we mean by mastitis, is there a need for redefinition? In: Proceedings of 38th Annual Meeting National Mastitis Council Inc. Arlington (VA). Madison (WI): National Mastitis Council; 1999, p. 200–1.
3. Roberson JR. Clinical mastitis perceptions of Kansas dairy producers. Dairy Day newsletter (Report of Progress 919). Manhattan (KS): Kansas State University Agricultural Experiment Station and Cooperative Extension Service; 2003. p. 30–5. Available at: http://hdl.handle.net/2097/6863. Accessed March 24, 2012.
4. Dube C, Goodell GM, Dinsmore RP, et al. Comparison of two clinical mastitis management protocols for predicting case outcome and cow survivability. In: Proceedings of 2nd Annual International Symposium on Mastitis and Milk Quality. Vancouver (British Columbia). Madison (WI): National Mastitis Council; 2001. p. 116–20.

5. Roberson JR. Clinical mastitis: The first eight days. In: Proceedings of 43rd Annual Conference American Association of Bovine Practitioners. Albuquerque (NM). Stillwater (OK): VM Publishing Company; 2010. p. 124–33.

6. Wenz JR, Garry FB, Lombard JE, et al. Short Communication: efficacy of parenteral ceftiofur for treatment of systemically mild clinical mastitis in dairy cattle. J Dairy Sci 2005;88:3496–9.

7. Lago A, Godden SM, Bey R, et al. The selective treatment of clinical mastitis based on on-farm culture results: I. Effects on antibiotic use, milk withholding time, and short-term clinical and bacteriological outcomes. J Dairy Sci 2010;94:4441–56.

8. Roberson JR, Warnick LD, Moore G. Mild to moderate clinical mastitis: efficacy of intramammary amoxicillin, frequent milk-out, a combined intramammary amoxicillin and frequent milk-out treatment versus no treatment. J Dairy Sci 2004;87:583–92.

9. Roberson JR. Treatment of severe clinical mastitis. In: Proceedings of American College of Veterinary Internal Medicine Forum; Seattle (WA). Ontario (Canada): Content Management Corp; 2007. p. 286–8.

10. Erskine RJ, Bartlett PC, VanLente JL, et al. Efficacy of systemic ceftiofur as a therapy for severe clinical mastitis in dairy cattle. J Dairy Sci 2002;85:2571–5.

11. Neeser NL, Hueston WD, Godden SM, et al. Evaluation of the use of an on-farm system for bacteriologic culture of milk from cows with low-grade mastitis. J Am Vet Med Assoc 2006;228:254–60.

12. Roberson JR. Apparent efficacy of blanket clinical mastitis treatment. In: Proceedings of 41st Annual Convention American Association of Bovine Practitioners. Charlotte (NC). Stillwater (OK): Frontier Printers Inc.; 2008. p. 288.

13. White ME, Glickman LT, Barnes-Pallesen FD, et al. Accuracy of clinicians in predicting the bacterial cause of clinical bovine mastitis. Can Vet J 1986;27:218–20.

14. Kamphuis C, Mollenhorst H, Hogeveen H. Sensor measurements revealed: Predicting the Gram-status of clinical mastitis causal pathogens. Comput Electronics Agri 2011;77:86–94.

15. Hess JL, Neuder LM, Sears PM. Rethinking clinical mastitis therapy. In: Proceedings of 42nd Annual Meeting National Mastitis Council Inc. Fort Worth (TX). Madison (WI): National Mastitis Council; 2003. p. 372–3.

16. Ruegg P, Godden S, Lago A, et al. On-farm culturing for better milk quality. In: Proceedings of 2009 Western Dairy Management Conference. Reno (NV). Manhattan (KS): Kansas State University; 2009. p. 149–59.

17. Anderson KL, Smith AR, Gustafsson BK, et al. Diagnosis and treatment of acute mastitis in a large dairy herd. J Am Vet Med Assoc 1982;181:690–3.

18. Ohtsuka H, Mori K, Hatsugaya A, et al. Metabolic alkalosis in coliform mastitis. J Vet Med Sci 1997;59:471–2.

19. Wenz JR, Barrington GM, Garry FB, et al. Bacteremia associated with naturally occurring acute coliform mastitis in dairy cows. J Am Vet Med Assoc 2001;219:976–81.

20. Erskine RJ, Wilson RC, Riddell MG, et al. Intramammary administration of gentamicin as treatment for experimentally induced Escherichia coli mastitis in cows. Am J Vet Res 1992;53:375–81.

21. Jones GF, Ward GE. Evaluation of systemic administration of gentamicin for treatment of coliform mastitis in cows. J Am Vet Med Assoc 1990;197:731–5.

22. National Mastitis Council (NMC). Laboratory handbook on bovine mastitis. Verona (WI): NMC; 1999. p. 212.

23. Hallberg JW, Watts JL, Wachowski MB, et al. Field efficacy and dose concentration study for an intramammary formulation of ceftiofur for the treatment of clinical mastitis in lactating dairy cattle. In: Proceedings of 2nd Annual International Symposium on Mastitis and Milk Quality. Vancouver (British Columbia). Madison (WI): National Mastitis Council; 2001. p. 238–41.

24. Dascanio JJ, Mechor GD, Grohn YT, et al. Effect of phenylbutazone and flunixin meglumine on acute toxic mastitis in dairy cows. Am J Vet Res 1995;56:1213–8.
25. McDougall S, Bryan MA, Tiddy RM. Effect of treatment with nonsteroidal antiinflammatory meloxicam on milk production, somatic cell count, probability of re-treatment, and culling of dairy cows with mild clinical mastitis. J Dairy Sci 2009;92:4421–31.
26. Lohuis JACM, Van Leeuwen W, Verheijden JHM, et al. Effect of steroidal antiinflammatory drugs on Escherichia-coli endotoxin-induced mastitis in the cow. J Dairy Sci 1989;72:241–9.
27. Ziv G, Shem-Tov M, Ascher F. Combined effect of ampicillin, colistin and dexamethasone administered intramuscularly to dairy cows on the clinico-pathological course of E-coli-endotoxin mastitis. Vet Res 1998;29:89–98.
28. Wenz JR, Barrington GM, Garry FB, et al. Use of systemic signs to assess disease severity in dairy cows with acute coliform mastitis. J Am Vet Med Assoc 2001;218:567–72.
29. Leininger DJ, Roberson JR, Elvinger F, et al. Evaluation of frequent milkout for treatment of cows with experimentally induced Escherichia coli mastitis. J Am Vet Med Assoc 2003;222:63–6.
30. Suojala L, Simojoki H, Mustonen K, et al. Efficacy of enrofloxacin in the treatment of naturally occurring acute clinical Escherichia coli mastitis. J Dairy Sci 2010;93:1960–9.
31. Ødegaard SA, Sviland S. Comparison of intramammary antibiotic preparations for the treatment of clinical bovine mastitis caused by bacteria sensitive to penicillin. In: Proceedings of 2nd Annual International Symposium on Mastitis and Milk Quality. Vancouver (British Columbia). Madison (WI): National Mastitis Council; 2001. p. 502–3.
32. Hektoen L, Ødegaard SA, Løken T, et al. Evaluation of stratification factors and score-scales in clinical trials of treatment of clinical mastitis in dairy cows. J Vet Med Assoc 2004;51:196–202.
33. Schukken YH, Grommers FJ, van de Greer D, et al. Incidence of clinical mastitis on farms with low somatic cell counts in bulk milk. Vet Rec 1989;125:60–3.
34. Erskine RJ, Bartlett PC. Assessing the success of clinical mastitis treatment: what are production medicine goals? Agri-Practice 1995;16:6–10.
35. Roberson JR. Managing gram-positive clinical mastitis. In: Proceedings 2004 Western States Veterinary Conference. Las Vegas (NV): Veterinary Software Publishing Inc; 2004. p. 540–2.
36. Hogan JS, Smith KL. Occurrence of clinical and subclinical environmental streptococcal mastitis. In: Proceedings of Udder Health Management for Environmental Streptococci. Guelph (Ontario). Madison (WI): National Mastitis Council; 1997. p. 36–41.
37. Cattell MB. An outbreak of Streptococcus uberis as a consequence of adopting a protocol of no antibiotic therapy for clinical mastitis. In: Proceedings of 35th Annual Meeting National Mastitis Council Inc. Nashville (TN). Madison (WI): National Mastitis Council; 1996. p. 123–30.
38. Wilson DJ, Sears PM, Gonzalez RN, et al. Efficacy of florfenicol for treatment of clinical and subclinical bovine mastitis. Am J Vet Res 1996;57:526–8.
39. Griffin TK, Dodd FH, Bramley AJ. Efficacy and financial value of antibiotic treatment of bovine clinical mastitis during lactation: a review. Br Vet J 1987;143:410–22.
40. Keefe G, Leslie K. Therapy protocols for environmental streptococcal mastitis. In: Proceedings of Udder Health Management for Environmental Streptococci. Guelph (Ontario). Madison (WI): National Mastitis Council; 1997. p. 75–86.

41. Hillerton JE, Kliem KE. Aggressive therapy of clinical Streptococcus uberis mastitis. In: Proceedings of 2nd Annual International Symposium on Mastitis and Milk Quality. Vancouver (British Columbia). Madison (WI): National Mastitis Council; 2001. p. 234-7.

42. Hillerton JE, Kliem KE. Effective treatment of Streptococcus uberis clinical mastitis to minimize the use of antibiotics. J Dairy Sci 2002;85:1009-14.

43. Cattell MB, Dinsmore RP, Belschner AP, et al. Environmental gram-positive mastitis treatment: In vitro sensitivity and bacteriologic cure. J Dairy Sci 2001;84:2036-43.

44. Krömker V, Paduch JH, Klocke D, et al. Efficacy of extended intramammary therapy to treat moderate and severe clinical mastitis in lactating dairy cows. Berl Munch Tierarztl Wochenschr 2010;123:147-52.

45. Milne MH, Biggs AM, Barrett DC, et al. Treatment of persistent intramammary infections with Streptococcus uberis in dairy cows. Vet Rec 2005;157:245-50.

46. Oliver SP, Almeida A, Gillespie BE, et al. Extended ceftiofur therapy for treatment of experimentally-induced Streptococcus uberis mastitis in lactating dairy cattle. J Dairy Sci 2004;87:3322-9.

47. Timms L. Field trial evaluation of extended pirlimycin therapy with or without vaccination for Staphylococcus aureus mastitis. In: Proceedings of 2nd Annual International Symposium on Mastitis and Milk Quality. Vancouver (British Columbia). Madison (WI): National Mastitis Council; 2001. p. 538-9.

48. Taponen S, Jantunen A, Pyörälä E, et al. Efficacy of targeted 5-day combined parenteral and intramammary treatment of clinical mastitis caused by penicillin-susceptible or penicillin-resistant Staphylococcus aureus. Acta Vet Scand 2003;44: 53-62.

49. Roberson JR. 2003. Treatment of E. coli & Klebsiella: Mild to moderate cases. In: Proceedings of North American Veterinary Conference 2003. Large Animal; Orlando (FL). Gainesville (FL): Eastern States Veterinary Association: 2003. p. 94-6.

50. Shpigel NY, Levin D, Winkler M, et al. Efficacy of cefquinome for treatment of cows with mastitis experimentally induced using Escherichia coli. J Dairy Sci 1997;80:318-23.

51. Sears PM, Ackerman CE, Crandall KM, et al. Treatment of persistent Escherichia coli mastitis on a large dairy. In: Proceedings of 37th Annual Convention American Association of Bovine Practitioners. Fort Worth (TX). Stillwater (OK): Frontier Printers Inc.; 2004. p. 188-9.

52. Roberson JR. Mastitis treatment: does anything really work? In: Proceedings of 18th Annual Central Veterinary Conference. Kansas City (MO). Lenexa (KS): Advanstar Veterinary Healthcare Communications; 2006. p. 806-10.

53. Hoeben D, Monfardini E, Burvenich C, et al. Treatment of acute Escherichia coli mastitis in cows with enrofloxacin: effect on clinical signs and chemiluminescence of circulating neutrophils. J Dairy Res 2000;67:485-502.

54. Poutrel B, Stegemann MR, Roy O, et al. Evaluation of the efficacy of systemic danofloxacin in the treatment of induced acute Escherichia coli bovine mastitis. J Dairy Res 2008;75:310-8.

55. Smith LK, Todhunter DA, Schoenburger PS. Environmental mastitis: cause, prevalence, prevention. J Dairy Sci 1985;68:1531-53.

56. Roberson JR, Kalck KA. Treatment of candidal mastitis in two Holstein cows: a case report and review. Bovine Pract 2010;44:52-8.

57. Motta RG, Ribeiro MG, Perrotti IBM, et al. Outbreak of bovine mastitis caused by Arcanobacterium pyogenes. Arquivo Bras Med Vet Zoo 2011;63:736-40.

58. Ziv G, Schultze WD. Influence of intramammary infusion of polymyxin B on the clinicopathologic course of endotoxin-induced mastitis. Am J Vet Res 1983;44: 1446-50.

59. Ziv G. Treatment of peracute and acute mastitis. Vet Clin North Am: Food Anim Pract 1992;8:1–15.
60. Varshney JP, Naresh R. Evaluation of a homeopathic complex in the clinical management of udder diseases of riverine buffaloes. Homeopathy 2004;93:17–20.
61. Varshney JP, Naresh R. Comparative efficacy of homeopathic and allopathic systems of medicine in the management of clinical mastitis of Indian dairy cows. Homeopathy 2005;94:81–5.
62. Hektoen L, Larsen S, Ødegaard SA, et al. Comparison of homeopathy, placebo and antibiotic treatment of clinical mastitis in dairy cows: methodological issues and results from a randomized-clinical trial. J Vet Med Assoc 2004;51:439–46.
63. Guterbock WM, Van Eenennaam AL, Anderson RJ, et al. Efficacy of intramammary antibiotic therapy for treatment of clinical mastitis caused by environmental pathogens. J Dairy Sci 1993;76:3437–44.
64. Krömker V, Zinke C, Paduch J, et al. Evaluation of increased milking frequency as an additional treatment of cows with clinical mastitis. J Dairy Res 2010;77:90–4.
65. Roberson JR. Frequent milk-out and oxytocin use. In: Proceedings of the North American Veterinary Conference 2003. Orlando. Gainesville (FL): Eastern States Veterinary Association; 2003. p. 105–9.

Assessment and Management of Pain in Dairy Cows with Clinical Mastitis

Kenneth E. Leslie, DVM, MSc[a],*, Christina S. Petersson-Wolfe, MSc, PhD[b]

KEYWORDS

- Mastitis • Assessment of pain • Management of pain • Perception of pain
- Treatment • Non steroidal anti-inflammatory agents

KEY POINTS

- Mastitis is a common and economically important problem. One of the major costs may be related to dairy cattle welfare, which remains largely unexplored.
- Pain is an unpleasant sensory and emotional experience associated with tissue damage. It is highly variable and difficult to quantify in dairy cattle.
- Both producers and veterinarians perceive severe clinical mastitis as being very painful but have varying views on the pain involved with mild and moderate cases.
- The public is concerned that the animal is feeling well, functioning well, and can live according to its nature, in addition to it having the five freedoms of animal welfare.
- Observations of both physiologic and behavioral changes should be considered when monitoring for disease.
- Behavioral responses related to pain and discomfort may include changes in activity, gait, mental state, vocalization, and posture.
- Novel tools for assessment of behavior include pedometry and position data loggers, weight distribution scales, pain pressure algometer, laser nociception tests, and rumination monitors.
- There is clear benefit to the use of nonsteroidal anti-inflammatory drugs for management of inflammation and alleviation of pain.
- Research conducted on lipopolysaccharide-induced, experimental-challenge models, and naturally occurring clinical mastitis cases has shown considerable benefit for pain management therapy.

INTRODUCTION

Despite the widespread implementation of mastitis control programs, clinical mastitis is a commonly occurring, and economically important, disease for the worldwide dairy

This work was supported by a grant from the Canadian Bovine Mastitis Research Network.
The authors have nothing to disclose.
[a] Department of Population Medicine, University of Guelph, 50 Stone Road East, Guelph, Ontario N1G 2W1, Canada; [b] Department of Dairy Science, Virginia Tech, 175 West Campus Drive, 2120 Litton Reaves Hall, Blacksburg, VA 24061, USA
* Corresponding author.
E-mail address: keleslie@uoguelph.ca

Vet Clin Food Anim 28 (2012) 289–305
http://dx.doi.org/10.1016/j.cvfa.2012.04.002
0749-0720/12/$ – see front matter © 2012 Elsevier Inc. All rights reserved.

industry.[1] In recent years, there has been a general decline in the incidence of clinical mastitis.[2] However, with an incidence rate of 23 cases per 100 cow years in Canadian herds,[1] a focus on research and extension on this issue is still greatly needed. Mastitis can be attributed to an annual economic loss of approximately $400 million for dairy producers in the United States.[3] Economic costs associated with mastitis include milk production losses, treatment costs, and potential long-term damage to the mammary gland as a result of inflammation.[3] Indirect costs from mastitis can include somatic cell count (SCC) penalties and increased culling rates.[4] In Britain, mastitis has been documented to be the leading cause of premature culling in dairy cattle.[5] In addition, an association between clinical mastitis and reduced reproductive performance in lactating dairy cattle has been reported; cows with clinical mastitis prior to being confirmed pregnant showed increased days to first service, days open, and services per conception.[6,7] In summary, clinical and subclinical intramammary infection is a major issue for the dairy industry, with broad-ranging impacts and consequences.

With the state of our knowledge on mastitis and its effects, it is understandable that intensive research has been conducted on the clinical, physiologic, immunologic, and molecular changes associated with mastitis. As such, our understanding of the biology and epidemiology of mastitis in dairy cattle has increased exponentially. Despite this increase in understanding, the effects of mastitis on cow behavior and welfare remain largely unexplored.[8] A wide variety of tools and techniques are now available and validated for the assessment of animal behavior and welfare. However, the assessment of pain due to mastitis has not been adequately studied. Many researchers contend that animals suffering from mastitis have compromised welfare and are in need of supportive pain management therapy.[8] Furthermore, some authors have asserted that appropriate analgesic treatment of clinical mastitis, to provide relief from suffering caused by pain, discomfort, and distress, should be mandatory.[9] Several nonsteroidal anti-inflammatory drugs (NSAIDs) are available as supportive therapies for clinical mastitis, even though documented evidence of efficacy and regulatory approvals for treatment of clinical mastitis are very limited.

This review will focus on our general understanding of pain, valid methods of assessment of pain in dairy cattle, as well as the state of our knowledge concerning the assessment, therapy, and effects of mastitis on cow behavior and welfare. Finally, the potential for increasing our knowledge in this area, through the incorporation of measures of cow behavior and welfare into mastitis research, will be discussed.

WHAT IS PAIN?

Pain is a term generally associated with human experience. This term is relatively subjective in context, depending on the individual's experience. The International Association for the Study of Pain defines *pain* as "an unpleasant sensory and emotional experience associated with actual or potential tissue damage, or described in terms of such damage."[10] This definition is extremely broad and open to interpretation. Individuals can construe pain in many different ways, making it extremely difficult to characterize. For example, humans can verbally describe their pain, while we rely on behavioral and physiologic reactions from animals to determine if they are experiencing pain. Furthermore, there are differences in pain responses between species, between individual animals, between different disease stages, and between acute versus chronic conditions. As such, defining pain can be a controversial problem.

Perception of Pain in Dairy Cattle

Cases of clinical diseases, as seen with severely lame cows or severe clinical cases of mastitis, are extremely easy to characterize as being painful.[11] In such cases, the animal shows visible signs of pain and discomfort, including depressed appearance, decreased milk yield, weight loss, and abnormal postures, to name a few.[12] On the other hand, mild and moderate cases of clinical disease are not as easily characterized as being painful.[11] Unfortunately, the mild and moderate cases of disease occur at a substantially greater frequency. Thus, there is considerable potential for a large number of animals to be experiencing pain that may be overlooked. In most cases, it is a lack of understanding of the behavioral changes indicative of animal pain. As previously mentioned, the assessment and detection of pain can be extremely difficult and are complicated by the stoic nature of dairy cattle.[11] This situation is exacerbated in that from an evolutionarily perspective, cattle are considered a prey species and are predisposed to avoid showing pain and vulnerability, even when exposed to harmful stimuli.[11,13] Although modern dairy production systems do not expose cattle to any forms of predation, the herd dynamic of a free-stall facility can provide an opportunity for similar behavioral responses. In other words, the expression of pain could result in a more dominant animal causing restriction from access to feed and optimal housing areas.[14] In these situations, pain can be extremely difficult to identify and characterize.

Dairy Producers' Perception of Pain in Dairy Cattle

In Norway, a pain assessment instrument was administered as a questionnaire using a visual analog scale. It was completed by 149 dairy producers to evaluate their opinions on pain associated with various conditions in dairy cattle.[15] It was found that a large proportion of the producers surveyed did agree that animals do experience physical pain (70%). Yet, there was a wide range of pain scores allocated for the 21 conditions presented, ranging from 2.4 to 8.6 (on a 10-point scale). Severe clinical mastitis received a score of 7.6, which was in the same range as conditions such as dystocia and distal limb fractures in calves. However, moderate clinical mastitis with clots received a score of 5.7, which was similar to eye infections and laminitis. It is evident that several factors about a disease can influence a producer's opinion on how much pain an animal is experiencing.

Veterinary Practitioners' Perception of Pain in Dairy Cattle

The attitudes and approaches of animal health professionals toward the recognition, prevention, and alleviation of potential causes of reduced animal welfare have been explored to identify how animals are being treated in the dairy industry. For example, at a veterinary conference in Scotland, clinicians were administered a survey on the subject of dairy cattle welfare.[16] It was found that 68% of the respondents identified that it would be useful to have a validated scoring system for pain in cattle. These respondents also indicated that mastitis was not as painful as other clinical conditions or procedures, such as castration, cesarean section, or lameness. Yet, it is noteworthy that the greatest variation among respondents was with respect to mastitis. It was concluded that the numerous causative agents involved, the range of environmental conditions, and the varying levels of severity of infection that occur with cases of clinical mastitis may have been responsible for the wide range in response.[16]

A larger survey performed in the United Kingdom was used to assess the attitudes of cattle veterinarians on the use of analgesics, and on pain in general.[17] The respondents were questioned about the severity of pain associated with a variety of cattle diseases, including mild clinical mastitis and severe endotoxic *Escherichia coli* mastitis. On a 10-point scale, respondents rated severe mastitis at a pain level of 7, comparable to a fracture or foot abscess. On the other hand, mild clinical mastitis was rated at a severity score of 3, similar to hair loss from hock abrasion or left displaced abomasum. There was a significant difference between male and female respondents. Women rated many of the clinical conditions to be significantly more painful than the rating assigned by men. Interestingly, even though the veterinarians who were surveyed recognized that there was pain associated with even mild cases of mastitis, the use of analgesics for this condition was not suggested. Yet, it is well documented that veterinarians have a responsibility to the producers and their animals to prevent both the pain and distress that result in altered behavior and physiologic changes from an animal's normal state.[18]

Recently, a survey conducted by Thomsen and colleagues attempted to quantify the use of analgesics in cows and calves by bovine practitioners in Scandinavian countries.[19] The results indicated that younger veterinarians who graduated in the 2000s, in comparison to older graduates, were more likely to agree that recovery time is faster when analgesics are used. This result is understandable, considering the evolution of the teaching of pain management in veterinary medical education, especially over the past 10 to 15 years. Another important finding of this survey was the lack of difference between the attitudes of male and female veterinarians, which had been previously documented in the literature. It was speculated that this discrepancy could be due to an overall increase in awareness of changes in national legislation that encompasses the use of anesthesia and analgesia for common husbandry practices in Scandinavia.[19]

Public Perception of Pain in Animals

The increase in research on the behavior and welfare of dairy cattle can be attributed to many reasons. One of the primary motivating factors may be public perception. Various public media are focusing increased attention on the treatment, and overall welfare, of livestock. Scientists are encouraged to understand the behavior of animals and how to optimize management practices to decrease any stress and pain that they are experiencing.[20,21] There are 3 major questions that the public will ask when they are assessing the welfare of animals within a livestock industry:

1. "Is the animal functioning well?"
2. "Is the animal feeling well?"
3. "Is the animal able to live according to its nature?"

In regard to clinical mastitis in dairy cattle, it is probable that the answer to all of these questions is "no." As such, response to these questions may affect the opinions of the general public that clinical mastitis compromises the welfare of dairy cattle. In the consideration of the basic principles of animal welfare, there are the "five freedoms of welfare."[22] Mastitis interferes with 4 of the 5 freedoms. The first 2, "freedom from discomfort" and "freedom from pain, injury or disease," are common effects with most cases of clinical mastitis. To avoid this situation, mastitis should be detected and assessed quickly, and therapy should be provided in a timely fashion, so the welfare of these animals is not jeopardized. The "freedom from fear and distress" can also be compromised with cases of clinical mastitis. Finally, the fourth freedom, "freedom to express normal behavior" can also be applicable with clinical mastitis, since the environment in commercial dairy facilities restricts the opportunity for the animal to exhibit sickness behaviors, compared to a cow's natural environment. Given the dramatic effect that mastitis, and disease in general, has on cow welfare, it is important to identify and treat clinical mastitis cases as quickly and effectively as possible.

Research on Pain in Dairy Cattle

Recently, animal science and veterinary research has placed increased emphasis on animal welfare. Specifically, quantifying and alleviating the effects of painful surgery, husbandry procedures, and lameness have been the focus of most research involving pain in cattle. However, there is relatively little published literature aimed at determining the severity of pain linked with other specific cattle diseases, and at quantifying the importance of pain mitigation on animal welfare. An increasing focus has been placed on pain and distress exhibited due to management practices and how it impacts the animal's affective state.[21] These practices include dehorning and tail docking. As intervention procedures, humans performing these practices should easily identify when the animal is in pain and is suffering. In addition, recent emphasis has also been placed on the health and biological functioning of the animal, including acute diseases or injuries, such as lameness, transition diseases, and dystocia.[21] In response, it is clear that these issues receive the most attention in prospective research on welfare and pain, as they are of importance to the industry.

PHYSIOLOGICAL AND BEHAVIORAL CHARACTERISTICS ASSOCIATED WITH ILLNESS IN DAIRY CATTLE

Illness results in physiologic and behavioral changes in dairy cattle. Physiologic changes are extremely useful in the diagnoses of illness. Producers and veterinarians can monitor deviations from normal physiologic levels with considerable accuracy. However, the early detection of clinical disease by dairy producers may also be enhanced through the identification of behavioral changes. Therefore, the monitoring of both physiologic and behavioral characteristics should be considered when monitoring disease.

Inflammation and pain in animals are associated with neural, endocrine, hematologic, immune, metabolic, and behavioral changes that aim to restore homeostasis within the animal.[21] The immune system and the brain form a bidirectional communication network, whereby the immune system informs the brain about events occurring within the body. Through this communication network, initiation of a response by the immune system produces physiologic, behavioral, affective, and cognitive changes that are jointly termed "sickness" or "sickness behavior."[23] Sickness behavior is a sophisticated response to infection and inflammation. This sickness response is manifested by a number of distinct physiologic and behavioral changes, including loss of appetite, adipsia, increased thermoregulatory behavior, decreased social activity, somnolence, and changed grooming behaviors.[24] In addition, sick animals may experience malaise, an affective state that involves negative feelings of depression, anhedonia, pain, and lethargy.[23] Sickness behavior is not a maladaptive state. It is actually a highly adaptive response that acts together with the immune system to facilitate recuperation from both injury and illness.[23,25]

Physiological and Behavioral Indicators Associated with Mastitis in Dairy Cattle

To effectively treat clinical mastitis, it is important to have reliable methods for the detection and classification of severity of infection. The implementation of a clinical evaluation system, which incorporates both local and systemic signs of disease, has been found to provide the most sensitive and precise classification system for clinical mastitis, with very few false-positive results.[26,27] However, clinical mastitis is still most often detected at milking, by direct observation of the milk and mammary gland. Yet, as farm sizes continue to increase and available labor continues to decrease, dairy producers need to rely more heavily on automated systems, rather than visual detection. Less time is spent on the individual observation of each cow, and there is a greater risk of missing or misdiagnosing a mild or moderate case of clinical mastitis.

Mild and moderate cases of clinical mastitis cases have previously been studied, observing pain thresholds, altered stance, heart rate, respiratory rate, and rectal temperature in affected cows, compared with control cows.[28,29] It was found that animals with cases of moderate clinical mastitis had significantly higher heart rates, rectal temperatures, and respiratory rates compared to cows with cases of mild clinical mastitis and with normal cows. Cortisol levels and SCC were also significantly higher in cows with mastitis compared to normal cows.[28] Cows with both mild and moderate cases of mastitis had significantly larger hock-to-hock distances compared to normal cows, thereby indicating an altered stance.[29] These affected animals also exhibited an increased sensitivity to a mechanical pressure stimulus on the leg closest to the affected mammary quarter, suggesting a change in pain information processing as a result of inflammation. In general, in the case of moderate or mild clinical mastitis, it is more difficult to determine whether dairy cattle experience pain and reduced welfare compared with cattle with severe cases of mastitis. Due to their stoic behavior, it is also difficult to determine if NSAIDs would be beneficial to aid in recovery, and mitigate pain, during these less severe cases of mastitis.

With the difficulties of characterizing a case, and accurately identifying the initiation of illness, in cases of naturally occurring clinical mastitis, models have been developed to induce intramammary in dairy cattle. Recently, behavioral and physiologic effects of lipopolysaccharide (LPS) endotoxin-induced mastitis cases were examined in 20 lactating Holstein cows, randomly assigned to receive an intramammary infusion of either LPS endotoxin or saline.[30] Cows receiving the LPS endotoxin had higher rectal temperatures, serum cortisol levels, and peak milk SCC in the challenged quarter in the first 24 hours after infusion compared with saline-infused cows. In addition, endotoxin-infused cows spent reduced time eating, cud chewing, and lying in their stalls compared with saline-infused cows. Furthermore, rumen contractions were reduced in endotoxin-infused cows at sample times, which corresponded with peak rectal temperatures. Results of this study suggest that endotoxin-induced mastitis affects both behavioral and physiologic responses in lactating dairy cows.[30] These interesting findings support the need for more investigation of responses in experiments that utilize challenge models with mastitis-causing pathogens, as well as with naturally occurring cases of clinical mastitis. Yet, preliminary conclusions could be drawn that the behavioral and physiologic changes found with severe and moderate clinical mastitis are indicative of pain. Furthermore, it could be concluded that NSAID therapy could provide very useful anti-inflammatory and antipyretic activity for these cattle, along with an analgesic effect, that would result in substantially improved animal welfare.

OBJECTIVE ASSESSMENT OF DISTRESS AND PAIN IN DAIRY CATTLE

Chronic pain, as observed in cases of mastitis, is generally regarded as a pathologic process.[31,32] Recent research has focused on behavioral observations and assessing physiologic parameters to objectively define if an animal is experiencing pain or distress.[33] Although research-based equipment is an ideal method for assessing discomfort as precise indicators of pain, some of the more traditional measurements can be applicable on-farm. For example, the most basic indicators of illness or pain are decreased dry matter intake (DMI), water consumption and milk production.[34]

Since cows generally have relatively consistent intakes and production, a decline in either measure is a good indicator that there may be a problem. Similarly, changes in milk quality can also be an indirect indicator of inflammation and potential pain. An elevated SCC is usually associated with inflammation and tissue damage, which can be indicative of pain.[35] Another milk component that can be objectively measured is L-lactate dehydrogenase, which is an enzyme in the milk that increases due to mastitis.[36] A biosensor to detect this component has become commercially available and can predict the onset of infection before it actually becomes clinical.[37] In terms of physiologic parameters, acute phase proteins, such as serum amyloid A and haptoglobin, have also been shown to be good indicators of infection, stress, inflammation, and pain.[38] All of these parameters can be successful in assessing the pain associated with mastitis. However, one of the most effective, but frequently unused, methods of assessing discomfort is observing the overall behavior of the animal.[39] Behavioral responses related to pain and discomfort may include changes in activity, gait, mental state, vocalization, and posture. Some of these behaviors are reflexive, whereas others are manifested to decrease the occurrence of tissue damage, reduce the recurrence of tissue damage, and promote overall recovery.[39,40]

Pedometry systems are available for activity monitoring in the dairy industry and have been used for the detection of lameness, estrus, and other conditions. There are many commercial pedometry systems currently available. Systems with monitors attached to the leg, rather than the neck or body, produce the most accurate representation of lying behavior.[41] A field study in Israel revealed that 92% of cows that developed clinical lameness had a decrease in pedometric activity of at least 15%.[42] Conversely, estrus causes an increase in physical activity and can increase the pedometric activity of free-stall housed cows by 4-fold.[43] Evidence is accumulating that cow activity increases significantly in the period immediately prior to calving. It has been suggested that this increased restlessness may be a result of discomfort or distress.[44,45] Huzzey and colleagues observed that in the 3 days before calving in dairy cows housed indoors, the number of standing bouts increased by 80%.[44] With the development of automated recording of activity data and the development of algorithms for its interpretation, there is considerable potential for pedometry activity measurements to be a beneficial on-farm tool for the early detection of clinical mastitis and, in turn, help to mitigate potential pain in cattle.

There have been some new research developments that show considerable potential for assessment of pain in dairy cows. These measures are extremely precise and automated, to easily identify subtle changes in cow behavior that may accurately detect pain. For example, electronic data loggers that measure the orientation of the animal (recumbent or upright) can be used to monitor lying and standing behavior. Specific measurements include time spent lying, time spent standing, and the frequency of lying bouts and lying laterality that the cow exhibits. Significant changes in these behaviors, such as decreased lying times, and increased lying bouts, can be an early indicator of discomfort. Recent research in cows with endotoxin-induced clinical mastitis showed decreased lying time and increased lying bouts in these cases.[46]

In other recent research, specialized weighing platforms have been used to identify lameness in dairy cattle. This weight scale system has the ability to calculate the weight distribution on each hoof independently, allowing the identification discomfort in dairy cows.[47] Similarly, research conducted by Pastell and colleagues looked at weight distribution in cattle and its ability to detect lameness and other hoof care issues.[48] This measure was proved to be sensitive for the detection of lameness in cows, and particularly those suffering from sole ulcers. However, this method was not useful in detecting cases of mild lameness. Combined with the use of other tools, this technology has the potential of being an extremely useful indicator of discomfort.

The pressure algometer is another technology that has been shown to accurately measure pain. This instrument is used to exert and measure pressure on an affected body region, and determine the *pain threshold*, which is defined as "the minimum intensity of a stimulus that is perceived as painful."[10] The algometer has been used successfully in dairy cattle research, specifically after the procedure of dehorning,[49] and in cases of lameness caused by integument lesions.[50]

Changes in nociceptive thresholds have been observed in situations of acute stress. These thresholds can be measured using a laser-based method to detect thermal nociception.[51,52] *Nociceptive pain* is defined as "pain that arises from actual or threatened damage to non-neural tissue and is due to the activation of nociceptors."[10] In this method, a laser beam is focused on the animal's lower limb. A change of behavior in response to the laser, such as kicking or tail flicking, can be used to identify discomfort. Research suggests that the behavioral responses elicited in response to laser stimulation are both valid and reliable as an indication of nociceptive responses in the cow.[52]

A decrease in rumination has been shown to be a good indicator of discomfort in cows with cases of mastitis.[53] It is possible that monitoring rumination may provide a reliable measure of pain or systemic discomfort in cases of clinical disease. It has been determined that when dairy calves were intravenously infused with LPS endotoxin, there was a reduction in their total rumination time simultaneously with peak fever response.[54] Similarly, it has been reported that a reduction in rumination time was associated with increased cortisol levels in cattle.[55] Although visual detection of rumination has proven to be a good method to monitor rumination patterns, as with any subjective measurement, it can sometimes be difficult to detect changes solely from visual observations, which necessitates an automated device to measure rumination. A recent technologically advanced tool has been developed and validated and become commercially available for dairy farm use. This new tool, rumination HR Tags (SCR Engineers Ltd, Netanya, IL), is an enhanced version of an activity monitoring tag for the measurement of rumination and can be used for monitoring and detecting changes in the daily rumination of dairy cattle.[56] It is evident that there are many instruments that can be used by both scientists and producers to successfully evaluate the pain associated with disease, such as with clinical mastitis.

THE USE OF NSAIDS IN CATTLE

Treatment of inflammation relies on relieving the pain and other systemic effects that commonly accompany inflammation, and slowing any further tissue damage. NSAIDs are commonly used in animals to reduce inflammation (anti-inflammatory), reduce pain (analgesic), reduce pain sensitivity (antihyperalgesic), and decrease overall body temperature (antipyretic). These drugs act by inhibiting cyclooxygenase, which in turn prevents prostaglandin synthesis (**Fig. 1**).

Around the world, commercially available NSAIDs are approved for anti-inflammatory and antipyretic indications. The actual intended pharmacologic effect of NSAID administration has not been documented, meaning that the frequency of use of NSAIDs in cattle with an intention to mitigate pain is not well understood. One survey performed by the Colorado Veterinary Medical Association (Denver, CO) determined that approximately 50% of veterinarians use NSAIDs for pain management following surgery.[57] A Canada-wide survey was conducted to describe the use of analgesics in cattle. Of the 309 veterinarians who reported treating acute toxic mastitis cases, 93% of them provided analgesia in the form of ketoprofen or flunixin meglumine as

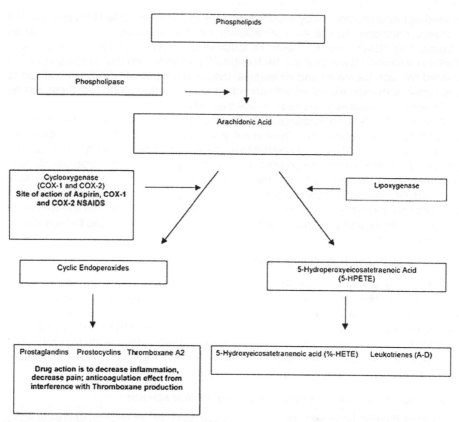

Fig. 1. The mechanism of action of NSAIDs. (*From* Summers S. Evidence-based practice part 1: pain definitions, pathophysiologic mechanisms, and theories. J Perianesth Nurs 2000;15:357–65; with permission.)

supportive therapy.[58] This Canadian study did not attempt to determine the distribution of use of analgesics in moderate versus severe clinical mastitis cases. It is noteworthy that of the 309 veterinarians questioned, 300 of them had graduated prior to 2001. Of those respondents, 27% had never participated in a continuing education program for pain management in animals. Yet, a large majority of the veterinarians that graduated prior to 2001 thought that their knowledge of pain management in dairy cattle was adequate. These veterinarians were asked to rank common dairy management procedures such as dehorning, displaced abomasum surgery, castration, toxic mastitis, etc, with respect to the amount of pain endured by the animal. None of the procedures were considered to be painless. It was therefore concluded that there is a need for continuing education opportunities for veterinarians with respect to pain identification and analgesic use in food animal species.[58]

A recent Canadian study evaluated the efficacy of a single administration of an NSAID at the onset of a naturally occurring case of neonatal calf diarrhea complex, in conjunction with oral rehydration therapy, and perhaps antibiotic treatment.[59] It was found that NSAIDs successfully reduced the behaviors associated with sickness and pain and significantly improved calf welfare. Calves treated with NSAIDs had a stronger appetite for milk during sickness, consumed more starter ration and water, gained significantly more body weight during the trial, and exhibited less pain-related behavior compared to calves that received placebo treatment.[59] Similarly, when investigating NSAID use for cases of induced diarrhea in calves, treatment with flunixin meglumine decreased the fecal output[60] and improved the clinical status[61] of treated animals. Bednarek and colleagues observed the use of NSAIDs in addition to antimicrobial therapy for calves with bronchopneumonia and found that there was an improvement in recovery rates with these treated animals.[62]

With the accumulated evidence, it is clear that there may be benefit to the use of NSAIDs for management of inflammation and alleviation of pain. As an example, research concerning the use of NSAIDs to manage pain in lame cows has been widely studied. By administering ketoprofen to lame cows, the resulting hyperalgesia was regulated on certain days following treatment, showing promising potential to reduce hyperalgesic effects.[63] Incorporating NSAID therapy into treatment protocols for a variety of clinical problems, including clinical mastitis, should improve the welfare of diseased animals and correspondingly decrease the economic losses to food animal producers.[64]

USE OF NSAIDs WITH CASES OF MASTITIS

Treatment decisions for animals with severe clinical mastitis most often involve veterinary intervention. Survey research has shown that both dairy producers and veterinarians generally agree that severe cases of mastitis can cause the animal significant pain and distress.[58] As such, it is common practice to provide the severely mastitic cow with NSAID therapy, in addition to antibiotics. Finally, there is mounting evidence for this use in both induced and naturally occurring cases of clinical mastitis, even though formal regulatory approval is rare.

NSAID Therapy in Cases of Endotoxin-Induced Clinical Mastitis

The use of NSAIDs has been shown to decrease rectal temperatures, decrease signs of inflammation, maintain rumen motility, and reduce heart rates in cows challenged with an intramammary infusion of LPS endotoxin to mimic early coliform mastitis compared with their nontreated counterparts.[30,65,66] Decreased heart rate could be interpreted as a result of a decrease in animal distress or alleviation of pain by the NSAID. There was also an observed reduction in fever of treated animals. As previously stated, fever is a strategy used by animals to combat infection. As such, it is unknown whether the reduction of fever is actually advantageous for animals with an early case of clinical mastitis. There is generally a lack of published literature supporting the beneficial or detrimental effects of reducing fever in these cases.

Milk measurements and behavioral activity was monitored to examine the effects of flunixin meglumine given 4-hour postinfection during endotoxin-induced clinical mastitis.[30] The frequency of rumen sounds were numerically increased in challenge animals, but DMI was not affected by the infection or treatment. The lack of difference in intake was likely due to the feeding management or the actual length of the infection time during the study. However, treated cows did show an increased eating time 9 to 12 hours after administration, as well as an increase in cud chewing compared to the nontreated control group. While infected cows spent less time lying in the first 12 hours after infection, flunixin treatment had no effect on the lying behavior.[30] This study was effective in showing the impact of flunixin administration against nontreated controls.

Ketoprofen is another NSAID used in the dairy industry.[11] Ketoprofen inhibits both of the cyclooxygenase pathways. The effectiveness of ketoprofen in experimental LPS-induced clinical mastitis cases has been evaluated. Three treatment groups were studied where 2 groups of experimental animals were inoculated with LPS and compared to an untreated group and served as the control group. The 2 groups of experimental animals were given ketoprofen either orally or intramuscularly 2 hours after LPS mastitis was induced.[67] Untreated control animals showed an increase in rectal temperature to an average of 40.5°C with differences between the groups seen at 6, 8, and 10 hours postchallenge. By 2 hours postchallenge, respiratory rates were increased. Yet, the respiratory rate–treated groups started to decline by 6 hours and were normal after 24 hours. Rumen contractions were reduced by 50% in the 2 hours postchallenge. But, within 6 hours, ketoprofen-treated animals began to recover, with full recovery by 24 hours; whereas the control group did not recover until day 7. As the udder of the animals was palpated, a visual analogue scale assessed the pain experienced. Ketoprofen allowed for a more rapid decline in pain scores compared to the untreated control. Further, milk thromboxane β_2 levels, an indicator of the general inflammatory status of an animal, were reduced at 6 hours postchallenge compared to 12 hours postchallenge in the control animals.

NSAID Therapy in Clinical Mastitis after Experimental Challenge

Anderson and Muir reviewed numerous articles concerning the use of NSAIDs in dairy cattle, which clearly demonstrated an improved response to treatment in affected animals after a variety of veterinary procedures.[18] These animals also returned to a normal physiologic state more quickly when an NSAID was administered prior to specific procedures. When cows were infused with *Escherichia coli* and given an NSAID prior to the development of clinical signs of infection, it was found that 2 NSAIDs almost entirely blocked febrile response and delayed the decrease in rumen activity of affected animals.[68] Other studies with experimentally induced coliform mastitis have also shown improved recovery in these treated animals.[69] Oral and intravenous NSAIDs provided equal systemic responses.[70] In a similar experiment, it was found that NSAIDs decreased mammary inflammation and rectal temperature but did not prevent milk production losses or appetite reduction.[71] In very recent research, the use of flunixin meglumine was evaluated during experimentally induced *E coli* mastitis.[72] It was concluded that *E coli* mastitis altered physiologic parameters, animal resting activity, DMI, and milk production, having a negative impact on animal well-being. There was improvement in DMI and milk production with flunixin therapy, providing evidence for using an NSAID as supportive therapy in alleviating the adverse effects associated with *E coli* mastitis.[72]

NSAID Therapy with Naturally Occurring Mastitis

The effect of NSAIDs on naturally occurring clinical mastitis is not well documented in the literature. As it is difficult to perform research on naturally occurring infections, most of the published literature reports on results obtained from experimentally induced infections. Both induced and naturally occurring infections result in increases in milk SCC, body temperature, and concentrations of tumor necrosis factor-α; mammary gland swelling; and a decrease in milk production.[73] Thus, there are many similarities between clinical symptoms for natural infections and experimentally induced infections. However, it may be inappropriate to directly compare cases of clinical mastitis resulting from LPS endotoxin infusion or even experimental challenge using live organisms with cases of naturally occurring mastitis. Early research in this area documented the administration of antibiotics and 1 intravenous treatment of NSAID at the time of first physical examination after the detection of severe endotoxic naturally occurring clinical mastitis.[74] These researchers found no difference in body temperature, milk production, or need for additional therapy between treatment groups, when monitoring animal responses every 24 hours.

Another early study evaluated the therapeutic usage of flunixin meglamine administered intravenously to animals with naturally occurring clinical mastitis, to determine whether cows with clinical mastitis suffered pain over time and if treatment with an NSAID would help with pain alleviation.[11] Cows with mild or moderate mastitis were given an NSAID, via either intramammary or intravenous route of administration. Pain thresholds were determined using a mechanical device that exerted pressure to the hind limb of each cow. Cows with mild and moderate cases of clinical mastitis showed a heightened responsiveness to pain that persisted for days or weeks after onset. The cows with mild clinical mastitis exhibited reduced sensitivity to pain when treated with an NSAID intravenously. A beneficial effect of the relief of pain was documented. However, similar results were not found with the moderate cases of clinical mastitis, which may have been attributed to the dosage of NSAID being too low. In addition, the observed pain relief by the NSAID in that study was short-lived, and it was recommended that repeated doses of intravenous NSAID might allow for more long-term pain relief.[11,75]

In a study in Israel, it was found that giving ketoprofen intramuscularly for 5 days allowed affected cows to return to 75% of their daily milk production recorded prior to their mastitis infection.[76] Upon initial diagnosis of clinical mastitis, the animals were given antimicrobials in combination with ketoprofen. A secondary portion of the study included ketoprofen treated versus a placebo-treated control group. The animals treated with ketoprofen had an average 93.5% recovery rate based on production parameters compared to the average recovery rate from the control groups of 78.4%. Furthermore, only 1 (3%) of 39 ketoprofen-treated cows were culled that lactation versus 9 (22%) of 41 control animals.

In another study, 100 dairy cows with both mild and moderate naturally occurring cases of mastitis were assessed for pain.[77] It was found that the respiratory rate, rectal temperature, and heart rate were all significantly higher in cases of moderate mastitis compared to mild clinical mastitis cases. Animals were administered the NSAID, meloxicam, in either a single- or a 3-dose regimen. Pain threshold levels were then measured. Animals treated with NSAIDs returned to their normal threshold levels for these outcome variables significantly faster than untreated animals. The effect was similar whether an animal received 1 or 3 doses of meloxicam. It was concluded that by promoting recovery of moderate or mild mastitis by alleviating pain associated with a case of mastitis, cattle welfare will be improved. Other studies that have treated cows with meloxicam have recorded the alleviation of pain and discomfort associated with mastitis, by reducing heart and respiratory rates and pain responses in lactating dairy cows.[78]

The use of NSAIDs for the treatment of mastitis has been most commonly prescribed for cases of severe endotoxic mastitis and has not been widely adopted as a standard treatment for cases of mild and moderate clinical mastitis. It is well recognized that for such cases, treatment decisions do not often directly involve veterinarians. Usually, the therapy of these cases at the time of their detection is up to the discretion of the dairy producer or farm manager. Farm personnel often follow a treatment protocol that is designed by both farm staff and the herd health advisory team. It is desirable to create a set of standard operating procedures as a treatment protocol for all cases of clinical mastitis, such as found with the Canadian Quality Milk On-Farm Food Safety Program,[79] and to consult with a veterinarian about how to carry these plans out efficiently. As such, there may be an opportunity for greater use of NSAID therapy in mild and moderate clinical mastitis cases.

In a field study conducted in New Zealand, treatment of mild and moderate clinical mastitis with a combination of meloxicam and a parenteral antibiotic (penethamate hydriodide) was evaluated for its effect on SCC, milk yield losses, clinical outcomes, and culling rates as compared with antibiotic therapy alone.[80] Cows were treated with 5 g of penethamate hydriodide daily for 3 days after the clinical detection of mastitis. Half of these cows were also treated with 250 mg of meloxicam and the other half were treated with a placebo vehicle (control group). It was found that there was no difference between treatment groups in the number of cows that were defined as treatment failures (ie, retreated within 24 days of initial treatment, died, or the treated gland stopped producing milk). There was also no difference in milk yield for the cows treated with meloxicam compared with the control cows. However, SCC was lower in the meloxicam-treated group compared with the control group after treatment (550 ± 48 vs 711 ± 62 ×1,000/mL, respectively) and fewer meloxicam-treated cows were removed from the herds (39 of 237 [16.4%] vs 67 of 237 [28.2%], respectively). It was concluded that treating cows with a combination of meloxicam and penethamate resulted in a lower SCC and a reduced risk of removal from the herd (culling) compared with the penethamate treatment alone.[80]

SUMMARY

It is clear that clinical mastitis has severe detrimental effects on the animal and negative economic impacts for dairy producers. However, pain associated with clinical mastitis, generally, is not measured and not treated. Attention to behavioral and physiologic indicators should be used to monitor animal health. New technologies may allow dairy producers to identify clinical mastitis in its very early stages, or even before clinical changes occur. Furthermore, automated measures of activity, such as step counts and lying time, show promise as predictors of clinical problems. These new technologies, in addition to other automated measures, have the potential for improving the screening methods for preclinical mastitis and accurately predicting the onset of a clinical mastitis event. With this opportunity for very early detection of infection, there is a potential for early intervention with NSAID therapy, which may allow for maximum efficacy from its use.

Despite which specific NSAID is used, it is clear that the benefits on temperature, rumen function, SCC, milk production, behavior, and pain sensitivity in animals during mastitis indicate that this therapy has a role throughout the dairy industry. As the health and well-being of dairy cattle continue to be scrutinized by consumer groups, it is essential that the alleviation of any perceived pain or discomfort associated with clinical mastitis should be addressed.

REFERENCES

1. Olde Riekerink RGM, Barkema HW, Kelton DF, et al. Incidence rate of clinical mastitis on Canadian dairy farms. J Dairy Sci 2008;91:1366–77.
2. Bradley AJ. Bovine mastitis: an evolving disease. Vet J 2002;164:116–28.
3. Fetrow J, Stewart S, Eicker S, et al. Mastitis: an economic consideration. In: National Mastitis Council Annual Meeting Proceedings. Madison (WI). Atlanta (GA): National Mastitis Council; 2000. p. 3–47.
4. Blowey R, Edmondson P. Mastitis control in dairy herds. 2nd ed. Oxfordshire (UK): CAB International; 2010.
5. Milne MH. Mastitis is a welfare problem. In: Proceedings of the British Mastitis Conference, Institute for Animal Health. Stoneleigh, Coventry. West Midlands (UK); 2005. p. 15–9.

6. Barker AR, Schrick FN, Lewis MJ, et al. Influence of clinical mastitis during early lactation on reproductive performance of Jersey cows. J Dairy Sci 1998;81:1285–90.
7. Schrick FN, Hockett ME, Saxton AM, et al. Influence of subclinical mastitis during early lactation on reproductive parameters. J Dairy Sci 2001;84:1407–12.
8. Leslie KE, Kielland C, Millman ST. Is mastitis painful and is therapy for pain beneficial? In: National Mastitis Council Annual Meeting Proceedings. Madison (WI). Albuquerque (NM): National Mastitis Council; 2010. p. 114–30.
9. Hillerton JE. Mastitis therapy is necessary for animal welfare. In: Bulletin of the International Dairy Federation (IDF). Brussels (Belgium): IDF; 1998. p. 4–5.
10. International Association for the Study of Pain (IASP). Pain terms. International Association for the Study of Pain. 2011. Available at: http://www.iasp-pain.org/Content/NavigationMenu/GeneralResourceLinks/PainDefinitions/default.htm#Pain. Accessed September 27, 2011.
11. Fitzpatrick JL, Young FJ, Eckersall PD, et al. Recognising and controlling pain and inflammation in mastitis. In: Proceedings of the British Mastitis Conference, Institute for Animal Health. Stoneleigh, Coventry. West Midlands (UK); 1998. p. 36–44.
12. Huxley JN, Hudson C. Should we control the pain of mastitis? Int Dairy Topics 2007;6:17–9.
13. Dobromylskyj P, Flecknell BD, Lascelles BD, et al. Pain assessment. In: Flecknell BD, Waterman-Pearson AE, editors. Pain management in animals. Philadelphia: Elsevier; 2000. p. 53–79.
14. Huzzey JM, Veira DM, Weary DM, et al. Prepartum behavior and dry matter intake identify dairy cows at risk for metritis. J Dairy Sci 2007;90:3220–33.
15. Kielland C, Skjerve E, Østerås O, et al. Dairy farmer attitudes and empathy toward animals are associated with animal welfare indicators. J Dairy Sci 2010;93:2998–3006.
16. Fitzpatrick JL, Nolan AM, Scott EM, et al. Observers perception of pain in cattle. Cattle Pract 2002;10:209–12.
17. Huxley JN, Whay HR. Current attitudes of cattle practitioners to pain and the use of analgesics in cattle. Vet Rec 2006;159:662–8.
18. Anderson DE, Muir WW. Pain management in cattle. Vet Clin North Am Food Anim Pract 2005;21:623–35.
19. Thomsen PT, Gidekull M, Herskin MS, et al. Scandinavian bovine practitioners' attitudes to the use of analgesics in cattle. Vet Rec 2010;167:256–8.
20. Fraser D, Weary DM, Pajor EA, et al. A scientific conception of animal welfare that reflects ethical concerns. Anim Welfare 1997;6:187–205.
21. von Keyserlingk MAG, Rushen J, de Passillé AM, et al. Invited review: the welfare of dairy cattle—key concepts and the role of science. J Dairy Sci 2009;92:4101–11.
22. Farm Animal Welfare Council (FAWC). Five freedoms. Farm Animal Welfare Council. 2009. Available at: http://www.fawc.org.uk/freedoms.htm. Accessed July 15, 2010.
23. Millman ST. Sickness behaviour and its relevance to animal welfare assessment at the group level. Anim Welfare 2007;16:123–5.
24. Hart BL. Biological basis of the behavior of sick animals. Neurosci Biobehav Rev 1988;12:123–37.
25. Aubert A. Sickness and behaviour in animals: a motivational perspective. Neurosci Biobehav Rev 1999;23:1029–36.
26. Wenz JR, Barrington GM, Garry FB, et al. Use of systemic disease signs to assess disease severity in dairy cows with acute coliform mastitis. J Am Vet Med Assoc 2001;218:567–72.
27. Wenz JR, Garry FB, Barrington GM. Comparison of disease severity scoring systems for dairy cattle with acute coliform mastitis. J Am Vet Med Assoc 2006;229:259–62.

28. Fitzpatrick JL, Nolan AM, Young FJ, et al. Objective measurement of pain and inflammation in dairy cows with clinical mastitis. In: Proceedings of the International Symposium on Veterinary Epidemiology and Economics, Breckenridge (CO); 2000. p. 73.
29. Milne MH, Nolan AM, Cripps PJ, et al. Preliminary results of a study on pain assessment in clinical mastitis in dairy cows. In: Proceedings of the British Mastitis Conference, Stoneleigh, Lancashire, North West England (UK); 2003. p. 117–9.
30. Zimov JL, Botheras NA, Weiss WP, et al. Associations among behavioural and acute physiologic responses to lipopolysaccharide-induced clinical mastitis in lactating dairy cows. Am J Vet Res 2011;72:620–7.
31. Muir WW, Woolf CJ. Mechanisms of pain and their therapeutic implications. J Am Vet Med Assoc 2001;219:1346–56.
32. Watkins LR, Maier SF. Immune regulation of central nervous system functions: from sickness responses to pathological pain. J Intern Med 2005;257:139–55.
33. Rutherford KMD. Assessing pain in animals. Anim Welfare 2002;11:31–53.
34. Weary DM, Niel L, Flower FC, et al. Identifying and preventing pain in animals. Appl Anim Behav Sci 2006;100:64–76.
35. Harmon RJ. Somatic cell counts: a primer. In: National Mastitis Council Annual Meeting Proceedings. Madison (WI). Atlanta (GA): National Mastitis Council; 2001. p. 3–9.
36. Chagunda MGG, Friggens NC, Rasmussen MD, et al. A model for detection of individual cow mastitis based on an indicator measured in milk. J Dairy Sci 2006;89:2980–98.
37. Hogeveen H, Kamphuis C, Steeneveld W, et al. Sensors and milk quality the quest for the perfect alert. In: Proceedings of the The First North American Conference on Precision Dairy Management. Toronto (ON). Madison (WI): Omnipress; 2010. p. 138–51.
38. Grönlund U, Sandgren CH, Waller KP. Haptoglobin and serum amyloid A in milk from dairy cows with chronic sub-clinical mastitis. Vet Res 2005;36:191–8.
39. Anil L, Anil SS, Deen J. Pain detection and amelioration in animals on the farm: issues and options. JAAWS 2005;8:261–78.
40. Molony V, Kent JE. Assessment of acute pain in farm animals using behavioral and physiological measurements. J Anim Sci 1997;75:266–72.
41. Ledgerwood DN, Winckler C, Tucker CB. Evaluation of data loggers, sampling intervals, and editing techniques for measuring the lying behavior of dairy cattle. J Dairy Sci 2010;93:5129–39.
42. Mazrier H, Tal S, Aizinbud E, et al. A field investigation of the use of the pedometer for the early detection of lameness in cattle. Can Vet J 2006;47:883–6.
43. Kiddy CA. Variation in physical activity as an indication of estrus in dairy cows. J Dairy Sci 1977;60:235–43.
44. Huzzey JM, von Keyserlingk MAG, Weary DM. Changes in feeding, drinking, and standing behavior of dairy cows during the transition period. J Dairy Sci 2005;88: 2454–61.
45. von Keyserlingk MAG, Weary DM. Maternal behavior in cattle. Horm Behav 2007;52: 106–13.
46. Cyples JA, Fitzpatrick CE, Leslie KE, et al. Short communication: the effects of experimentally-induced E. coli clinical mastitis on lying behavior of dairy cows. J Dairy Sci 2012;95:2571–5.
47. Chapinal N, de Passillé AM, Rushen J, et al. Short communication: measures of weight distribution and frequency of steps as indicators of restless behavior. J Dairy Sci 2011;94:800–3.

48. Pastell M, Hänninen L, de Passillé AM, et al. Measures of weight distribution of dairy cows to detect lameness and the presence of hoof lesions. J Dairy Sci 2010;93:954–60.
49. Heinrich A, Duffield TF, Lissemore KD, et al. The effect of meloxicam on behavior and pain sensitivity of dairy calves following cautery dehorning with a local anesthetic. J Dairy Sci 2010;93:2450–7.
50. Dyer RM, Neerchal NK, Tasch U, et al. Objective determination of claw pain and its relationship to limb locomotion score in dairy cattle. J Dairy Sci 2007;90:4592–602.
51. Veissier I, Rushen J, Colwell D, et al. A laser-based method for measuring thermal nociception of cattle. Appl Anim Behav Sci 2000;66:289–304.
52. Herskin MS, Müller R, Schrader L, et al. A laser-based method to measure thermal nociception in dairy cows: short-term repeatability and effects of power output and skin condition. J Anim Sci 2003;81:945–54.
53. Siivonen J, Taponen S, Hovinen M, et al. Impact of acute clinical mastitis on cow behaviour. Appl Anim Behav Sci 2011;132:101–6.
54. Borderas TF, de Passillé AM, Rushen J. Behavior of dairy calves after a low dose of bacterial endotoxin. J Anim Sci 2008;86:2920–7.
55. Bristow DJ, Holmes DS. Cortisol levels and anxiety-related behaviors in cattle. Physiol Behav 2007;90:626–8.
56. Schirmann K, von Keyserlingk MAG, Weary DM, et al. Technical note: validation of a system for monitoring rumination in dairy cows. J Dairy Sci 2009;92:6052–5.
57. Wagner AE, Hellyer PW. Survey of anesthesia techniques and concerns in private veterinary practice. J Am Vet Med Assoc 2000;217:1652–7.
58. Hewson CJ, Dohoo IR, Lemke KA, et al. Canadian veterinarians' use of analgesics in cattle, pigs, and horses in 2004 and 2005. Can Vet J 2007;48:155–64.
59. Todd CG, Millman ST, McKnight DR, et al. Nonsteroidal anti-inflammatory drug therapy for neonatal calf diarrhea complex: effects on calf performance. J Anim Sci 2010;88:2019–28.
60. Roussel AJ Jr, Sriranganathan N, Brown SA, et al. Effect of flunixin meglumine on Escherichia coli heat-stable enterotoxin-induced diarrhea in calves. Am J Vet Res 1988;49:1431–3.
61. Barnett SC, Sischo WM, Moore DA, et al. Evaluation of flunixin meglumine as an adjunct treatment for diarrhea in dairy calves. J Am Vet Med Assoc 2003;223:1329–33.
62. Bednarek D, Zdzisin'ska B, Kondrackid M, et al. Effect of steroidal and non-steroidal anti-inflammatory drugs in combination with long-acting oxytetracycline on non-specific immunity of calves suffering from enzootic bronchopneumonia. Vet Microbiol 2003;96:53–67.
63. Whay HR, Webster AJF, Waterman-Pearson AE. Role of ketoprofen in the modulation of hyperalgesia associated with lameness in dairy cattle. Vet Rec 2005;157:729–33.
64. Barrett DC. Non-steroidal anti-inflammatory drugs in cattle: should we use them more? Cattle Pract 2004;12:69–73.
65. Anderson KL, Smith AR, Shanks RD, et al. Efficacy of flunixin meglumine for the treatment of endotoxin-induced bovine mastitis. Am J Vet Res 1986;47:1366–72.
66. Wagner SA, Apley MD. Effects of two anti-inflammatory drugs on physiologic variables and milk production in cows with endotoxin-induced mastitis. Am J Vet Res 2004;65:64–8.
67. Banting A, Banting S, Heinonen K, et al. Efficacy of oral and parenteral ketoprofen in lactating cows with endotoxin-induced acute mastitis. Vet Rec 2008;163:506–9.

68. Lohuis JACM, Van Leeuwen W, Verheijden JHM, et al. Effect of steroidal anti-inflammatory drugs on Escherichia coli endotoxin-induced mastitis in the cow. J Dairy Sci 1989;72:241–9.

69. Vangroenweghe F, Duchateau L, Boutet P, et al. Effect of carprofen treatment following experimentally induced Escherichia coli mastitis in primiparous cows. J Dairy Sci 2005;88:2361–76.

70. Odensvik K, Magnusson U. Effect of oral administration of flunixin meglumine on the inflammatory response to endotoxin in heifers. Am J Vet Res 1996;57:201–4.

71. Morkoç AC, Hurley WL, Whitmore HL, et al. Bovine acute mastitis: effects of intravenous sodium salicylate on endotoxin-induced intramammary inflammation. J Dairy Sci 1993;76:2579–88.

72. Yeiser EE, Leslie KE, McGilliard ML et al. The effects of experimentally induced Escherichia coli mastitis and flunixin meglumine administration on activity measures, feed intake, and milk parameters. J Dairy Sci 2012, in press.

73. Van Oostveldt K, Tomita GM, Paape MJ, et al. Apoptosis of bovine neutrophils during mastitis experimentally induced with Escherichia coli or endotoxin. Am J Vet Res 2002;63:448–53.

74. Dascanio JJ, Mechor GD, Gröhn YT, et al. Effect of phenylbutazone and flunixin meglumine on acute toxic mastitis in dairy cows. Am J Vet Res 1995;56:1213–8.

75. Fitzpatrick JL, Young FJ, Eckersall PD, et al. Mastitis: a painful problem? Cattle Pract 1999;7:225–6.

76. Shpigel NY, Chen R, Winkler M, et al. Anti-inflammatory ketoprofen in the treatment of field cases of bovine mastitis. Res Vet Sci 1994;56:62–8.

77. Milne MH, Nolan AM, Cripps PJ, et al. Preliminary results on the effects of meloxicam (Metacam) on hypersensitivity in dairy cows with clinical mastitis. In: Proceedings of the World Buiatrics Congress, Quebec City (Quebec); 2004.

78. Banting A, Schmidt H, Banting S. Efficacy of meloxicam in lactating cows with E.coli endotoxin-induced acute mastitis. J Vet Pharmacol Ther 2003;(Suppl 1):23.

79. Dairy Farmers of Canada (DFC). Canadian quality milk on-farm food safety program: reference manual. Ottawa (Ontario): Agriculture and Agri-Food Canada (AAFC); 2010.

80. McDougall S, Bryan MA, Tiddy RM. Effect of treatment with the nonsteroidal antiinflammatory meloxicam on milk production, somatic cell count, probability of retreatment, and culling of dairy cows with mild clinical mastitis. J Dairy Sci 2009;92:4421–31.

The Role of the Milking Machine in Mastitis Control

Graeme A. Mein, BAgrSc, MAgrSc, PhD

KEYWORDS

- Machine milking • New infection rate (NIR) • New infections (NIs) • Teatcup action

KEY POINTS

- Most new infections (NIs) are caused by factors other than the milking machine.
- Direct and indirect milking machine effects may account for up to 20% of NIs in some herds and, perhaps, only about 10% in an "average" herd nowadays—provided the machine settings are right.
- Mastitis risk is reduced by keeping bacterial numbers low on or near the teat-ends, especially if machine settings and/or milking management practices are less than ideal.
- Healthy teat-ends are critical to the maintenance of low numbers of infected quarters.
- NI rates are reduced by pulsation characteristics which provide effective teat massage.
- Machine or management conditions that lead to a sudden, transient inrush of air through a teatcup will increase the risk of NIs. The main risk factors are liner slips, rough cluster removal, or clusters kicked off, especially at or near the end of milking.
- Vacuum fluctuations in the milkline or receiver are too slow to increase the NI rate unless they increase the frequency of liner slips or cluster falling.
- New research during the past 20 years has shown there is no need to leave clusters on cows in an attempt to empty the udder completely at every milking.

The contribution of mechanical milking to mastitis incidence is often misunderstood. Machine-related effects usually are smaller and less important than the effects of milking management, herd management, and cow or teat characteristics in most herds. Nevertheless, powerful physical forces are applied by the milking machine to a cow's teats for 4 to 10 minutes, 2 or 3 times every day. The inside of a teatcup is where the business-end of a complex machine meets and interacts with biological tissues—where the rubber meets the teat. If things go wrong, then udder health specialists and machine technicians need to know what to look for, how to resolve problems quickly, and how to minimise future risks. The main purposes of this article are to clarify some of the mysteries or misconceptions about the machine and to describe its likely contributions to new infection rates (NIRs) in commercial herds. This

The author has nothing to disclose.
20 K Road, Werribee South, Victoria 3030, Australia
E-mail address: mein@netspace.net.au

Vet Clin Food Anim 28 (2012) 307–320
http://dx.doi.org/10.1016/j.cvfa.2012.03.004
0749-0720/12/$ – see front matter © 2012 Published by Elsevier Inc.

is an edited and updated version of a 2004 article, co-authored with Doug Reinemann, Norm Schuring, and Ian Ohnstad.[1]

Five main milking-related mechanisms of mastitis infection were proposed in 1987 by an International Dairy Federation (IDF) Group of Experts.[2] These mechanisms, summarized later, provide a convenient starting point. Although most of the IDF information remains relevant today, new information and some new perspectives on older information are available to either strengthen or modify the conclusions of that IDF Group.

MAIN MILKING-RELATED MECHANISMS OF MASTITIS INFECTION (FROM REF 2)

1. Changing numbers of pathogens on teat skin or teat orifice.
2. Changing the resistance of the teat canal to invasion by mastitis pathogens.
3. Providing forces to overcome the resistance of the teat canal to bacterial invasion.
4. Dispersing pathogens within the udder.
5. Frequency and/or degree of udder evacuation.

1. Changing Numbers of Pathogens on Teat Skin or the Teat Orifice

A superb review on the significance of levels of exposure to pathogens by the late Frank Dodd was re-published in 2003.[3] Dodd listed the following examples to support his conclusion that frequency of new infections (NIs) increases with increasing level of exposure to mastitis pathogens.

- Milking-time hygiene lowers bacterial exposure and also reduces the NI rate.
- Reducing levels of infection in a herd results in lower subsequent rates of NI.
- Rates of NI in uninfected quarters of cows with no infected quarters are lower than in the uninfected quarters of cows with one or more infected quarters.
- Infection rates are increased when teat lesions, colonised by mastitis pathogens, are common.
- Data from artificial challenge experiments indicate that NI rates are much greater than those normally occurring in herds that are subjected to natural levels of exposure to pathogens.

As Dodd pointed out, not all of these observations demonstrate a direct (causal) relationship between NI and level of exposure but, overall, they provide strong support for the likelihood of a causal relationship. According to Smith,[4] the same logic applies to environmental streptococci. Smith concluded that the level of exposure is the major risk for environmental streptococcal mastitis in today's dairy herds and we need to continually learn ways to keep cows clean, dry, cool and comfortable.

Clearly, pathogen concentration in or near the environment of the teat orifice has a dominant influence on rates of new mastitis infection. Nevertheless, direct effects of milking machine function (or malfunctions) on increasing the degree of contamination, at or near the teat orifice, are likely to be quite low compared with the influence of milking procedures and herd management. The most obvious sources of cross-contamination within the milking machine are the claw and teatcup liners. Cross-contamination does not necessarily lead to NIs, however. Furthermore, NI rates often remain quite low in the presence of high bacterial challenge. The implication is that factors other than the simple transfer of bacteria from a given teat to the skin of another teat of the same cow, or to the external surfaces of another cow's teats, may play an important role.

2. *Changing the Resistance of the Teat Canal to Invasion by Mastitis Pathogens*

The conclusions of the IDF Group of Experts[2] on the effects of teat reaming to remove keratin, of management factors such as overmilking, and of machine effects such as vacuum level and pulsation failure are well known. Their conclusions support Dodd's view[3] that the main way that milking machines will influence [mastitis risk] is likely to be their direct effect on the health of the teat duct and teat skin.

Up until the early 1990s, this view was widely assumed to apply only—or mainly—to contagious mastitis pathogens. Jane Lacy-Hulbert was, perhaps, the first to demonstrate a clear link between a milking machine "fault" and higher NI risk for *Streptococcus uberis*, an organism previously regarded as an environmental pathogen.[5(p59)] She reported a significantly higher rate of clinical infections (7 vs 0) in identical twin cows milked without pulsation and subjected to a bacterial challenge (2.6 × 10^9 colony-forming units [cfu]/mL *S uberis*). Lacy-Hulbert suggested that "reducing the keratin removal rate, such as by pulsationless milking, leads to a significant reduction in the keratin growth rate."

The late Murray Woolford's thoughtful reviews of progress in understanding the effects of the milking machine on udder health included the following points on teat canal keratin.[6,7]

- About 10% to 20% of the mature keratin cells lining the teat canal are lost during a single milking without pulsation, whereas mechanical reaming of the teat canal removes up to 80% of the keratin.
- Both the above treatments increase the new infection rate, relative to milking with normal pulsation.
- Up to 40% of the keratin cells lining the teat canal are lost during a single milking with normal pulsation.
- These results suggest that regular removal of keratin during the milking process is desirable but that the degree of removal should be neither too much nor too little. Too much depletion of keratin (eg, 80%) will expose immature keratin cells that may be slower to slough off and, thereby, remove any entrapped bacteria. Too little depletion (eg, 10%-20%) may fail to remove the surface layers of keratin, together with any adherent bacteria, and may slow the rate of turnover of keratin.
- Cyclic opening and closing of the liner promote fracturing of the mature keratin layers within the teat canal, thereby increasing the effective shear forces acting on the keratin during milking.
- Periodic flushing of the canal during milking removes sufficient keratin (about 40%) to remove any bacteria trapped in, or adhering to, the surface folds of keratin.

The results of both research herd studies and field observations confirm that, if pulsation is effective, new infection rates usually remain low despite the application of other practices or machine settings regarded as harmful or undesirable. Effective pulsation is achieved when the combined actions of the pulsator and liner provide an adequate milk/rest time on the teat with optimum milk flow rates and minimal tissue changes evident after milking.

Pulsation is ineffective if teats are too long to allow complete collapse of the liner below the teat[8] or too short to be compressed by the closed liner.[9,10] Field studies summarized by Reinemann and colleagues[11] confirm that increasing liner compression increases the degree of teat-end hyperkeratosis and that liner overpressure (OP) appears to be a better predictor of teat-end hyperkeratosis than either the average claw vacuum or the liner Touch Point or the Residual Vacuum available for Massage.

To summarize this section, the risk of NIs by contagious as well as environmental pathogens such as *S uberis* is increased by machine-induced changes in teat-end condition. Such changes may include:

- Increased congestion and edema in the teat wall, which results in slower closure of the teat canal and/or hypoxia in teat tissues[9]
- Slower rate of removal and regrowth of teat canal keratin[5,7]
- Greater degree of openness of the teat canal orifice after milking[12]
- Increased hyperkeratosis of the teat-end.[11,13,14]

Relatively slow rates of growth and removal of teat canal keratin soon after calving could, perhaps, be one of many factors contributing to the typically high rates of new infection in most herds during early lactation.

3. *Providing Forces to Overcome the Resistance of the Teat Canal to Bacterial Invasion*

The IDF Group of Experts[2] provided a comprehensive review of the extensive scientific literature on irregular and cyclic vacuum fluctuations and liner slips, published during the previous 25 years. My intention is to highlight the main results and to offer some new interpretations (see Mein and colleagues[1] for further background information).

Two Irish researchers were the first to show that inadequate vacuum pump capacity (albeit in the very small milking systems, which were the norm in Ireland during the 1960s) was associated with higher bulk milk cell counts.[15] They also produced the first research herd evidence to show that unstable vacuum was linked to an increase in new infection rate.

Subsequently, a series of bacterial challenge experiments in the United Kingdom in the 1970s showed that 30% to 65% of udder quarters became infected when exposed to very high "cyclic" vacuum fluctuations, averaging over 40 kPa (12 inHg), in combination with experimentally-induced, large but relatively slow "irregular" fluctuations. In marked contrast, only 2% to 12% of quarters became infected when exposed to these astonishingly high cyclic fluctuations alone, or to large irregular fluctuations in combination with relatively small cyclic fluctuations, or to small cyclic plus small irregular fluctuations.[16,17] The main mechanism of infection was thought to be "impacts"—a term coined to describe the rapid upward movement of small droplets or slugs of milk from the short milk tube (SMT) toward the teat orifice. NI risk was higher if impacts occurred at or near the end of milking.[17]

Meanwhile, in Ireland, O'Shea, O'Callaghan, and Meaney became famous for their research herd studies on effects of liner slips on new mastitis infection rate.[18,19] Their conclusion was that the sudden inrush of air through one teatcup, if it slips or falls during milking, drives droplets of milk through the claw and up into the adjacent teatcups. Cows may become infected if bacteria-laden milk droplets strike the ends of adjacent teats with sufficient force to carry pathogens into or through the teat canal, beyond the reach of a post-milking teat disinfectant.

The effect of a "high" versus a "low" slip liner on NIR was assessed in the United States using a 160-cow research herd under conditions of natural exposure and post-milking teat disinfection.[20] Slips were recorded whenever a vacuum drop of 10 kPa or more occurred within a time of 0.25 second or less. The "high slip" liner averaged 7.6 major slips per cow-milking, compared with 3.1 for the "low slip" liner. NIRs were 0.49 per 100 cow-days for high slip compared with 0.27 for the low slip liner, which, interestingly, is about 1 NI per 2500 liner slips for both the high and low slip liners. NIR was higher in cows that had one or more quarters already infected (1500–1850 slips per NI) compared with the rate for previously uninfected cows (>6000 slips per NI).

The common factor in published studies of machine-induced bacterial penetration of the teat canal has been an abrupt drop in vacuum within the teatcup or cluster. Thompson and colleagues[21] calculated that a pressure difference of 25 to 40 kPa (7.5 to 12 inHg) between the claw and liner barrel was needed to generate air speeds within the SMT high enough to constitute a significant risk of infection by impacts. This critical pressure difference is markedly higher than the threshold of 10 kPa (3 inHg) set by Baxter and colleagues[20] for recording liner slips.

Thiel and colleagues[22] demonstrated that a stream of liquid containing endotoxin could penetrate the teat canal when directed toward the teat from a nozzle mounted in a teatcup 50 mm (2 in) below the teat orifice. Penetration of endotoxin into the teat sinus occurred at jet speeds of 6.2 or 9.8 m/s (20 or 32 ft/s) but not at 1.9 m/s (6.2 ft/s). The lowest jet speed (1.9 m/s) was just sufficient to keep the end of the teat wetted.

Such results beg the question: "What forces are available to generate air speeds of 2 m/s (6.5 ft/s) or more upwards through the SMT?" Spencer[23] measured speeds of movement for 9 different liners. Liner opening speeds ranged from 33 to 75 mm/s (mean 53.6 mm/s) while closing speeds were 112 to 235 mm/s (mean 166.7 mm/s). Thus, the average speed of movement when the liner is opening is only about 0.05 m/s (ie, <0.2 km/h or about 0.1 mile/h), which is about 40 times slower than the walking speed of a relaxed adult! Such slow rates of cyclic liner movement are unlikely to generate impact speeds high enough to cause bacterial penetration of the teat canal. Clearly, other conditions are required.

Factors such as low pump capacity, poor vacuum regulation, or limited capacity of milklines cannot (directly) generate transient pressure differences, within a cluster, that are capable of driving milk droplets at speeds greater than 2 m/s toward the teat orifice. Such factors might have an indirect influence, but only if they contribute to an increase in frequency of liner slips.

The additional driving force required to impel milk droplets into a teat canal can be generated by sudden air leakage past one or more teats as a result of liner slips, vigorous machine stripping (only if slips occur), or abrupt cluster removal. Such events can produce very rapid, transient rates of vacuum change within the liner (see O'Shea and O'Callaghan, **Fig. 2**,[18] for example) and high transient air speeds within the SMT.[24] By fitting a calibrated orifice, 7.5 mm (0.3 in) in diameter, into the SMT, Woolford and colleagues[24] measured average air inflow speeds of 6 to 8.3 m/s (20–7 ft/s) resulting from a simulated liner slip timed to occur as the liner opened. In the absence of a simulated liner slip, peak air speed through the orifice was only 1.9 m/s. Presumably, those air speeds would be halved by increasing the tube diameter from 7.5 mm (0.3 in) to 11 mm (0.43 in).

In light of these results and calculations, the physical basis for the droplet "impact" theory seems clearer now. We can conclude that:

- A sudden, high inflow of air through a SMT toward the teat-end is not, by itself, sufficient to cause an infection because the air speed must, inevitably, fall quickly as the air enters the dead-end space beneath the teat-end.
- Some additional energy (eg, the momentum of slugs or milk droplets picked up in the claw or lower end of the SMT) is needed to penetrate the defenses of the teat canal.

- The 1987 IDF Group of Experts[2] concluded, correctly indicates that the "impact" mechanism is an inertial effect for droplets of macroscopic size. Macroscopic droplets may be picked up in the claw bowl by sudden air admission from one SMT, carried into adjacent claw inlets, then accelerated up the lower part of the SMT. If a milk droplet has reached a sufficient velocity, its inertia could carry it toward the teat end after the air inflow has decelerated and stopped.
- This effect is unlikely to be true for microscopic droplets, however, because they are effectively "embedded" in the air stream. Although they may reach the same high speed as the air moving up the SMT, they *must* slow down and then stop when they enter the dead space beneath the teat-end.[24]

Reverse Pressure Gradients (RPGs)

Woolford and colleagues[25] observed what they described as "reverse flow" at or near the end of milking in their studies with a Swinging Vacuum Single-Chambered milking system. Importantly, their observations of reverse flow occurred in the absence of a liner to compress and close the teat canal.

Transient RPGs have been measured at the time of attachment of a liner to an empty teat, at the instant of teatcup removal, or, occasionally, at times when air is admitted suddenly into a teatcup via the SMT.[26,27] High risk factors for RPG[27,28] include:

- Teats with little or no milk to fill the teat sinus or to maintain a clear, continuous milk pathway between the udder cistern and teat sinus.
- Use of liners having a small mouthpiece lip relative to the teat diameter.
- Manipulation of empty teats before milking (and, presumably, during reattachment of a slipping teatcup or a fallen cluster near the end of milking).
- Detachment with liners stopped in their closed position (although detachment, with liners pulsating normally or stopped in their open position, is not risk-free).

To date, however, the RPG hypothesis remains unproved as a significant contributor to new mastitis infections. Based on physical principles, it seems unlikely that small transient RPGs can produce enough energy to penetrate the teat canal under normal milking conditions. In all situations where a 2-chambered teatcup is used with effective pulsation, bacterial penetration of the teat canal has been demonstrated only in association with extreme pressure events and the likely presence of macroscopic droplets or slugs of milk.

4. Dispersing Pathogens Within the Udder

Cinefilm and cine-radiographic studies as well as ultrasonic techniques have shown that about one third of the milk volume present in a teat sinus, just before the liner starts to close, is "pumped" back up into the udder cistern by the closing liner. Nevertheless, the practical importance of dispersing bacteria within the udder has not been established according to the 1987 IDF Group.[2]

Perhaps the only new information that can be added to this conclusion is derived from a radiographic study by Williams (reported in Mein and colleagues[14]). Williams showed that the closing liner compresses and closes the teat canal first in the region 30% to 50% of the canal length above the teat orifice. Williams' elegantly simple study provides a further demonstration of the value of an effective liner and pulsation in minimizing the risk of moving any pathogens, which may have contaminated the teat-end, into or through the teat canal under normal milking conditions.

5. *Frequency and/or Degree of Udder Evacuation*

Compared with NIRs in the early dry period or when normal milkings are omitted, the NIR is relatively low in cows that are milked regularly 2 or more times per day. Thus, machine milking has a positive effect in reducing the risk of new mastitis infection. In general, the clinical symptoms of mastitis are decreased as milking frequency is increased—provided that teat-end condition is not compromised by milking too many times per day.

Since the dawn of mechanical milking in the late 1800s, up until about 1970, most cows were either hand-stripped or machine-stripped routinely to ensure that all of the "available milk" was extracted from udders at any given milking. Most of the older publications reviewed by O'Shea and colleagues[2] concluded that mastitis increased when machine stripping was omitted. However, the results of recent research on raising the threshold setting for automatic cluster removers,[29] in conjunction with setting a maximum time limit for milking slow cows,[30,31] have opened up new possibilities for milking herds more quickly with minimal—or no—apparent adverse effects on milk yield, somatic cell count, or clinical mastitis.

In Rasmussen's pioneering study,[29] milking time was reduced by 0.5 minute per cow with no loss of milk yield and no increase in mastitis when the end-of-milking setting for automatic cluster removers was raised from 0.2 kg/min to a flow-rate threshold of 0.4 kg/min (0.9 lb/min). Subsequent studies[31,32] indicated that early termination of milking had no significant effects on incidence of clinical mastitis or average somatic cell count in healthy quarters or in quarters subclinically infected with either *Staphylococcus aureus* or *S uberis*. These relationships have not been examined in *S agalactiae* herds.

DISCUSSION

At the 1987 International Mastitis Symposium in Montreal, Canada, a panel of speakers was invited to answer the question: "What percentage of all infections are due to milking machine factors?" The responses from various speakers were "We don't really know"; "Probably quite low"; "Anywhere between 0% and 100%." A more definitive answer can be given now. My estimate of the direct and indirect milking machine contributions to the overall NIR was roughly 20% during the last 30 years of last century but, now, is much less than 20% on most farms—for reasons outlined next.

Insights From Studies Involving High Bacterial Challenge

The extreme effects of mechanisms 1 to 3, described earlier, are illustrated in **Fig. 1.** (adapted from Grindal and Hillerton[33]). These data are the combined results of a series of short, intensive studies in the United Kingdom during the 1970s and 1980s in which cows' teats were dipped, immediately before or after milking, in a concentrated broth of mastitis pathogens.

- The lower curve, representing the extreme effect of mechanism 1, confirms that NIRs can remain remarkably low despite a high pathogen challenge and the complete absence of teat disinfection—as long as the machine settings are "correct."
- The middle curve, representing an extreme effect of one aspect of mechanism 2 (the complete failure of pulsation in all milking units!), confirms the importance of effective pulsation.

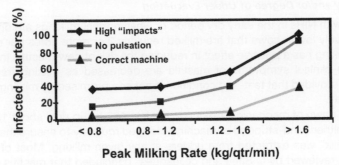

Fig. 1. Extreme effects of 3 mechanisms of infection: (1) high bacterial challenge in conjunction with "correct" milking conditions; (2) absence of pulsation; (3) high frequency or severity of "impacts" against the teat-end. To give readers a clearer appreciation of the flow-rate values along the x-axis, about 95% of North American cows probably have peak milking rates of 1.1 to 1.4 kg/quarter/min (ie, about 10–12.5 lb/min/cow). (*Adapted* from Grindal RJ, Hillerton E. Influence of milk flow rate on new intramammary infection in dairy cows. J Dairy Res 1991;58:263.)

- The upper curve, representing mechanism 3, confirms that machine or management conditions that increase the frequency or severity of impacts will increase the risk of NIs.
- The steep rise in all 3 curves at the high end of this range of peak flow rates is, perhaps, a warning signal for dairy breeding organisations. Peak milking rates have risen during the past 30 to 40 years (partly due to genetic selection for faster milking). The implication is that teat canals have become more patent, thereby increasing the risk of infection—not only during lactation but also during the dry period.

Insights From Field Studies in Commercial Herds

The economic importance of "impacts" can be inferred from field studies with deflector shields or one-way valves fitted between the teat-end and claw. Field experiments using deflector shields in Britain and Australia produced an overall reduction in new intramammary infections of about 10%—from 20.6% to 18.4% of eligible quarters.[34] Similar results were obtained in field experiments with deflector shields in Norway[35] or using a special claw fitted with one-way valves in Britain.[36]

It is likely that these devices prevented all or most of the effects of liner slip, vigorous machine stripping, and abrupt cluster removal on NIRs. The implication is that these direct machine effects contributed about 10% of the new mastitis infections on "typical" farms in the 1980s. However, NIRs due to these direct machine effects probably have fallen in most herds since then because:

- The average bore of SMTs has been increased (from about 7 mm for many clusters in the early 1980s to a more sensible 10–11 mm in many present-day clusters), thereby improving their drainage characteristics and reducing the peak speed of air flowing through these tubes.
- Average claw volume has been increased (up to a more sensible effective volume of 150 mL or more), thereby reducing the likelihood that milk slugs or macroscopic droplets can be transferred across the claw bowl from one milk inlet to another.

- Manufacturers generally pay more attention to designing liners that slip less frequently.
- Vigorous machine-stripping is a thing of the past on almost all modern dairy farms.
- Most farmers are aware of the need to remove teatcups gently at the end of milking.
- The proportion of NIs due to contagious pathogens has fallen during the past 30 years, while the proportion due to environmental pathogens has increased markedly in most dairying nations.

There has been at least one opposing trend, however. The process of genetic selection in dairy herds has lead to a significant shortening of teats over the past 30 to 40 years. We know that liners tend to slip more frequently on shorter teats—and that liner slip is a major cause of higher NIs. Furthermore, shorter teats have shortened teat canals—and the risk of NI is known to be higher for teats with short teat canals.

Turning to the indirect machine effects (mechanism 2), the value of effective pulsation has been demonstrated in both research herd and field experiments as well as in field observations. It is clear that:

- NIRs are higher if a liner is absent or if pulsation is deliberately omitted.
- NIRs are higher if pulsation fails or if pulsator settings are outside acceptable limits.
- Pulsation fails (either partially or completely) if teats are too long or too short to allow the liner to collapse and compress the end of the teat.

These indirect effects (including effects on the health of the teat canal, teat tissues, and skin) might account for another 10% of NIs in an average herd. It is difficult to go beyond these broad-brush estimates, however, because of the lack of published data from controlled experiments in commercial herds. We need to keep in mind that correlation does not imply causation and that attempts to correlate single-factor effects with poor teat condition or udder health often lead to misconceptions. Thus, I agree with the conclusion of Woolford[6(p3)] that "further quantification of the overall contribution of the milking machine is difficult and elusive because of the multi-factorial nature of the disease."

Despite these elusive difficulties, it is clear that the majority of NIs are caused by factors other than the milking machine. A significant reduction in machine-related infections might account for a change in the overall NIR of about 10%. In a herd with a NIR of 10 per 100 cows per month, for example, the number of NIs would be reduced by 1 cow per 100 cows per month.

SUMMARY

Most NIs are caused by factors other than the milking machine. Direct and indirect milking machine effects may account for up to 20% of NIs in some herds and, probably, not much more than about 10% in an "average" herd these days—provided that machine settings are right. Thus, proper maintenance and operation of any milking system is a key aspect of successful milking.

Contamination

- Mastitis risk is reduced by keeping bacterial numbers low on or near the cows' teat-ends, especially if machine settings and/or milking management practices are less than ideal.

- Herd management and milking management practices probably have overriding effects compared with the potential contribution from milking machines.

Teat Health and Teat Canal Integrity

- Healthy teat ends are critical to the maintenance of low numbers of infected quarters.
- NIR is reduced by pulsation characteristics that provide effective teat massage. My "default" recommendation for pulsation settings these days is a rate of 50 to 55 c/min and a ratio (a + b phase) of 65%.
- "Effective pulsation" involves much more than the present industry preoccupation with recording and analyzing pulsator rate and ratio, or the individual a, b, c, and d phases of pulsation.
- The key additional factor is the cyclic overpressure applied by the closed liner to the teat tissues to overcome the dilating and congesting effects of the milking vacuum.
- The main variables affecting the cyclic overpressure applied to a teat are:
  - Average vacuum beneath the teat during the d phase of pulsation.
  - Geometry and mounting tension of the liner.
  - Physical properties of the liner material.
  - Teat size and shape.
- As a guide, a cyclic overpressure of about 12 kPa (3.5 inHg) above atmospheric pressure appears to be a good compromise between fast and gentle milking conditions for cows. This overpressure should be applied for about 20% or 200 ms within each pulsator cycle.
- Claw vacuum is the best and most direct measure of the effects of vacuum in the milking system on the cow. As a guide for adjusting system vacuum, Reinemann and Mein[37] recommended the following simple classification for describing/setting the average claw vacuum level.

High:	42 ± 2 kPa	$(12.5 \pm 0.6$ inHg).
Moderate:	38 ± 2 kPa	$(11.2 \pm 0.6$ inHg).
Low:	34 ± 2 kPa	$(10 \pm 0.6$ inHg).

If the system vacuum is adjusted to achieve a "high" claw vacuum, for example, the expectation is that average claw vacuum will fall to about 40 kPa during the period of peak milk flow, rising to about 44 kPa near the end of milking for most cows in the herd.

Penetration of the Teat Duct

- The risk of NIs (due to liner slips, rough cluster removal, clusters kicked off) is much higher near the end of milking.
- Air speeds greater than 2 m/s (6.5 ft/s) up the SMT may assist bacterial penetration into or through the teat canal.
- Normal liner movement is much too slow to generate air speeds greater than 2 m/s in SMT.
- The real action takes place within an individual cluster due to a sudden, transient air inrush through a teatcup when:
  - A liner slips or squawks loudly.
  - A cluster is kicked off or detached abruptly.
  - A cow is machine-stripped vigorously enough to break the seal between a teat and the liner mouthpiece.

- Such events can produce acute irregular vacuum fluctuations. As illustrated in **Fig. 2**, these are: large, transient drops in claw vacuum (15–30 kPa; 4.5–9.0 inHg), often lasting less than 1 to 2 seconds, with very fast rates of change (150–300 kPa/s; 45–90 inHg/s).
- The resulting high transient pressure gradients between the claw and adjacent liners can increase the NIR by accelerating milk droplets to speeds greater than 2 m/s toward the teat-ends in adjacent teatcups within the same cluster.
- High cyclic fluctuations in cluster vacuum (up to 20 kPa; 6 inHg) are unlikely to generate air speeds greater than 2 m/s in the absence of sudden, unplanned airflow into 1 (or 2) teatcups.
- Vacuum fluctuations in the milkline or receiver are too slow to increase the NIR (as illustrated in **Fig. 3**, for example) unless they increase the frequency of liner slips or cluster falling.
- Correlations linking unstable milkline or receiver vacuum with increased mastitis are likely to be associative rather than cause-effect relationships. That is:
  - NIR is increased by sudden air admission through one or more teatcups.
  - Air admission through teatcups is the primary cause of transient vacuum fluctuations in milklines.
- The "RPG" hypothesis remains unproved. It is unlikely that small transient RPGs can produce enough energy to penetrate the teat canal.
- Eliminating the common claw (as in Automatic Milking Systems) should reduce the NIR. Do not expect miracles with automatic milking, however, because:
  - Even a 20% reduction in NIR would mean, for example, 4 instead of 5 NIs per month per 100 cows. Other factors may mask this modest potential improvement.
  - Probably the widespread use of more stable clusters, larger-bore short milk tubes, and larger, free-draining claw bowls has already reduced the potential gain from eliminating the claw in many milking systems.

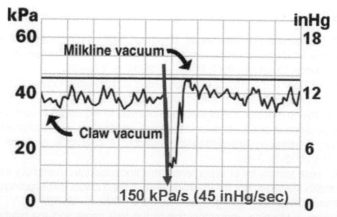

Fig. 2. Sudden air inflow into a teatcup due to rough cluster removal or a liner slip, for example, can produce very rapid rates of change in vacuum within the claw. Such high, transient airflows may cause milk droplets or small milk slugs to be thrown against the teat-end with sufficient force to penetrate the teat canal. Such "impacts" are a common cause of machine-induced mastitis. Usually, such transient air inflows are too brief to cause any measureable fluctuation in milkline vacuum.

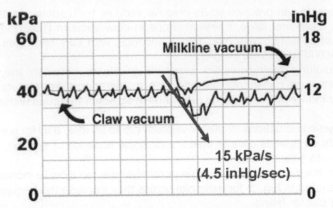

Fig. 3. Large, unplanned air inflows into a milking system due to a cluster falling off, for example, can produce a measureable drop in the milkline vacuum and a consequent fall in claw vacuum in other milking clusters. However, the resulting rate of change in claw vacuum is much too slow to have any direct effect on mastitis risk.

Dispersing Pathogens Within the Udder

The practical importance of dispersing bacteria within the udder has not been established.

Frequency and/or Degree of Udder Evacuation

NIRs are lower during lactation than in the early dry period. This implies that regular milking may have positive benefits in helping to keep teat canals and teat-ends clean.

New research during the past 20 years has shown there is no need to leave clusters on cows in an attempt to empty the udder completely at every milking. Furthermore, there are significant practical advantages (eg, better teat condition, calmer cows, quicker herd milking) to be gained from early removal of clusters.

REFERENCES

1. Mein GA, Reinemann DJ, Schuring N, Ohnstad I. Milking machines and mastitis risk: a storm in a teatcup. In: Proceedings of the 43rd Annual Meeting of the National Mastitis Council; Charlotte, (NC); Feb 1–4, 2004. p. 176–88.
2. International Dairy Federation. Machine milking factors affecting mastitis: a literature review. Bulletin 215, Machine Milking and Mastitis, 1987. p. 2–32.
3. Dodd FH. Bovine mastitis: the significance of levels of exposure to pathogens. Paper originally presented at an obscure retirement symposium. Re-published in International Dairy Federation Newsletter 25, Sweden: A colleague of Frank Dodd. IDF Bulletin 318:2003. p. 3–6.
4. Smith KL. Risk factors for environmental streptococcal intramammary infections. In: Udder Health Management for Environmental Streptococci, proceedings of symposium, Ontario Veterinary College; Canada; June 1997. p. 42–50.
5. Lacy-Hulbert J. Physical characteristics of the teat canal and the relationship with infection. In: Proceedings of the 37th annual meeting of the National Mastitis Council; 1998. p. 54–61.
6. Woolford MW. Milking machine effects on mastitis progress 1985-1995. In: Saran A, Soback S, editors. Proceedings of the 3rd IDF International Mastitis Seminar; Israel: Kimron Veterinary Institute; Book II, Section 7; May 28–June 1, 1995. p. 3–12.

7. Woolford MW. Perspectives on mastitis from "downunder." Proceedings of the 36th Annual Meeting of National Mastitis Council; 1997. p. 56–64.

8. Mein GA, Brown MR, Williams DM. Effects on mastitis of overmilking in conjunction with pulsation failure. J Dairy Res 1986;53:17–22.

9. Hamann J, Osteras O, Mayntz M, et al. Functional parameters of milking units with regard to teat tissue treatment. International Dairy Federation Bulletin No. 297. 1994.

10. Rasmussen MD, Frimer ES, Kaartinen L, et al. Milking performance and udder health of cows milked with two different liners. J Dairy Res 1998;65:353–63.

11. Reinemann DJ, Bade R, Zucali M et al. Understanding the influence of machine milking on teat defense mechanisms. In: Lam TJGM, editor. Mastitis Control: From Science to Practice International Conference Proceedings; The Hague; Wageningen, Netherlands: Wageningen Academic Publishers; 30 Sept–2 Oct, 2008. p. 323–31.

12. Mein GA, Neijenhuis F, Morgan WF, et al. Evaluation of bovine teat condition in commercial dairy herds: 1. Non-infectious factors. In NMC-AABP International Symposium on Mastitis and Milk Quality; Vancouver, BC, Canada; Sept 2001. p. 347–51.

13. Neijenhuis F, Mein GA, Britt JS, et al. Evaluation of bovine teat condition in commercial dairy herds: 4. Relationship between teat-end callosity or hyperkeratosis and mastitis. In NMC-AABP International Symposium on Mastitis and Milk Quality; Vancouver, BC, Canada; Sept 2001. p. 362–6.

14. Mein GA, Williams DM, Reinemann DJ. Mechanical forces applied by the teatcup liner and responses of the teat. In: Proceedings of the 42nd annual meeting of NMC; Fort Worth, (TX); Jan 2003. p. 114–23.

15. Nyhan JF, Cowhig MJ. Inadequate milking machine reserve and mastitis. Vet Rec 1967;81:122–4.

16. Thiel CC, Cousins CL, Westgarth DR, et al. Influence of some physical characteristics of the milking machine on rate of new mastitis infections. J Dairy Res 1973;40:117.

17. Cousins CL, Thiel CC, Westgarth DR, et al. Further short-term studies of influence of the milking machine on new mastitis infections. J Dairy Res 1973;40:289.

18. O'Shea J, O'Callaghan E. Milking machine effects on new infection rate. In: Proceedings of the International Symposium on Machine Milking, 17th Annual Meeting of National Mastitis Council; Louisville (KY); Feb 1978. p. 262–8.

19. O'Shea J, O'Callaghan E, Meaney B. Liner slips and impacts. In: Proceedings of the International Mastitis Symposium; Montreal, Canada; 1987. p. 44–65.

20. Baxter JD, Rogers GW, Spencer SB, et al. The effect of milking machine liner slip on new intramammary infections. J Dairy Sci 1992;75:1015–8.

21. Thompson PD, Schultze WD, Sauls JN, et al. Mastitis infection from abrupt loss of milking vacuum. J Dairy Sci 1978;61:344.

22. Thiel CC, Thomas CL, Westgarth DR, et al. Impact force as a possible cause of mechanical transfer of bacteria to the interior of the cow's teat. J Dairy Res 1969;36:279.

23. Spencer SB. Defining the wave form of liner wall movement. IDF World Dairy Summit: Proceedings of IDF Centenary Seminar 100 Years With Liners and Pulsators in Machine Milking; Belgium; Sept 2003. p. 515–519.

24. Woolford MW, Williamson JH, Phillips DSM. Aspects of milking machine design related to intramammary infection. In: O'Shea J, editor. Proceedings of IDF International Workshop on Machine Milking and Mastitis, Moorepark, Ireland, 1980. p. 5–59.

25. Woolford MW, Phillips DSM, Twomey A. A comparison of mastitis infection rates using a conventional intermittent milk flow and a continuous milk flow under conditions of an elevated standard bacterial challenge. Proceedings of the International Symposium on Machine Milking, 17th Annual Meeting of National Mastitis Council; Louisville, (KY); Feb 1978. p. 275–90.

26. Galton DM, Aneshansley DG, Petersson LG, et al. Pressure gradients across the teat canal during machine milking. Proceedings of Milking System Management, PA. Northeast Reg. Agric. Eng. Service; Ithaca (NY); 1988. p. 114.

27. Rasmussen MD, Frimer ES, Decker EL. Reverse pressure gradients across the teat canal related to machine milking. J Dairy Sci 1994;77:984.

28. Rasmussen MD. The movement of bacteria by reverse pressure gradients across the teat canal. In: Saran A, Sobach S, editors. Proceedings of the 3rd IDF International Mastitis Seminar, Israel. Kimron Veterinary Institute; Israel; Book II, Section 7; 1995. p. 13.

29. Rasmussen MD. Influence of switch level of automatic cluster removers on milking performance and udder health. J Dairy Res 1993;60:287–97.

30. Clarke T, Cuthbertson EM, Greenall RK, et al. Milking regimes to shorten milking duration. J Dairy Res 2004;71:419–26.

31. Jago J, Burke J. Williamson J. Does reducing cups-on time affect milk production, clinical mastitis, somatic cell count or teat condition? In Hillerton JE, editor. Proceedings of the 5th IDF Mastitis Conference; Christchurch (NZ). March 2010. p. 468–72.

32. Clarke T, Cole D, Greenall RK. Shorter Milking Times research program: Technical information package for advisers, December 2006. Department of Primary Industries, 1 Spring St., Melbourne, 3000. ISBN 978-1-74199-065-2.

33. Grindal RJ, Hillerton E. Influence of milk flow rate on new intramammary infection in dairy cows. J Dairy Res 1991;58:263.

34. Griffin TK, Mein GA, Westgarth DR, et al. Effect of deflector shields to reduce intramammary infection by preventing impacts on the teat ends of dairy cows during machine milking. J Dairy Res 1980;47:1–9.

35. Binde M, Melby HP, Ask A, et al. Effect of a shielded liner on new mastitis infection. J Dairy Res 1989;56:55–9.

36. Griffin TK, Grindal RJ, Bramley AJ. A multi-valved milking machine cluster to control intramammary infection in dairy cows. J Dairy Res 1988;55:155–9.

37. Reinemann DJ, Mein GA. Claw vacuum is the most direct measure of milking system's effect on the cow. US NMC Newsletter Oct-Nov 2008;31.

Stray Voltage and Milk Quality
A Review

Douglas J. Reinemann, PhD

KEYWORDS

- Stray voltage • Stray current • Mastitis • Milk quality • Electrical exposure
- Immune Function

KEY POINTS

- There have been no studies in the large body of research that support the hypothesis that stray voltage exposure of up to 8 V will result in increased somatic cell count or incidence of mastitis.
- The first mild behavioral responses for dairy cows in farm-like conditions occurs at 2.5 mA of current for the 5% most sensitive cows, 4.8 mA for the 50th percentile, and 8.5 mA for 95% of cows for 60 Hz current measured as root-mean-square (rms) values.
- The current levels required to cause aversive behaviors are 2 to 3 times higher than these values.
- These current levels can be converted into cow contact voltage levels by using Ohm's law and a value of the worst case (lowest) cow + contact resistance of 500 Ω, representative of a low-resistance cow environment, or 1000 Ω, representative of a more typical resistance value in dairy barns.
- The results of several studies showed that somatic cell counts and the incidence of mastitis were not increased at exposure levels sufficient to produce aversive behavior in dairy cows.

The term "stray voltage" describes a special case of voltage developed on the grounded neutral system of a farm and is defined as less than 10 V measured between 2 points that can be contacted simultaneously by an animal.[1] Some level of voltage between grounded metallic objects and the earth will always be present as a normal consequence of the operation of properly installed electrical equipment. Contact voltages less than 10 V are not lethal to cows or people. Contact voltages in excess of 10 V may be indicative of a major electrical fault that could pose an

The author has nothing to disclose.
Biological Systems Engineering, University of Wisconsin-Madison, 460 Henry Mall, Madison, WI 53706, USA
E-mail address: djreinem@wisc.edu

Vet Clin Food Anim 28 (2012) 321–345
http://dx.doi.org/10.1016/j.cvfa.2012.03.008
0749-0720/12/$ – see front matter © 2012 Elsevier Inc. All rights reserved.

electrocution hazard on a farm and are treated differently from the low-level contact voltages defined as stray voltage. The terms "earth current" or "ground current" are sometimes used to refer to stray voltage. These currents flowing in the earth or on grounded metal objects will only affect cows if sufficient voltage potential is developed between cow contact points and the same cow contact measurement methods should be used to assess these currents.

Stray voltage first came to the attention of the North American dairy professionals in the 1970s following research conducted in New Zealand in the 1960s.[2] Early work included surveys of dairy managers to determine their perceptions of the effects of stray voltage on dairy cows. Among the symptoms attributed to stray voltage were an increased incidence of mastitis and elevated bulk milk somatic cell counts (SCCs), reduced milk production, changes in milking performance, and changes in animal behavior.[3] There is a considerable body of research that has tested the hypotheses that stray voltage can cause these symptoms. This article will provide a brief overview of the studies conducted on behavioral responses to stray voltage exposure and a detailed review of studies that were designed with the primary objective to investigate the effects of stray voltage exposure on mastitis as well as those behavioral studies that also included measures of mastitis, such as individual cow or group SCC and other physiologic responses related to stress.

BASIC CONCEPTS OF VOLTAGE, CURRENT, AND RESISTANCE

Impedance is a measure of the resistance to current flow in alternating current (AC) circuits and includes elements of resistance, capacitance, and inductance. There are some situations in which the capacitance and inductance are important, such as when considering high-frequency AC circuits. "Impedance" is a more technically specific term for AC circuits, but "resistance" will be used here for simplicity unless otherwise noted. Voltage and current flow in AC circuits alternate between positive and negative values in a sinusoidal form 60/s (60 Hz) or 50 Hz in European power systems. The most common way to express voltage and current in AC circuits is with the root-mean-square (rms) average over the alternating cycle. References to voltage and current will be expressed as 60 Hz, rms averages in this review unless otherwise noted. The relationship between voltage exposure and current conducted through the animal is described by Ohm's law. Ohm's law expresses the relationship between voltage, current, and resistance in an electrical circuit:

Current = Voltage/Resistance or Amps = Volts/Ohms

This simple relationship has been a source of much confusion and resulting controversy in the stray voltage debate. Ohm's law indicates that if the voltage (across animal contact points) is increased, the current flowing through the animal will increase. Likewise, if the resistance (of contact points) is increased, the current flowing through the animal will decrease. The current measure used in most studies is milliamps (mA) or 1/1000th of 1 amp. The standard measurement circuit used for field investigations uses a 500 Ω resistor to simulate the combined resistance of a cow's body *plus* a conservative estimate of the resistance of the 2 contact points (cow + contact, or shunt resistor). A cow contact voltage of 1 V is equivalent to a cow contact current of 2 mA when using a cow + contact resistance of 500 Ω.

While the contact voltage is often used to describe animal exposure conditions, it is the resulting current flowing through animals' bodies that determines the "dose" and the resulting type and degree of nerve stimulation.[4] It is critically important to use a realistic value of animal resistance to relate voltage exposures to the level of current conducted through an animal and the resulting effects on nerve stimulation, sensation, and behavioral reaction. A competent field investigation will include voltage measurements at cow contact locations measurements both with a shunt resistor and without (open circuit). These 2 measurements are required to determine the "source resistance" of the electrical parts of the circuit [NB: source resistance is different from the cow contact resistance[1]].

The body resistance of dairy cows has been measured in several studies. The value of an animal's body resistance depends on the pathway between the 2 contact points (eg, muzzle-hoof or hoof-hoof) and the way in which the contact is made including factors such as the area over which the contact is made, pressure applied to the contact, and use of conductive liquids or gels on the measurement connection. The lowest body resistance values have been reported when the skin of the animal was pierced using needles. The next lowest category of body resistances includes measurement electrodes affixed to shaved patches of skin. The majority of body resistance measurements have been made with cows coming into contact with metallic devices. Some of the most common examples include cows standing on a metal plate or mesh, a metallic bit in the mouth, or a metallic clip applied to the nose.

It is clear from several studies as well as physical principles that real-world contact resistances have enormous variability. The lowest contact resistances would be expected if a clean, wet body part (eg, a cow's muzzle) comes into contact with a clean, wet, metallic object with a substantial mutual contact area and substantial contact pressure. The accepted practice by researchers and regulators has been to assume worst-case (lowest practical values) for contact resistances. Studies done to measure more typical body + contact resistances that would occur on farms[1,5,6] have shown that 500 Ω is a reasonable value to use in a measurement circuit to estimate the current that would flow through a cow's body. Although the resistance of the cow's body is typically less than 500 Ω for the muzzle to hoof pathway (other pathways have a higher resistance), it has been shown to be a "worst case" or minimum resistance value for the combination of a dairy cow's body + real-world contact resistance in the farm environment. Contact resistance in dry environments can be several orders of magnitude above these worst-case values.

THE BIOMECHANICS OF NERVE STIMULATION

The biomechanics of electrical nerve stimulation in humans has been widely studied for beneficial medical purposes (cardiac stimulators and pacemakers, relief of chronic pain, and muscle contraction for therapeutic purposes) as well as to set thresholds to avoid pathologic exposures that may result in injury or death.[7] This body of literature has been used as the basis to establish cause-effect relationships between various types of voltage and current exposure and behavioral responses in dairy cows. Both sensory neurons (producing sensations) and muscle neurons (producing muscle contraction) can be elicited with electric currents conducted through the skin. Sensory effects are elicited with lower current dose than are motor effects. Nerve stimulation is characterized by a current threshold. Current applied below the threshold will not produce nerve excitation, and hence no sensation, motor response, or behavioral response can occur. At the current level just above the threshold of sensory nerve excitation, the current will be perceptible but not painful. As the current level is increased earlier, the sensory nerve threshold motor neurons will begin to activate and involuntary muscle contraction begins to occur. This lower margin of muscle contraction is not generally perceived to be painful. Pain can be experienced as current exposures are increased further due to both increased sensory stimulation and more intense muscle contraction. Behavioral responses are the result of nerve

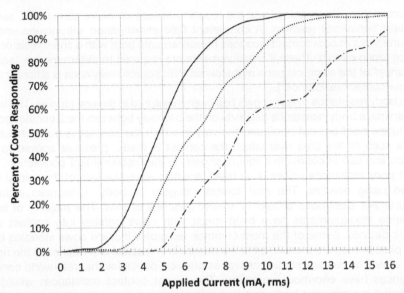

Fig. 1. Summary of behavioral response thresholds for dairy cows exposed to ascending series of 60-Hz current exposures. Current is expressed in equivalent 60-Hz rms values. Note: 60-Hz rms current values correspond to 60-Hz rms voltage values for a typical value of 1000 Ω for cow + contact resistance, such as 4 mA rms = 4 V rms. To obtain 60-Hz rms values for a worst case 500-Ω cow + contact resistance, divide 60-Hz rms current values by 2 (eg, 4 mA = 2 V). —, First behavioral response threshold for 365 cows; . . ., discomfort or involuntary muscle contraction threshold for 133 cows; -.-.-, aversion threshold for 36 cows.

stimulation that elicits a sensation and/or muscle contraction in an animal. Levels of current exposure just above the nerve excitation threshold will result in mild behavioral reactions in cows, such as the blink of an eye, which tend to become less pronounced over time as animals become accustomed to the sensation. As current exposure is increased above this threshold, behavioral responses in cows become more pronounced and more persistent, indicative of annoyance, pain, or involuntary muscle contraction (twitches).

REVIEW OF RESEARCH ON BEHAVIORAL RESPONSES TO VOLTAGE EXPOSURE

The most common type of research on stray voltage has been to identify the lowest thresholds of voltage or current exposure that could result in nerve stimulation and behavioral responses. An extensive review of the research literature on the behavioral responses of dairy cows to 60 Hz voltage exposure was conducted for the Ontario Energy Board as part of the process of developing rules and regulations in Canada.[8]

A summary of research results on individual animal behavioral response thresholds is shown in **Fig. 1**. These studies all applied known levels of current, in an ascending series, through an individual cow until a predefined behavioral response was observed and thus allowed for the specification of a response threshold for individual cows.[9–24]

The first behavioral response for this sample of 355 cows was 2.5 mA for the 5% most sensitive cows 4.8 mA for the 50th percentile, and 8.5 mA for 95% of cows. Many of the research groups noted rapid acclimation to the current levels just sufficient to produce subtle behavioral responses and increased current exposure levels in order to obtain a more repeatable response, often noted by researchers as indicative of discomfort or involuntary muscle contraction. The threshold of involuntary muscle contraction would be expected to occur at higher current does levels than the threshold of sensory stimulation and would also be expected to be a more repeatable threshold indicator as acclimation would not reduce the reaction to the stimuli. The threshold of discomfort and/or involuntary muscle contractions for 125 cows was 3.5 mA for the 5% most sensitive cows 6.5 mA for the 50th percentile, and 11 mA for 95% of cows. Thresholds for aversive response thresholds (primarily a delay to drink water) and those studies in which researchers identified thresholds at which cows appeared to be in pain (36 cows) were 5.5 mA for the 5% most sensitive cows, 8.5 mA for the 50th percentile, and 16 mA for 95% of cows. These results show remarkable repeatability and consistency in the response of dairy cows to 60 Hz current exposure in farm-like conditions across 15 separate experiments, by 9 research groups, across 31 years and 2 continents.

TRANSIENT AND HIGH FREQUENCY AND EXPOSURE

In addition to the steady 60- or 50-Hz voltages developed by the use of electrical power, there are also transient voltages that may occur at higher frequencies. The responses to electrical exposures to alternating current with frequencies above 60 Hz have also been studied and are explained well by neuroelectric models.[1,9,10,19,20,25] Studies on high-frequency current exposure clearly indicate that as the duration of a current pulse gets shorter (or the frequency increases >60 Hz), more voltage and current is required to cause a behavioral response (**Fig. 2**).

Momentary 60 Hz events (several AC cycles) can be generated by starting electric motors. The starting current of the motor and the resistance of the farm neutral determine the magnitude of a motor starting transient for 120 V motors and the primary neutral for 240 V motors. The most common short-duration electrical pulses on farms are produced by is improperly installed electric fences and electrified crowd gates. These devices are designed to produce a powerful electric impulse that is used to control animal behavior. Improper installation of these devices can cause these pulses to appear in unintended areas on the farm. Another source of high-frequency events are switching transients that occur when electrical equipment is turned on or off. These high-frequency pulses decay quickly, do not travel far from their source, and extremely rarely reach exposures levels that are problematic to animals.

REVIEW OF RESEARCH ON STRAY VOLTAGE, MASTITIS, AND STRESS

A summary of all published studies in which mastitis, SCC and physiologic responses of cows was monitored are presented for constant voltage exposure (**Table 1**) and for constant current exposure (**Table 2**). Details of these studies are presented in this section. In an early experiment conducted by US Department of Agriculture scientists the endocrine response of 6 cows exposed to 5 mA of current applied through electrocardiographic patches applied to the skin of the udder and hock starting 10 minutes before milking and continuing through the milking and continuing for a total of 20 minutes was investigated.[14] Cows were exposed to both continuous current and to current applied in an intermittent pattern (5 of every 30 seconds). Prolactin concentration decreased and milk yield decreased by 11% to 17% by intermittent current but neither was reduced by continuous current. Neither treatment appeared to have an effect on norepinephrine or prolactin levels. Both exposures increased oxytocin responses. The authors noted that cows seemed to adapt to the stimulation.

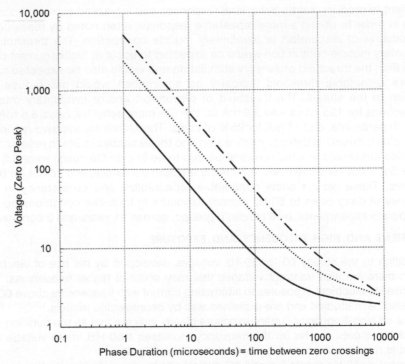

Fig. 2. Summary of behavioral response thresholds for the 5% most sensitive dairy cows. Voltages are expressed in zero to peak rather than rms values for conveinience in reading an oscilloscope screen for monophasis and biphasic waveforms. The voltage levels assume a 500-Ω cow + contact resistance. The phase duration is the time between zero-crossings foralternating waveforms. —, Multiple cycle sine wave; . . ., monophasic sine; -.-.-, biphasic sine wave.

A team of researchers at the University of Minnesota measured the electrical resistance of milking machine components and found that milk hose resistances were inversely proportional to milk flow rates with minimum values of about 30,000 Ohms for a low line and 80,000 Ohms for a high line milking system.[26] The minimum resistance from the claw through the cow to the floor was 3000 Ω. It was estimated that over 25 V across a low-line or 50 V across a high-line milking system would be required to obtain perception level currents through a cow.

Six nonpregnant cows were milked while being exposed to current levels of 0 mA, 4 mA, or 8 mA, applied from udder to 4 hooves.[13] Each treatment was applied during the entire milking period with an intermittent pattern (5 seconds on, 5 seconds off), twice per day for 7 days. Each cow was exposed to all 3 exposure levels. Cows showed behavioral responses to the 4 mA and 8 mA treatments. There was an increase in blood cortisol concentration and a trend of increased prolactin and oxytocin concentrations at the 8 mA treatment level. There was no difference in SCC, fat, protein, milk yield, residual milk peak milk flow rate, time to achieve peak milk flow, or milking duration between any of the treatments.

Six nonpregnant Holsteins were exposed to 4 mA (60 Hz rms) of current 10 seconds before udder preparation and during the entire milking period at every-other-morning milking on 6 consecutive days.[13] Current was applied through subdermal

Table 1
Summary of constant voltage exposures reported by exposure level

Refs.	n	Exposure Level	Exposure Pathway	Exposure Pattern and Duration	Negative Response (No Statistically Significant Change)	Nonsignificant Trends Noted	Significant Responses
30	6	0.5 V	Metallic water bowl→rear hooves	21 d, when drinking	SCC, clinical mastitis, milk conductivity, body temperature, reproduction		
30	6	1 V	Metallic water bowl→rear hooves	21 d, when drinking	SCC, clinical mastitis, milk conductivity, body temperature, reproduction		
33	10	1 V	Metallic water bowl→rear hooves	Full lactation when drinking	SCC, incidence of mastitis, milk, fat%, prot%, feed, water, hoof problems, body weight, days to first breeding, days open, service per conception, calving interval, visible abortion, calves born dead		
36	4	1 V	Metallic water bowl→rear hooves	7 d	SCC, S aureus-infected quarters, immune gamma-globulins,[a] cortisol, blood chemistry,[b] milk, fat%, prot%, water, feed	+0.7 ng/mL cortisol	
37	4	1 V	Metallic water bowl→rear hooves	7 d S uberis challenge after milking (2×)	SCC, S uberis-infected quarters, milk, fat%, prot%, feed, water		

34,35	30	1 V	Metallic water bowl→hooves	56–84 d, 0.3 V cont w/two 3-h periods of 1 V	Treatment and carryover effects: SCC, milk, FCM, fat KG, prot KG, lact KG, prot%, feed, water, behavior, breeding, milking duration	Treatment: +0.12 fat%, +0.06 lactose% Carryover: +0.2 lactose%
31	7	2 V	Teat cups electrodes→rear hooves	During 1 milking	SCC, milk, fat%, prot%, Rmilk fat%, Rmilk prot%, behavior, milking duration	−fat%, −prot%, +Rmilk fat%, in 1L cows; +fat%, +prot%, −Rmilk fat%, +Rmilk prot% in 2L cows
30	6	2 V	Metallic water bowl→rear hooves	21 d, when drinking	SCC, clinical mastitis, milk conductivity, body temperature, reproduction	
33	10	2 V	Metallic water bowl→rear hooves	Full lactation, when drinking	SCC, incidence of mastitis, milk, fat%, prot%, feed, water, hoof problems, body weight, days to first breeding, days open, services per conception, calving interval, visible abortion, calves born dead	Delay to drink
36	4	2 V	Metallic water bowl→rear hooves	7 d	SCC, S aureus-infected quarters, immune gamma-globulins,[a] cortisol, blood chemistry,[b] milk, fat%, prot%, water, feed	+0.8 ng/mL cortisol Delay to drink

(continued on next page)

Table 1 (continued)

Refs.	n	Exposure Level	Exposure Pathway	Exposure Pattern and Duration	Negative Response (No Statistically Significant Change)	Nonsignificant Trends Noted	Significant Responses
37	4	2 V	Metallic water bowl→rear hooves	8 d w/S uberis challenge after milking (2×)	SCC, S uberis-infected quarters, milk, fat%, prot%, feed, water	+2% water intake	
34,35	30	2.5 V	Metallic water bowl→hooves	56–84 d, 0.75 V cont w/two 3-h periods of 2.5 V	SCC, milk, FCM, fat KG, prot KG, lact KG, fat%, prot%, lact%, feed, water, behavior, breeding (treatment and carryover effects)		+12 s milking duration, carryover effect +42 s milking duration
31	15	4 V (4.1 mA aver, 2 mA–7 mA range)	Teat cups electrodes→rear hooves	During 1 milking	SCC, milk, fat%, Rmilk fat% milking duration	1L cows; −fat%, −prot%, +Rmilk fat% 2L cows +fat%	1L cows; behavior changes. 2L cows; +0.1% prot%, +0.2% Rmilk prot%, −1.4 Rmilk fat%
30	6	4 V	Metallic water bowl→rear hooves	21 d, when drinking	SCC, clinical mastitis, milk conductivity, body temperature, reproduction		
33	10	4 V	Metallic water bowl→rear hooves	Full lactation, when drinking	SCC, incidence of mastitis, milk, fat%, prot%, feed, water, hoof problems, body weight, days to first breeding, days open, services per conception, calving interval, visible abortion, calves born dead		Delay to drink, 1 cow and 1 heifer refused to drink for 36 h, 1 place-holder heifer, no grain for 36 h

36	4	4 V	Metallic water bowl→rear hooves	7 d	SCC, S aureus-infected quarters, immune gamma-globulins,[a] cortisol, blood chemistry,[b] milk, fat%, prot%, water, feed	+1.2 ng/mL cortisol	Delay to drink
37	4	4 V	Metallic water bowl→rear hooves	9 d, S uberis challenge after milking (2×)	SCC, S uberis-infected quarters, milk, fat%, prot%, feed, water	+3% water intake	
34,35	30	5 V	Metallic water bowl→hooves	56–84 d, 0.75 V cont w/two 3-h periods of 5 V	SCC, milk, FCM, fat%, feed, milking duration, behavior, breeding. Treatment and carryover effects except as noted		Treatment effect; −0.05 prot%, −8% water. Carryover effects; −0.8 kg milk, +0.1 prot%, −1 kg FCM, −0.1 prot KG, −0.2 lact KG
31	15	8 V (9.1 mA aver, 4–14 mA range)	Teat cups electrodes→rear hooves	During 1 milking	SCC, milk, fat%, Rmilk fat%, Rmilk prot% in 1L cows, milking duration	1L cows; −fat%, −prot%, +Rmilk fat%. 2L cows; +fat%, +prot%, −Rmilk fat%	Behavior changes, 1 heifer kicked milking unit off; +0.1% Rmilk prot% in 2L cows
31	8	16 V	Teat cups electrodes→rear hooves	During 1 milking	SCC, milk, fat%, prot%, Rmilk fat%, Rmilk prot%, milking duration	1L cows; −fat%, −prot%, +Rmilk fat%. 2L cows; +fat%, +prot%, −Rmilk fat%, +Rmilk prot%	Behavior changes, 2 cows kicked milking unit off

Some groups were part of the same experiment that used several different treatment levels.

Abbreviations: fat%, milk fat percentage; fat KG, kilograms of fat produced per day; FCM, fat corrected milk; feed, feed intake; L1, 1st lactation cows; L2, 2nd or more lactation cows lact%, milk lactose percentage; lact KG, kilograms of lactose produced per day; milk, milk yield; n, number of cows in the treatment group; prot%, milk protein percentage; prot KG, kilograms of protein produced per day; Rmilk, residual milk harvested after machine milking; water, water intake.

[a] IgG, IgA, IgM.

[b] Sodium, potassium, chloride, bicarbonate, anion gap, urea, creatinine, calcium, phosphate magnesium total protein, albumin, globulin, glucose, alkaline phosphatase, AST/PSP, SDH, hGGT, indirect, direct and total bilirubin, CK, iron, and TIBC.

Table 2
Summary of constant current exposures reported by exposure level

Refs.	n	Exposure Level	Exposure Pathway	Exposure Pattern and Duration	Negative Response (No Statistically Significant Change)	Nonsignificant Trends Noted	Significant Responses
39	12	1 mA	Front→rear hooves	14 d 10 min on, 10 min off	Cortisol, lymphocyte blastogenesis,[a] immunoglobulin production, oxidative burst (chemiluminescence PMA), standing and lying behavior		Lymphocyte blastogenesis response to S aureus mitogen
38	48	1 mA	Front→rear hooves	During 1 milking	Milk, average milk flow rate, maximum milk flow rate, activity, strip yield		
22	8	1 mA–5.3 mA	Front→rear hooves	5-min exposures w/ ascending series of 4 levels	Cortisol (Note: significant cortisol increase observed during hoof trimming)		Some behaviors
15	7	2.5 mA	RR hock→RF knee, ECG patch	10 s	Heart rate, prolactin, norepinephrine, epinephrine, glucocorticoids		

28	3.6 mA	RR hock→RF knee, ECG patch	7 d at milking (2×) 5 s on, 25 s off	Wisconsin Mastitis Test, milk, milking duration		Behavior, +3 beats/min heart rate, +time to peak oxytocin, +peak milk flow, +peak prolactin, + prolactin curve
13	4 mA	Udder→hooves	3 d, intermittent 5-s bursts during milking (2×)	SCC, cortisol, prolactin, oxytocin, milk, fat%, prot%, Rmilk, peak milk flow, time to peak milk flow, milking duration		Some behavior changes
13	4 mA	Subdermal electrodes	3 d, during morning milking	SCC, milk, fat%, prot%, feed, water	−1% milk	+Heart rate, carotid arterial blood pressure, mammary blood flow, behaviors in first 30 s of exposure
27	4 mA	Subdermal electrodes	4 d, with 5 min of intermittent exposure (5 s on, 5 s off), 6 ×/d	SCC, milk, fat%, prot%, feed, water	−1% milk	Some behavior changes with acclimation
29	4 mA	Udder→hooves	7 d, for 5 min before milking and during milking (2×), 5 s on 25 s off	SCC, prolactin, oxytocin, cortisol, milk, prot%, fat%, milking duration, peak milk flow, duration of peak milk flow, Rmilk	−SCC, +milk,	Some behavioral changes with acclimation

(continued on next page)

Table 2
(continued)

Refs.	n	Exposure Level	Exposure Pathway	Exposure Pattern and Duration	Negative Response (No Statistically Significant Change)	Nonsignificant Trends Noted	Significant Responses
5	6	4.9–9.5 mA	Metallic water bowl→hooves	21 d, 1 per s, while drinking, BRT[c]	SCC, milk, water, feed		
31	8	5 mA	Teat cup electrodes→rear hooves	3 d, 6 milkings, L1 cows	SCC, milk, fat%, prot%, behavior	+SCC, −milk	−1 min milking duration
14	6	5 mA	Udder→hock ECG patch	20 min continuous, 2 milkings	Norepinephrine, prolactin, milk		+Blood oxytocin, behaviors with acclimation
14	6	5 mA	Udder→hock ECG patch	20 min intermittent (5 s on 20 s off), 2 milkings	Norepinephrine		−Milk yield, −prolactin, +oxytocin
15	7	5 mA	RR hock→RF knee, ECG patch	10 s	Heart rate, prolactin, norepinephrine, epinephrine, glucocorticoids		
28	6	6 mA	Udder→hock ECG patch	7 d at milking (2×) 5 s on, 25 s off	Wisconsin Mastitis Test, milk, time to peak oxytocin, milking duration		Behavior (1 cow removed for severe behavior) +3 beats/min heart rate, +peak milk flow, +peak prolactin, +prolactin curve
5	6	6.0–9.5 mA	Metallic water bowl→hooves	21 d, 1 per s, while drinking, BRT[c] + 1 mA	SCC, milk, water, feed		

5	6	6.4–12 mA	Metallic water bowl→hooves	21 days, 1 per s, while drinking, BRT^c +2 mA	SCC, milk, water, feed		
15	7	7.5 mA	RR hock→RF knee, ECG patch	10 s	Heart rate, prolactin, norepinephrine, epinephrine, glucocorticoids		
5	6	7.8–14 mA	Metallic water bowl→hooves	21 days, 1 per s, while drinking, BRT^c × 1.5	SCC, milk, water, feed on days 4–21 of exposure		–Water, –feed, –milk; first 3 d of exposure
31	8	8 mA	Teat cups electrodes→rear hooves	3 days, 6 milkings, 2L cows	SCC, milk, fat%, prot%, milking duration, behavior	–SCC, –milk	–Cortisol 2 min prior and 6 min after milking began, similar at other times
13	6	8 mA	Udder→hooves	3 days, Intermittent 5 second bursts during milking (2x)	SCC, milk, fat%, prot%, Rmilk, peak milk flow, time to peak milk flow, milking duration	+Prolactin, +oxytocin	Some behavior changes, +cortisol
29	6	8 mA	Udder→hooves	7 d, for 5 min before and during milking (2×), 5 s on 25 s off	SCC, prolactin, oxytocin, cortisol, milk, prot%, fat%, milking duration, peak milk flow, duration of peak milk flow, Rmilk	–SCC, +milk, +cortisol, +milking duration	+Cortisol, delayed oxytocin, some behavioral changes with acclimation

(continued on next page)

Table 2
(continued)

Refs.	n	Exposure Level	Exposure Pathway	Exposure Pattern and Duration	Negative Response (No Statistically Significant Change)	Nonsignificant Trends Noted	Significant Responses
15	7	10 mA	RR hock→RF knee, ECG patch	10 s	Heart rate, prolactin, norepinephrine, glucocorticoids		+Heart rate immediately after shock, epinephrine doubled in 2o exceptional cows
15	7	12.5 mA	RR hock→RF knee, ECG patch	10 s	Heart rate, prolactin, norepinephrine, epinephrine, glucocorticoids		+Heart rate immediately after shock

Some groups were part of the same experiment that used several different treatment levels.

Abbreviations: ECG, electrocardiographic; fat%, milk fat percentage; FCM, fat corrected milk; feed, feed intake; L1, 1st lactation cows; L2, 2nd or more lactation cows; milk, milk yield; n, number of cows in the treatment group; PMA, phorbol myristate acetate; prot%, milk protein percentage; RF, right front; Rmilk, residual milk harvested after machine milking; RR, right rear; water, water intake.

[a] Response to mitogens, concanavalin A, phytohemagglutinin, pokeweed.

[b] IgG serum, IgG in vitro, IgA serum, interleukin (IL)-1 serum, IL-1 in vitro, IL-2 serum, IL2 in vitro.

[c] BRT, predetermined behavioral reaction threshold.

electrodes placed in the lumbar region of spinal column approximately 15.2 cm apart (targeting the sensory nerves to the udder). Current exposure resulted in an increase in heart rate, increased carotid arterial blood pressure, and increased mammary blood flow.

Eight pregnant Holstein cows from 16 to 20 weeks in second lactation were exposed to 4 mA of current for 96 hours with current administered once every 4 hours in an intermittent pattern (30 seconds on, 30 seconds off for 5 minutes) using a semirandomized exposure scheme.[27] Current was applied through subdermal electrodes placed in the lumbar region of spinal column approximately 15.2 cm apart (targeting the sensory nerves to the udder). Some behavioral changes were noted during the first 30 seconds of exposure and a slight (1%) but not statistically significant reduction in milk yield. There were no significant differences in SCC, milk fat, milk protein, feed intake, or water consumption.

Seven cows were exposed to 3.6 mA and 6 cows to 6.0 mA applied through electrocardiographic patches applied to shaved skin on the right rear hock and right front knee during milking (2 times) with an intermittent pattern (5 seconds on, 25 seconds off) for 7 days.[28] The number of behavioral events increased with a greater increase in the 6.0 mA group. One cow had to be removed from the 6.0 mA group because of severe behavioral responses. Heart rate was elevated (+3 beats/min) only in response to the initial 1-minute exposure during udder preparation. Time to peak oxytocin response was delayed in the 3.6 mA group. Peak milk flow increased slightly and peak prolactin and area under prolactin response curves increased similarly for both groups. Wisconsin Mastitis Test scores, milk yield, and milking duration were not affected. The author concluded that any negative effects of electrical shock on milk production or mammary health most likely are not related directly to shock (physiologic responses to shock were minimal and milk yield was maintained); however, the behavioral responses to 6 mA would result in management problems for some cows.

Six cows were exposed to 0 mA, 4 mA, or 8 mA of current applied from udder to hooves during 14 consecutive milkings using a changeover design over 3 consecutive 1-week periods.[29] Current was applied as 60 Hz square waves of 5-second duration applied every 30 seconds and began 5 minutes before milking and continued until milking unit removal. Behavioral responses to current were noted but decreased with time. Blood cortisol concentration increased and oxytocin release was delayed for the 8 mA exposure. Neither treatment affected SCC, milk yield, protein, fat, milking duration, peak milk flow rate, duration of peak milk flow, residual milk yield, or prolactin.

Seven cows were exposed to an ascending series of 60 Hz currents of 0, 2.5, 5.0, 7.5, 10, then 12.5 mA, applied through electrocardiographic patches applied to shaved skin on the right rear hock and right front knee.[15] Currents were applied for 10-second intervals. As the current dose increased, cows became more agitated and 2 cows were not shocked at 12.5 mA due to severe behavioral responses. Heart rate immediately after shock increased at 10 mA and 12.5 mA treatments while prolactin, norepinephrine, and glucocorticoids were unaffected. Epinephrine doubled in 2 exceptional cows at 10 mA. Dramatic behavioral responses displayed by cows at the higher current exposures were not correlated with significant or prolonged physiologic responses and electrical exposure was not considered a reliable way to induce "stress" in cows.

Fourteen multiparous cows (8 second, 5 third, 1 fourth lactation) and 14 first lactation cows were enrolled in an 7-week experiment with 14-day pretreatment, 21-day treatment, and 14-day posttreatment periods.[30] Cows were randomly assigned to 0 V, 0.5 V, 1 V, 2 V, or 4 V treatment groups. The current flow path was from the mouth (drinking cup) to rear hooves (metal grid). There were no statistically significant differences in SCC or milk conductivity within each treatment voltage across periods or within each period across voltages for either group of cows. Some cows developed clinical mastitis during the experiment: 5 in the pretreatment period, 4 during treatment (1 at 0 V, 0 at 0.5 V, 1 at 1 V, 1 at 2 V, and 1 at 4 V), and 4 during posttreatment. The incidence of mastitis was evenly distributed across control and treatment groups with no consistent pattern between clinical mastitis and voltage levels, leading the authors to conclude that both the incidence of the disease and type of infecting bacteria were not related to voltage level. There were also no significant relationships found between level of voltage and body temperature or reproductive problems.

AC currents were delivered to lactating cattle through the milk during milking.[31] The current flow path was between electrodes placed at the top of each short milk tube to a metal grid on which the cows' rear hooves stood. In trial 1, 4 voltage levels were selected for the first lactation (0, 2, 4, and 8 V) and 8 multiple lactation (0, 4, 8, and 16 V) cows using a Latin square design on 4 over consecutive milkings. Behavioral changes were noticeable at voltages greater than and equal to 4 V for first lactation cows and 8 V for multiple lactation cows and corresponded to average currents of 4.1 mA (range 2–7 mA) for first lactation cows and 9.1 mA (range 4–14 mA) for multiple lactation cows. Only at 8 V for first lactation cows and 16 V for multiple lactation cows did some cows kick off machines. Currents associated with kicking the machine off were 5 to 12.5 mA for first lactation cows and 8 to 18 mA for multiple lactation cows. There were no consistent significant differences in milking duration, milk yields, or composition (milk fat, milk protein, or SCCs) of primary milk and residual milk. For the 8 multiple lactation cows, milk protein increased by 0.1% for the 4 V, but not the 8 V or 16 V, treatments, and protein in residual milk increased by 0.2% at the 4 V and 0.1% at the 8 V, but not at the 16 V treatment. Fat in residual milk also decreased by 1.4% for these cows at the 4 V, but not for the 8 V or 16 V treatments. Milking durations were generally longer (0.4–1.0 minute, with an increasing trend with voltage levels), but these differences were not statistically significant.

A second trial was conducted in which currents selected were just below those that caused cows to kick milking machines (5 mA for first lactation cows and 8 mA for multiple lactation cows) and was delivered for 6 consecutive milkings to 8 first lactation cows and 8 multiple lactation cows in the same manner as in the first trial.[31] No undesired behaviors were observed for either group of cows. There was no significant change in SCC, milk yield, milk fat, or milk protein. SCC was lower for the multiple lactation cows and higher for the first lactation cows when currents were applied, but neither was significantly different. Milking duration was 1 minute less in first lactation cows but did not differ in multiple lactation cows. Serum cortisol concentrations were lower in multiple lactation cows 2 minutes prior to and 6 minutes after milking began and were similar at other times. Milk yield showed a slight (0.1–0.5 kg) but not significant increase in both groups of cows during milkings in which current was applied. The authors concluded that a voltage greater than 125 V on the milk line and voltage greater than 5 V on the claw of the milking cluster would be required to produce 5 mA of current through the milk to the cow and that the milking machine does not appear to provide a significant risk because of the magnitude of the voltage and currents needed to create economic effects.

Four groups of 10 Holstein cows each were exposed to 0 V, 1 V, 2 V, or 4 V between waterers and a metal grid throughout an entire lactation.[32,33] Cows could not drink without placing their front hooves on the metal grid. The test pens had 10 cows in them at all times. Herd cows or "placeholders" were replaced by test cows as fresh cows became available from the herd. All of the test cows completed their entire lactation in the treatment pens. Although there were some behavioral changes on the first day of exposure, feed and water intakes of test cows were not affected by any of the voltage treatments. One cow and 1 heifer refused to drink from their water bowls for 36 hours when bowls were electrified at 4 V. All other cows that were subjected to voltage on the water bowl drank after some delay during the first 24 hours. The delay was directly proportional to the voltage level. However, within 48 hours, those cows were consuming the same amount of water as during the pretest period. One first lactation cow, of a total of 51 cows placed in the 4 V pen, had to be removed. This cow was a herd cow. Her milk yield decreased rapidly, and she was not consuming grain during her first 36 hours in the pen. This was the only cow in this experiment that showed a dramatic reduction in feed intake and milk production. Milk yield for the full 305-day lactation test group showed no significant differences between groups exposed or unexposed to the voltage treatment levels. SCC, milk fat, and milk protein in the test cows showed no significant differences between groups exposed or unexposed to voltage. Voltage treatments did not significantly influence cow health or reproductive performance as measured by mastitis, hoof problems, changes in body weight, days to first breeding, days open, and services per conception, calving intervals, visible abortion, and calves born dead.

Three switch back experiments (30 cows each) were conducted to determine the effects of the 3 different levels of voltage applied from muzzle (water bowls) to hooves (the cow platform).[34,35] The 112 day experiment was divided into 4 periods of 28 days, and cows were randomly assigned to 6 treatment groups with voltage and no-voltage treatments applied in different patterns across the 4-week periods. A continuous low-level voltage was interrupted by 2 periods of 3 hours of higher levels at 5 a.m. and 5 p.m., to simulate higher loads during milking that occur on many dairy farms. The first experiment used 1 V with a background voltage of 0.3 V, the second experiment used 2.5 V with a background level of 0.75 V, and the third experiment used 5 V with a background voltage of 0.75 V. The parameters measured were daily milk production, milking time, milk composition (% butterfat, % protein, % lactose, and SCC), water consumption, and feed consumption. Dates of estrus and breeding were recorded, and behaviors (urination, defecation, drinking, lying time, standing time, and any abnormal behavior) of each cow were observed for 25% of each day. The effects of each outcome variable were analyzed for effect during the treatment period as well as for carryover effects occurring 1 or 2 periods after the treatment. Exposed cows had significantly higher milk fat percentage (31.2 vs 30.6 kg/cow/d) in the first experiment (1 V). Milking time was longer (8.5 vs 8.3 minutes) for the second experimental group (2.5 V). There was a carryover effect on milk yield 2 periods after the treatment for the third group (5 V). In addition, less water (97.6 vs 100 L/cow/d) was consumed by the treatment group. No differences in SCC were detected at any of the exposure levels, nor were any carryover effects observed. The authors concluded that exposures up to 5 V in well-managed tie-stall dairy operations were unlikely to cause observable changes in cow milk production or behavior.

Sixteen Holstein cows with a history of subclinical mastitis (cultured positive for *Staphylococcus aureus*) were used to determine whether exposure to steady state voltages could trigger clinical mastitis or result in compromised health or reduced immune function in cows predisposed to mastitis.[36] Cows were divided into 4 treatment groups of 4 cows each with constant voltage treatments of 0 V, 1 V, 2 V, and 4 V applied continuously between water bowls and metal floor mats for 7 days. Water intake, milk yield, feed consumption, milk composition, somatic cell counts, and milk microbiology and cortisol were monitored before during and after 7-day exposures to voltages. Blood samples were taken from each cow every other day throughout each period prior to milking via tail vein venipuncture. Samples were allowed to clot and serum was isolated. Serum was analyzed for (1) bovine panel (sodium, potassium, chloride, bicarbonate, anion gap, urea, creatinine, calcium, phosphate, magnesium, total protein, albumin, globulin, glucose, alkaline phosphatase, Aspartate aminotransferase pyridoxal 5' phosphate (AST/P5P), Sorbitol dehydrogenase (SDH), gamma glutamyl transferase (hGGT), indirect, direct and total bilirubin, creatine kinase (CK), iron, and total iron-binding capacity (TIBC)); (2) gamma-immunoglobulins (Ig) IgG, IgA, and IgM; and (3) blood serum cortisol. Animals perceived voltages as evidenced by delays in drinking, which increased with voltage. There was no significant difference in milk production, milk composition, SCC, feed consumption, blood chemistry, milk microbiology, and serum cortisol when the treatment period was compared to the 1-week pre- and post-treatment periods. The number of S aureus–infected quarters did not increase across treatments. The quarters showing high SCCs were consistently high throughout the experimental periods, and those noninfected quarters within those animals remained uninfected with S aureus organisms throughout the experiment. A nonsignificant trend existed for higher cortisol levels as voltage levels increased (+1 ng/mL at 4 V). The absolute level of milk production, SCCs, milk fat and protein, and IgM levels were higher in the 2 V group, but these differences were also present in the pre- and post-treatment periods and the authors noted that this was likely caused by the subclinical S aureus infections present in the cows at the start of experimentation.

Sixteen lactating Holstein cows (8 cows receiving bovine somatotropin [bST] and 8 bST-free cows) were exposed to 0 V, 1 V, 2 V, or 4 V applied from a metallic water bowl to a metallic plate under the rear hooves for a period of 7 days.[37] Microbial analysis revealed that no cows were infected with Streptococcus uberis at the beginning of the experiment. All cows were exposed to S uberis, as a post teat dip after milking. Milk samples were aseptically collected and cultured for bacteria. Voltages did not significantly influence SCCs, feed intake, water intake, milk yield, milk fat, or milk protein. Of the 16 cows studied, no cows developed clinical mastitis. The authors concluded that steady state voltages of up to 4 V, applied to water bowls, for 7 days, did not promote clinical mastitis in dairy cattle during or after direct exposure of live bacteria to teat ends and that bST treatment did not result in mastitis in cows subjected to these conditions. The authors noted that this experiment is supported our previous work that steady state levels of up to 4 V on water bowls do not lower the immune resistance of cows, consequently making them more prone to mastitis, and further demonstrates there is no physiologic causal relationship between steady state stray voltage exposure of up to 4 V and mastitis in dairy cattle.

Milking performance of cows subjected to electrical current during milking and 2 common milking machine problems were documented.[38] The first experiment used 32 cows in a 2 × 2 factorial design with exposure to 1 mA of electrical current from front to back hooves during milking and a pulsation failure (no massage phase) as treatments. A second experiment used 16 cows in a 2 × 2 factorial design with exposure to 1 mA of electrical current from front to back hooves during milking and excessively aged milking machine liners as treatments. The main effect of current exposure was not statistically significant for milk yield, average milk flow rate, maximum milk flow rate, cow activity, and strip yield. The main effect of pulsation failure was significant for cow activity (−5.8 weight shifts during a milking). The main effect of aged liners was significant for milk yield (+2.2 kg), average flow rate (0.3 kg/min reduction), maximum flow rate (−1.2 kg/min), and liner slips per milking (+26) The significance of some interactive effects appeared to indicate that current exposure had a mitigating effect on the changes caused by the milking machine problems. However, these interactions were not consistent across experiments and in some cases were highly influenced by a few observations. This study adds further evidence to the body of literature showing that exposure to low-level step potential resulting in less than 1 mA rms of 60 Hz electrical current during milking is not a cause of cow discomfort or poor milking performance.

A series of experiments was performed to measure behavioral responses and changes in blood cortisol concentration of cows exposed to 60 Hz electrical current applied from front to rear hooves.[22] The current flow pathway was between 1 front hoof and 2 rear hooves. The current exposure levels administered in an ascending series using 0.5, 0.75, 1.0, and 1.5 times the previously determined behavioral reaction threshold for each cow resulting in currents ranging from 1 mA to 5.25 mA. The time between current exposures was 10 minutes. Cortisol levels did not increase in response to 5-minute current exposure at levels up to 150% of the behavioral reaction threshold but serum cortisol concentrations did increase in response to hoof trimming. The authors concluded that these results confirm several previous studies indicating that behavioral changes are a more sensitive indicator of response to short-term electrical current exposure than blood cortisol levels.

Twelve mid-lactation dairy cattle were subjected to intermittent low electrical currents (1 ± 0.1 mA) from front to rear of stall for a period of 14 days.[39] Twelve additional cows were housed in identical stalls with no treatment. Feed intake, water intake, milk production, and rectal temperature were monitored daily and were unaffected by treatment. Behavioral measurements, including percentage of time lying and time to reenter stalls after milking, were unaffected by treatment. Immune function was assessed by analyzing blood samples taken twice a week for 13 different response variables. The measures for lymphocyte blastogenesis (concanavalin A and phytohemagglutanin mitogens) and oxidative burst (phorbol myristate acetate [PMA]-induced chemiluminescence) were chosen a priori as the best indicators of immune function response. Immunoglobulin production and interleukins 1 and 2 were also assessed. There was no statistically significant difference between control and treatment cows for any of the main response variables. The difference between the control and treatment cows was statistically significant for one of the secondary response variables (lymphocyte blastogenesis for S aureus mitogen). The authors concluded that collectively, these results suggest that exposure to 1 mA of current for 2 weeks had no significant effect on the immune function of dairy cattle.

Four groups of 8 cows each were divided into a control group (n = 2) and treatment groups (n = 6) and monitored for a 14-day pretreatment period followed by a 21-day treatment during which a single-cycle, 60 Hz transient current was applied to water bowls once every second and a 14-day post-treatment period.[5,18] Cows in these experiments were exposed to the transient current whenever they attempted to drink. Exposure levels were set relative to the sensitivity of individual animals to short-duration exposure to take into account the wide range of sensitivities among cows. The exposure levels ranged from 4.9 to 7.8 mA rms for cows exposed at their behavioral reaction threshold (n = 6), 6.0 to 9.5 mA rms for cows exposed to 1.1 mA rms above their behavioral reaction threshold (n = 6), 6.4 to 12 mA rms for cows exposed to 2.2 mA above their behavioral reaction threshold (n = 6), and 7.8 to 14 mA rms (n = 6) to cows exposed to 150% above their behavioral reaction threshold. Animals showed an acclimation to the transient current exposure with avoidance behaviors most prominent immediately after exposure and reduced avoidance response with increasing exposure time. Significant reductions in water and feed intake, and milk production were measured on the first 3 days of exposure for cows exposed to 150% of their reaction threshold current level. The current level required to elicit this short-term reduction in water and feed intake and milk production was thus considerably higher than that required to produce a behavioral response. Average changes in feed and water intake and milk production during the 21-day treatment period were not significant compared with the 14-day pretreatment period. No changes in SCC or linear score were found. Three cows experienced an elevated SCC and were treated for mastitis during the experiment. Two of the cows affected by mastitis were the control cows, and one incident of mastitis occurred during the pre-treatment period for a cow that was later exposed to current at the behavioral response threshold. All 3 of the mastitis incidents were for cows in test stall number 3. This was cleaned and disinfected and the cow housed in that stall for the final block did not experience an elevated SCC. This study confirms results of previous studies and field observations noting rapid acclimation to voltages as well as changes in animal behaviors with no measurable decline in water or feed intake or milk production and no increase in SCC or incidence of mastitis.

The effects of permanent or random exposure to stray voltage applied to the water trough were evaluated on milk production and stress physiology of 74 Holstein cows[6] that were assigned during two 8-week experimental periods to 1 of 3 treatments: permanent exposure (1.8 V, n = 23), random exposure of 36 hr/wk (1.8 V, n = 25), and no voltage (C, n = 26). Voltage was applied between metallic water bowls and a metallic plate on the floor. The average cow + contact resistance was measured as 516 Ω, and the current applied was 3.6 $\pm$ 0.08 mA. The absence of differences between treatments for SCC was verified after the cows were assigned to their groups. On the first day of voltage exposure, permanently exposed cows had higher activity levels than control cows (9.8 vs −2.3 periods of movement/h). During the eighth week of exposure, randomly exposed cows had higher activity levels than control cows (4.2 vs −7.7 periods of movement/h). The randomly exposed cows had higher milk cortisol concentration (0.21 ng/mL) than the permanently exposed cows (0.14 ng/mL) during the 8th week of exposure, but neither group was different than the control group (0.15 ng/mL) and no difference in plasma cortisol concentration was observed between groups. There was a transient decrease in milk yield on the second day of exposure in permanently cows (−1.4 kg) and on the third day of exposure in randomly exposed cows (−3.5 kg) compared with control cows. No differences were observed between treatments for cortisol response after an adrenocorticotropic hormone challenge during the 7th week of exposure. No effects of voltage exposure were observed on daily water intake or SCC. The authors concluded that stray voltage exposure at these levels could be considered a mild chronic stressor in dairy cows, especially when it was unpredictable, with only slight modifications in stress physiology accompanied by changes in activity and no impairment of milk production or SCC.

SUMMARY

If animal contact voltage reaches sufficient levels, animals coming into contact with grounded devices may receive a mild electric shock that can cause a behavioral response. At voltage levels that are just perceptible to the animal, behaviors indicative of perception (eg, flinches) may result with little change in normal routines. At higher exposure levels, avoidance behaviors may result. The direct effect of animal contact with electrical current can range from:

- Mild behavioral reactions indicative of sensation, to
- Involuntary muscle contraction, or twitching, to
- Intense behavioral responses indicative of pain.

The indirect effects of these behaviors can vary considerably depending on the specifics of the contact location, level of current flow, body pathway, frequency of occurrence, and many other factors related to the daily activities of animals. There are several common situations of concern in animal environments:

- Animals avoiding certain exposure locations, which may result in:
  - Reduced water intake if exposure is required for animals to access watering devices,
  - Reduced feed intake if exposure is required for animals to accesses feeding devices or locations.
- Difficulty of moving or handling animals in areas of voltage/current exposure
- The physiologic implications of the release of stress hormones produced by contact with painful stimuli.

The severity of response will depend on the amount of electrical current (measured in milliamps) flowing through the animal's body, the pathway it takes through the body, and the sensitivity of the individual animal. The results of the combined current dose-response experiments, voltage exposure response experiments, and measurements of body and contact resistances is consistent with the lowest (worst case) cow + contact resistance as low as 500 Ω as estimated by Lefcourt[1] that may occur in some unusual situations on farms (firm application of the muzzle to a wet metallic watering device and hoof contact on a clean, wet, contoured metallic plate on the floor). These studies on responses of dairy cows to electrical exposure agree well with each other and with predictions from neuroelectric theory and practice. There is a high degree of repeatability across studies in which exposures and responses have been appropriately quantified.

For confirmation, a potential of 2 to 4 V (60 Hz, rms) must be measured between 2 points that an animal might contact (or animal contact measurement), and some animals should exhibit signs of avoidance behavior. The animal contact voltage measurement with an appropriate shunt resistor value provides the only reliable indication of exposure levels. Voltage readings at cow contact points should be made with a 500- or 1000-Ω resistor across the 2 measuring leads to the cow contact points in addition to open circuit measurements.

The only studies that have documented adverse effects of voltage and current on cows had both sufficient current applied to cause aversion and forced exposures (ie, animals could not eat or drink without being exposed to voltage and current) and all of the indirect responses (reduced water or intake and milk production) were behaviorally mediated. It is typical for voltage levels to vary considerably at different locations on a farm. Decreased water and/or feed intake or undesired behaviors result only if current levels are sufficient to produce aversion at locations that are critical to daily animal activity, such as feeders, waterers, and milking areas. If an aversive current occurs only a few times per day, it is not likely to have an adverse effect on cow behavior. The more often an aversive voltage occurs in areas critical to cows' normal feeding, drinking, or resting, the more likely it is to affect cows.

A number of studies have been done to investigate potential detrimental physiologic responses that may result from animals' exposure to voltage and current. The literature review presented here summarizes 46 research trials on groups of cows exposed to know levels of voltage and/or current. Many of these were part of the same experiment but exposed cows at different levels of voltage or current. None of these trials or experiments (some using aggressive exposure of cows to mastitis organisms) showed a significant effect of voltage/current exposure on SCC or the incidence of mastitis. Many of these studies showed behavioral modification and some showed minor changes in milk yield, milk composition, or stress hormones (especially cortisol). These studies have shown that increased concentrations of the stress hormone cortisol do not occur at levels below behavioral response levels and only become apparent in some, but not all, cows at substantially higher voltage/current exposures than the threshold required for behavioral modification. This body of research indicates that while exposure to stray voltage at levels of 2 V to 4 V may be a mild stressor to dairy cows, it does not contribute to increased SCC or incidence of mastitis or reduced milk yield.

REFERENCES

1. Lefcourt AM, editor. Effects of electrical voltage/current on farm animals: how to detect and remedy problems. USDA Handbook 696. Washington, DC: US Department of Agriculture; 1991.
2. Phillips DSM. Production of cows may be affected by small electric shocks from milking plants. N Z J Agri 1962;105:221–5.
3. Appleman RD, Gustafson RJ. Sources of stray voltage and effect on cow health and performance. J Dairy Sci 1985;68:1554–67.
4. Reilly JP. Transient current effects in stray voltage exposure: biophysical principles and mechanisms. ASAE Annual International Meeting. Atlanta (GA), December 13–16, 1994. Paper No. 94-3594.
5. Reinemann DJ, Stetson LE, Laughlin NK. Water, feed, and milk production response of dairy cattle exposed to transient currents. Trans ASABE 2005;48:385–92.
6. Rigalma K, Duvaux-Ponter C, Barrier A, et al. Medium-term effects of repeated exposure to stray voltage on activity, stress physiology, and milk production and composition in dairy cows. J Dairy Sci 2010;93:3542–52.
7. Reilly JP. Applied bioelectricity: from electrical stimulation to electropathology. New York: Springer-Verlag; 1998.
8. Reinemann DJ. Literature review and synthesis of research findings on the impact of stray voltage on farm operations. Report prepared for the Ontario Energy Board, March 31, 2008. Available at: http://www.ontarioenergyboard.ca/OEB/_Documents/EB-2007-0709/report_Reinemann_20080530.pdf. Accessed March 24, 2012.
9. Aneshansley DJ, Southwick LH, Pellerin RA, et al. Aversive response of dairy cows to voltages/currents on waterers at frequencies of 60 Hz and above. ASAE Annual International Meeting. Minneapolis (MN), August 10–14, 1997. Technical Paper No. 97-3109.
10. Aneshansley DJ, Gorewit RC. Sensitivity of Holsteins to 60 Hz and other waveforms present on dairy farms. ASAE Annual International Meeting. Toronto, Ontario (Canada), July 18–21, 1999. Technical Paper No. 99-3152.
11. Craine LB. Effects on mammals of grounded neutral voltage from distribution power lines. New York (NY): IEEE Rural Electric Power Conference; 1975. Paper No. 75-303-3-IA.
12. Currence HD, Steevens BJ, Winter DF, et al. Dairy cow and human sensitivity to short duration 60 Hertz currents. Appl Eng Agri 1990;6:349–53.
13. Gorewit RC, Scott NR, Henke-Drenkard DV. Effects of electrical current on milk production and animal health. ASAE Annual International Meeting. New Orleans (LA), December 11–14, 1984. Technical Paper No. 84-3502.
14. Lefcourt AM. Behavioral responses of dairy cows subjected to controlled voltages. J Dairy Sci 1982;65:672–4.
15. Lefcourt AM, Kahl S, Akers RM. Correlation of indices of stress with intensity of electrical shock for cows. J Dairy Sci 1986;69:833–42.
16. Norell RJ, Gustafson RJ, Appleman RD. Behavioral studies of dairy cattle sensitivity to electrical currents. Trans ASAE 1983;26:1506–11.

17. Reinemann DJ, Stetson LE, Laughlin N. Response of dairy cattle to transient voltages and magnetic fields. IEEE Trans Ind Appl 1995;4:708.
18. Reinemann DJ, Stetson LE, Laughlin NK. Water, feed and milk production response of dairy cattle exposed to transient currents. ASAE Annual International Meeting. Chicago (IL), June 18–23, 1996. Technical Paper No. 95-3276.
19. Reinemann DJ, Stetson LE, Riley JP, et al. Dairy cow sensitivity and aversion to short duration transient currents. ASAE Annual International Meeting. Phoenix (AZ), July 14–18, 1996. Technical Paper No. 96-3087.
20. Reinemann DJ, Stetson LE, Riley JP, et al. Dairy cow sensitivity to short duration electrical currents. Trans ASAE 1999;42:215–22.
21. Reinemann DJ, Thompson PD, Forster C. Sensitivity testing results: EPRI PEAC sponsored pulsed current impact assessment tests, University of Wisconsin-Madison, 2003.
22. Reinemann DJ, Wiltbank MC, Sheffield LG, et al. Comparison of behavioral and physiological response of cows exposed to electric shock. Trans ASAE 2003;46:507–12.
23. Whittlestone WG, Mullord MM, Kilgour R, et al. Electric shocks during machine milking. N Z Vet J 1975;23:105–8.
24. Woolford MW. Small voltage in milking plants. Second Seminar on Farm Machinery and Equipment Proceedings3. Hamilton (NZ): New Zealand Department of Agriculture; 1972.
25. Gustafson RJ, Sun ZY, Brennan TM. Dairy cow sensitivity to short duration electrical currents. ASAE Annual International Meeting. Chicago (IL), December 13–16, 1988. Technical Paper No. 88-3522.
26. Gustafson RJ, Christiansen GS, Appleman RD. Electrical resistance of milking system components. Trans ASAE 1983;26:1218–21.
27. Gorewit RC, Scott NR, Czarniecki CS. Responses of dairy cows to alternating electrical current administered semi randomly in a non-avoidance environment. J Dairy Sci 1985;68:718–25.
28. Lefcourt AM, Akers RM, Miller RH, et al. Effects of intermittent electrical shock on responses related to milk ejection. J Dairy Sci 1985;68:391–401.
29. Henke-Drenkard DV, Gorewit RC, Scott NR, Sagi R. Milk production, health, behavior, and endocrine responses of cows exposed to electrical current during milking. J Dairy Sci 1985;68:2694–702.
30. Gorewit RC, Zhao X, Aneshansley DJ, et al. Effects of neutral-to-earth voltage on animal health and reproduction in cattle. ASAE Annual International Meeting. Baltimore (MD), June 28–July 1, 1987. Technical Paper No. 87-3035.
31. Aneshansley DJ, Gorewit RC, Price LR. Cow sensitivity to electricity during milking. J Dairy Sci 1992;75:2733–41.
32. Aneshansley DJ, Price LR. Effects of voltages on cows over a complete lactation: 1, milk yield and composition. J Dairy Sci 1992;75:2719–25.
33. Gorewit RC, Aneshansley DJ, Price LR. Effects of voltages on cows over a complete lactation: 2, health and reproduction. J Dairy Sci 1992;75:2726–32.
34. Gumprich PS. Stray voltage effects on dairy cattle. New Liskeard (Ontario): New Liskeard College of Agricultural Technology; 1992.
35. Gumprich PS, Giesen L. Stray voltage effect on somatic cell count of dairy cows. Proceedings of the annual meeting of the National Mastitis Council. Madison (WI): National Mastitis Council; 1993.
36. Gorewit RC, Anesansley DJ. Effects of steady state voltages on Holstein cows with histories of subclinical mastitis. ASAE Annual International Meeting. Minneapolis (MN), August 10–14, 1997. Technical Paper No. 97-3110.

37. Gorewit RC, Aneshansley DJ. Effects of steady state voltages on mastitis. ASAE Annual International Meeting. Toronto, Ontario (Canada), July 18–21, 1999. Technical Paper No. 99-3151.
38. Reinemann DJ, Rasmussen MD, LeMire SD. Milking performance of dairy cows subjected to electrical current and induced milking machine problems. Trans ASAE 2003;45:833–8.
39. Reinemann DJ, Rasmussen MD, Sheffield LG, et al. Dairy cow response to electrical environment: part III, Immune function response to low-level electrical current exposure. Report to the Minnesota Public Utilities Commission, June 30, 1999. Available at: http://www.puc.state.mn.us/portal/groups/public/documents/pdf_files/000669. pdf. Accessed March 24, 2012.

Using Mastitis Records and Somatic Cell Count Data

David A. Rhoda, DVM[a],*, José C.F. Pantoja, MV, MS, PhD[b]

KEYWORDS

- Mastitis • Milk quality • Records • Software

KEY POINTS

- The use of on-farm records is essential for managing mastitis in dairy herds. Mastitis records are a useful tool for caring for an individual cow, to monitor compliance of farm personnel working with groups of animals, to understand the epidemiology of mastitis in the herd, to ensure responsible drug utilization, and to document accountability in our care of the cow.

- It is important to plan what data to record, when to capture it, and how to enter it into a cow's permanent record. Essential information to record include a clinical mastitis remark with symptomatic data and treatment decisions, milk culture information, somatic cell count results, and mastitis outcomes at the completion of the case.

- Once information is recorded, customized reports should be produced to create a records plan for clinical and subclinical mastitis. The records plan includes cow-side and herd-level reports.

- Cow-side reports can be used to manage current cases of mastitis. Herd-level reports include cohorts of cows and are useful for evaluation of treatment protocols, environmental risk factors, milking performance, and monitoring performance indexes of the group.

- Reports should be reviewed in a frequent basis as part of a mastitis control plan.

Mastitis is an infection of the udder that can either be clinical or subclinical in presentation. Although new diagnostic tests such as in-line milk sensors have been developed to improve the detection of clinical mastitis (CM),[1] diagnosis by means of physical examination of the milk, udder, and cow is still critical for managing this disease. Diagnosis of subclinical mastitis (SM) has been performed using somatic cell count (SCC), for which a threshold of 200,000 cells/mL has been universally accepted

The authors have nothing to disclose.
[a] College of Agriculture and Life Sciences, University of Wisconsin-Madison, 1675 Observatory Drive, Madison, WI 53706, USA; [b] Departamento de Higiene Veterinária e Saúde Pública, Faculdade de Medicina Veterinária e Zootecnia, Universidade Estadual Paulista, Campus de Botucatu, Distrito de Rubião Júnior, S/N, Botucatu, São Paulo, Brazil
* Corresponding author.
E-mail address: drhoda@wisc.edu

Vet Clin Food Anim 28 (2012) 347–361
http://dx.doi.org/10.1016/j.cvfa.2012.03.012
0749-0720/12/$ – see front matter © 2012 Elsevier Inc. All rights reserved.

to define a case.[2] Both forms of mastitis have a measurable economic importance[3,4] and are usually managed as separate groups.

The use of on-farm records is essential for managing mastitis in dairy herds. In the field we need to be aware of the patterns of mastitis within herds for management decisions, but also be prepared to make sound individual animal decisions based on reliable medical history coupled with an examination. In addition to their role in the care of individual cows, records have even greater value to (1) ensure compliance of farm workers with farm protocols, (2) allow veterinarians to understand epidemiology of mastitis in the herd, (3) ensure responsible drug utilization, and (4) document accountability of our care of the cow.

The gathering of data is a process that requires planning and should be efficient, easy, and accurate because gathering treatment and examination data is not a popular task for busy farm personnel. Data that are available as individual cow medical history can be collated to generate key performance indicators (KPIs). Records are used in many forms such as the standard operating procedures (SOP) for daily processes such as milking and health care or for use in managing SM and CM. Records are also useful for writing protocols that define a specific condition or situation and provide detailed treatment instructions to ensure medically appropriate drug use and food safety. Finally, treatment records have value for building the medical history for individual cows to aid in making management decisions and are used as a check and balance for identifying management deficits and biological shifts on the dairy.

IMPORTANCE OF MASTITIS RECORDS FOR MONITORING DRUG USE
The Veterinarian-Client-Patient-Relationship

The potential of drug interventions mandates the development of a veterinarian–client–patient relationship (VCPR).[5] In the United States, many of the antibiotics used on a dairy are administered by farm personnel and the majority of farm-based antibiotic use is for the management of udder health,[6] which makes the relationship of the people involved in mastitis decisions a priority. Communication for the mutual benefit of the people represented in the VCPR needs a foundation based on recorded cow-level data.

Mastitis records are fundamental for integrating the people involved in the VCPR:

1. *The patient:* Farm personnel need to accurately record the information about the conditions that will demonstrate the disease patterns, the care given to the affected animal, and convalescence data. Use of records helps farm workers stay on protocol and can also prevent critical mistakes such as failure to discard milk produced by cows receiving drugs.
2. *The client:* Client in this context is represented as the person (owner or manager) who has the responsibility to oversee the health care given by others and the processes and protocols they follow. Use of accurate records ensures that processes are followed.
3. *Attending or referral veterinarians* who have the responsibility of overseeing drug usage need the records to develop protocols, detect animals that need customized therapy, and oversee animals receiving specific protocols. The care of the individual animal is the first obligation, but understanding the herd-level epidemiology is critical for planning the herd health care plan.

Besides the VCPR team, there are multiple people working to ensure milk quality, food safety, and animal care. Not everyone on the team has the same responsibilities, so there is a need to use records to develop KPIs that can be shared by everyone involved as an indicator of management achievement.

The examples of records used in this chapter will be from use of DairyComp 305 (DC305) (Valley Agricultural Software, Tulare, CA). Nonetheless, the principles can be applied to other forms of records. DC305 is a herd management program that stores individual cow information, test day production, and SCC data and allows the production of customized reports. The reports can be used to display the history of an individual cow or summarized to display patterns of mastitis for specific cohorts of animals.

The objective of this report is to describe a records plan that can be used to monitor mastitis at the herd level, aid in the management of the decision-making process for individual cows, and improve drug use on dairy herds. First, some critical pieces of udder health data that can be entered on the farm are suggested and discussed. Last, records plans based on such data for both CM and SM are described including the interpretation of cow- and herd-level customized reports.

UDDER HEALTH DATA ENTRY

The first step is organizing the data to record including when to capture it and how to enter it into a cow's permanent record. It is difficult to write a universal template that all dairies must follow because of the unique needs of specific veterinarians and their clients. Managing herd and cow-level data is obviously dependent on first entering the data into a records system. As a basic package of information, it is recommended that the following data be recorded: (1) a CM entry or remark with symptomatic data and treatment decisions; (2) culture information for both clinical and subclinical cases; (3) SM information as represented by SCC levels (both pre- and post-CM); and (4) data about mastitis outcomes at the completion of the case or within a defined time period.

Entry of Clinical Mastitis Data

The reports used as examples use the mastitis remark of DC305, which recorded severity, affected quarter, and treatment administered (usually intramammary drug). DC305 limits the space that is available for each case to 8 characters, thus forcing the use of acronyms. When other programs are used, more information may be useful to record. These data are recorded at the cowside when the treatment decision is reached at the onset of the case. Planning the order that information will be recorded in the remark helps users to prioritize the importance of each piece of data. Severity of the case is one of the most important monitors of detection policies in the herd and treatment protocols always reference severity.[7,8] Other information that is useful to manage the case is also included. **Fig. 1** illustrates a recording form to ensure the data and structure of the recording. Many veterinarians are focused on management of severe cases, but the management of mild cases is actually where the opportunity for improved treatment protocols is most dramatic. DC305 and some other programs have a protocol module for automatically entering a predefined treatment protocol at the time the mastitis event is entered. In the reports demonstrated, the remark begins with a severity score abbreviated as the first 2 characters; quarters can use the next 4 characters, and drug protocol in the last 2 characters (see **Fig. 1**).

Culture Results

Culturing CM samples is a key management practice for many mastitis control programs.[9] A recording form that ensures accuracy of abbreviations is important in

Mastitis Examination Form				Examination
				1) Severity[1] 2) CMT[2] 3) Culture[3]
				4) Medical history[4] (for treatment decision)
	Mastitis Remark[6]			**Definitions:**
ID	Date	Severity, Quarter, Protocol		**Severity**
3	10/1/11	SE LR	SP	Mild (mi) = abnormal milk
4	10/1/11	MI LR RF	NT	Moderate (mo) = abnormal milk and udder
				Severe (se) = abnormal milk, udder, and cow
				Quarter[5] : RR, RF, LR, LF, all
				Protocol: name or treatment

Fig. 1. Example of a recording form for information to enter in permanent record plus a reminder of the examination standard operating procedures and definition of information desired.[1] Assessment of severity of clinical cases (defined in the form).[2] California Mastitis Test for quarters not clinically affected.[3] Milk culture for assessment of the causal pathogen.[4] Medical history including SCC, previous cases of clinical mastitis and other diseases, and productive information such as parity, reproductive status, and milk production.[5] Up to 4 characters to indicate the quarter or quarters affected.[6] Cow 3 had a severe case (SE) affecting the left-rear (LR) quarter that was treated with Ceftiofur (SP = Spectramast; Pfizer). Cow 4 had a mild (MI) case affecting both the left-rear and right-front quarters. No treatment (NT) was used.

order to be able to sort cases by cause and assess outcomes of therapies for specific pathogens. In herds with on-farm culture capabilities, this may be part of the protocol for making the initial treatment decision. In DC305 or other software, culture results from both CM and SM can be entered and will collate into permanent records to be used as part of customized reports. The column CULTR in the reports presented lists milk culture results using abbreviations for various mastitis pathogens (eg, STREP = streptococci; G– = gram-negative bacteria; NG = no growth). As an example in, **Fig. 2**, streptococci and gram-negative bacteria were isolated from the milk of cows 5 and 7, respectively.

Somatic Cell Count Data

Mastitis is a disease that often fluctuates between the subclinical and clinical states. Cows with SM are more likely to develop CM than are uninfected cows.[10,11] A history of SM preceding CM has been suggested to decrease the likelihood of successfully treating a clinical case.[12] Therefore, review of both clinical and subclinical data allows not only improvement of treatment decisions but also the assessment of treatment outcomes. In most herds, evaluation of mastitis can be improved by recording SCC data from both before and after CM. In this chapter, the linear score (LS) is used, but raw SCC counts could be used. Following convention of most DHI processors, LS greater than 4 or SCC of 200,000 cells/mL represents likely SM. For the plan presented here, the following pieces of SM information should be entered: (1) pre-mastitis LS; (2) post-mastitis LS; and (3) an SM remark as described next.

Pre-mastitis LS refers to the Dairy Herd Improvement (DHI) test before a case of CM and in most herds can be captured automatically through data downloads or manually by reviewing monthly DHI SCC records. Recording test day LS for the cow 30 to 60 and 60 to 90 days post CM is also useful. Because test days are not always evenly spaced, there will be no data for some cows. A specifically defined time reference after mastitis is more logical than recording the first and second tests after mastitis, and enough cows will fit into the time windows to assess outcomes on subclinical status for representative subsets of clinical cases.[13] The pre-mastitis SCC

ID	LACT	DIM	SCREM	CULTR	DSMST	PRMLG	MASRM	TMAST	MASRB	MINT
1	1	39	STRLFRRP	-	0	0	-	0	-	
2	1	21	STRLFLRP	-	0	0	-	0	-	
3	2	97	-	-	0	1.9	SELRS5	1	-	
4	2	29	-	STREP	0	9.3	MILRRFNT	2	MORFS3	11
5	1	237	-	STREP	1	2.4	MOLRS5	1	-	
6	3	106	-	G-ECO	2	6.6	MOLFRFS5	2	MORFS3	27
7	2	390	-	G-	2	3.2	SERRS5	3	MIALLNT	41
8	3	161	-	STREP	3	8.1	MILRS5	1	-	
9	1	239	-	G-/STAPH	3	7.9	SEALLS3	1	-	
10	1	299	-	G-/STAPH	4	1.5	SELFS3	1	-	
11	1	314	-	NG	6	6.1	MIALLNT	3	MILFRFNT	34
12	1	137	-	G-	8	0.4	SEALLS3	1	-	
13	4	294	-	G-K	11	2.0	SELRS3	1	-	
14	2	121	-	STREP/G-	13	7.7	MOLFS5	2	SEALLS5	21
15	1	324	-	STAPH	16	6.9	MIRRNT	2	MIRRNT	162

Fig. 2. Cow-side report produced with DC305 of cows currently under treatment organized by days since mastitis so information important for making the treatment decision is cow-side and information about severity, quarter, and protocol are available for monitoring convalescence. CULTR, remark of culture for cases of clinical mastitis (eg, STREP = streptococci, G– = gram-negative bacteria, NG = no growth); DIM, days in milk; DSMST, days since clinical mastitis; ID, identity; LACT, lactation number (parity); MASRB, remark of previous case of clinical mastitis (moderate (MO) clinical mastitis of the right front (RF), treated with Spectramast); MASRM, remark of current clinical mastitis case (eg, cow 3 had severe [SE] clinical mastitis affecting the left rear [LR] treated with Spectramast [S] for 5 days [5]); MINT, interval between the 2 cases of clinical mastitis (11 days); PRMLG, pre-mastitis linear score; SCREM, remark of SCC work (eg, STRLFRRP = *Streptococcus* spp cultured from the left front and right rear quarters treated with Pirsue); TMAST, number of clinical mastitis cases in current lactation (2 cases for cow 4).

information is an indicator of likelihood of a successful post-treatment outcome and is a significant piece of information when making the treatment decision for cows that have a high SCC before treating.

Cows diagnosed with SM may also be examined to determine the quarter involved and be cultured to identify the pathogen, and a decision is made to prescribe a treatment protocol that may or not include the use of intramammary antimicrobial treatment. Therefore, a separate event (ie, SCCWORK) can be created for recording SM data using the same intent as is used for recording data for CM. Capturing 3 distinct types of data (the culture result, affected quarter, and treatment) for SM completes the SM data and allows the use of both clinical and subclinical data when making herd and individual cow management decisions.

Mastitis Exit Remark

There is an opportunity at the completion of the CM case to add post-mastitis information to the cow's permanent record containing information to be used for assessing outcomes and accountability of withdrawal compliance. In the reports (eg, Fig. 3) presented as examples for management of CM on a dairy, the number of days out of the tank (days of milk discard due to CM) is used to demonstrate the entry of post-mastitis data. Of all the possibilities of information that could be gathered at the end of a treatment, days out of the tank is one of the most valuable for managing the economics of mastitis therapy and the flow of cows through the treatment pen.[4,12] Recording days out of the tank raises awareness, which potentially leads to the management of this key data point. It is important to note that data entry is a continually evolving process; whatever is considered valuable for managing mastitis should be considered and can be added to the records plan.

ID	LACT	DIM	SCCTX	SCREM	MASTX	CULTR	MASRM		PRMLG	LGSCC	MILK	RPRO	DOOT
1	1	421			365	G-	MIRF	NT	0.4	6.8	86	NO BRED	3
2	3	210	4	ALLPIRSU	168	G-/STAPH	MORF	NT	3.8	5.4	87	NO BRED	7
3	5	68	2	ALLS	15	STREP	MIRR	NT	0	2.5	95	FRESH	9
4	3	49	26	STRNT	4	-	MI	NT	0	3.8	113	FRESH	1
5	7	199			156	STREP	SERFLFSP		6.5	2.8	115	OK/OPEN	10
6	2	85			55	G-K	SERRLRSP		1.8	6.2	97	BRED	6
7	2	96			42	NG	SERR	SP	0.2	1.8	104	BRED	6
8	1	174	3	PIRSUELR	134	STAPH/G-	MORR	SP	4.8	5.3	99	BRED	6
9	2	125	3	LRPIRSUE	69	NG	MILR	NT	0.1	5.1	119	BRED	3
10	1	325	3	PIRSRRRF	287	-	BLOODY		0.4	1.1	88	PREG	2
11	1	301			258	STAPH	MILF	NT	2.8	2.0	65	PREG	2
12	1	173			115	STREP	MILFLRSP		2.0	2.9	67	PREG	10
13	5	175			132	STREP	SEALL	SP	0.7	7.0	95	PREG	8
14	1	289			249	G-	SERF	SP	0.9	3.1	66	PREG	8
15	1	303			290	G-	MIALL	NT	4.6	0	0	DRY	3
16	1	304			258	G-	SELF	SP	1.0	1.5	47	DRY	6
17	2	295			278	G-/STREP	MILF	NT	4.9	0	0	DRY	3
18	2	289			276	G-STAPH	SEALL	SP	5.5	0	0	DRY	6
19	4	238			210	STREP	MIALL	NT	7.7	8.4	69	SLD/DIE	6
20	3	225			197	STREP	MIRF	NT	7.1	7.8	64	SLD/DIE	6

Fig. 3. A list of cows that had their first case of mastitis (number of cases desired to review determines the period of time) and are presented to monitor for changes in pattern, oversight of drug use, and individual cows of concern. The cohort shown is 20 primary cases that were used to monitor the epidemiology pattern of cases by age, stage of lactation at first case, cause, subclinical history, and severity. The flow of cows through the treatment pen is assessed as days out of tank. CULTR, remark of culture for cases of clinical mastitis (a gram-negative bacterial species was cultured from cow 1); DIM, days in milk; DOOT, days out of tank (days of milk discard); ID, identity; LACT, lactation number (parity); LGSCC, current linear score (cow 1 is currently at 6.8 linear score); MASRM, remark of current clinical mastitis case (cow 1 had a mild case of right rear and received no antibiotics); MASTX, DIM at first case of clinical mastitis in current lactation (cow 1 had the first case at 365 DIM); MILK, current milk production; PRMLG, pre-mastitis linear score (pre-mastitis linear score of cow 1 was 0.4); RPRO, breeding group; SCCTX, days in milk at SCCWORK; SCREM, remark of SCC work (eg, all quarters of cow 2 were subclinically infected and were treated with Pirsue at 4 days in milk).

CLINICAL MASTITIS

While the SOP and written treatment plans are reference documents created and revised periodically in collaboration with veterinarians, the use of CM records is a dynamic system actively used on the farm. The CM records plan described here (**Fig. 4**) consists of cow-side and herd-level reports, which can be used to develop a medical history for the cow at the time of CM examination, provide information used to monitor the progress of CM cases (eg, evolution of clinical signs), allow efficient supervision of ongoing cases by veterinarians, and eventually generate permanent information at the herd-level.

Cow-Side Reports for Cases of Clinical Mastitis

It is well documented that several factors are associated with the efficacy of CM antibiotic therapy. Cow factors associated with treatment efficacy include age (parity), stage of lactation, effectiveness of the cow's immune response, SCC, number of infected quarters, chronicity of infection, and severity of the case.[12,14,15] Pathogen factors include inherent characteristics of the pathogen, duration of infection, and pathogen response to antimicrobial therapy.[14,15] As part of a mastitis records plan, 2 cow-side reports can be used to manage current cases of CM: (1) cow-side recording form (see **Fig. 1**), which serves as an aid and reminder for the examination and recording policies, and (2) cow-side report (see **Fig. 2**), which includes cows undergoing CM and contains critical medical history for the treatment decision and convalescent monitoring of the cows.

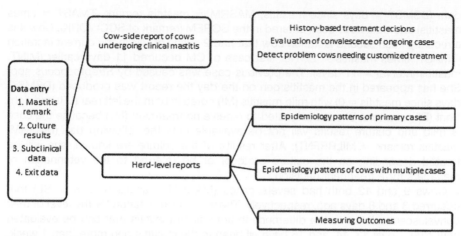

Fig. 4. Organization of a clinical mastitis records plan.

An examination of CM cases for severity, detection of any additional subclinically infected quarters (ie, using the California Mastitis Test), culturing of milk to diagnose the pathogen involved, and using the cows' records allows an informed treatment decision to be made. The objective is for farm workers to astutely recognize symptoms that will lead to a defined treatment protocol or identify information that can be used to qualify risk of treatment failure. The recording form (see **Fig. 1**) is a strategy to ensure that important information is added to the permanent record of a cow using a predictable format.

Fig. 2 is a management list of treated cows sorted by days since CM was diagnosed. This list demonstrates a method of presenting significant information captured by the cow-side examination integrated with known risk factors for potential treatment failure. The report includes a cow identification (ID), parity (LACT), stage of lactation (DIM), SM data (SCREM = remark from subclinical work; PRMLG = pre-mastitis LS), culture results (CULTR = remark of culture entry), information about CM (DSMST = days since mastitis; MINT = interval between cases; TMAST = times mastitis), the mastitis remark (MASRM; with severity, quarter, and treatment information), and information about previous cases of CM (MASRB = previous mastitis remark). Treatment decisions can now be much more informed and protocols can be based on culture results and historical information.

The cow-side report is organized by number of days since mastitis was detected, and it can also be used for monitoring convalescent progress. Convalescence can be monitored relative to expected response for each cow given her own previous medical history. Treatment failures can be detected and farm personnel can provide oversight of all cows currently receiving therapy. Compliance with SOP and protocols can be determined. The data selected for the report present the udder health history of individual cows by integrating current and past data about CM and SM. The report can also be customized for individual farms to include other relevant information such as production and fertility data.

For example, cows 1 and 2 (see **Fig. 2**) are fresh first lactation heifers selected for subclinical treatment for an intramammary infection caused by *Streptococcus* spp (as noted by the SCC work remark, please see legend in **Fig. 2**). The subclinical nature of the infection can be determined because there are no data in the fields that record CM data (DSMST = days since mastitis, MASRM = mastitis remark, TMAST = times mastitis) and data have been entered in the SCREM (remark of SCCWORK). Cow 4 is a recently fresh second lactation cow that had 2 cases of CM in the current lactation (TMAST, times mastitis = 2). Her first case of CM occurred 11 days earlier (MINT, mastitis interval = 11 days). The previous case was caused by *Streptococcus* spp. She has appeared in the mastitis pen on the day the report was produced (DSMST, days since mastitis = 0) with mild mastitis (MI) noted in both the left rear (LR) and right front (RF) quarters. She is designated to receive no treatment (NT) because the case is mild and culture results will not be available until the following day (MASRM, mastitis remark = MILRRFNT). After results of the culture are known, she will be treated depending on the culture protocol or be referred to the veterinarian or managers for a treatment decision.

Cows 9 and 12 both had severe cases (MASRM, mastitis remark = SE) that occurred 3 and 8 days ago, respectively. There is an expectation for the level of their convalescent relative to the difference in time since mastitis that can be evaluated cow-side. Cows 13, 14, and 15 have all been in the mastitis pen more than 1 week, which is unexpected and should be investigated.

The generation of this type of report allows efficient and timely oversight of the hospital group, which leads to hands-on timely training that can be appropriately targeted for individual farm circumstances. The report helps prioritize management decisions in that cows in need of a treatment decision are listed first.

Herd-Level Reports for Interpretation of Epidemiology, Compliance, and Evaluation of Effectiveness of the Mastitis Plan

The information used by farm personnel for making treatment decisions can be collated into herd-level reports for defined cohorts of cows to monitor and manage mastitis. **Figs. 3**, **5**, and **6** demonstrate the generation of reports for specific cohorts

ID	LACT	CULTR	PRMLG	MASRM		MASRB		TMAST	MINT	MILK	RPRO
1	5	G-/STAPH	8.7	MIALL	NT	MIRR	S5	2	221	26	PREG
2	2	STREP/G-	7.3	MIALL	NT	MIALL	S5	3	27	98	PREG
3	1	G-/STAPH	2.2	MILF	NT	MORR	S3	2	65	58	PREG
4	6	NG	6.0	MILF	NT	MOLRLFS3		3	37	77	NO BRED
5	3	G-	9.2	MILF	NT	SERR	S5	2	193	71	NO BRED
6	1	NG	8.8	MILR	P5	MILR	NT	2	50	71	BRED
7	4	NG	4.4	MILR	NT	MOALL	S3	4	25	78	NO BRED
8	3	NG	1.3	MIRF	NT	MILRRFNT		2	26	101	PREG
9	1	NG	4.6	MIRF	S3	MORF	S3	2	26	64	PREG
10	4	NG	5.8	MIRR	NT	MILR	NT	2	62	126	OK/OPEN
11	1	G-/STREP	2.8	MIRR	SP	MIRR	NT	2	107	73	PREG
12	3	G-	3.8	MOALL	S5	MIRFRRNT		2	34		DRY
13	4	G-		MOALL	S3	MIRR	NT	4	15	74	NO BRED
14	2	STREP	8.2	MOLRRRS3		MILR	NT	2	32	74	NO BRED
15	2	NG		MORF	S5	MIRF	NT	4	25	111	BRED
16	1	STAPH/G-	3.1	MORR	S3	MIRR	S3	2	89	103	BRED
17	2	G-	2.6	MORR	S3	SELR	S3	2	67		DRY
18	1	NG	2.4	SEALL	S3	MIRR	NT	3	13	65	NO BRED
19	1	NG		MYCO+		MOALL	S3	2	14	88	SLD/DIE
20	2	G-	4.0	SERFLRS		MOLRLFS3		2	144	49	SLD/DIE

Fig. 5. Cows that have had multiple cases of clinical mastitis this lactation (number of cases desired to review determines the period of time). Epidemiology by age, stage, cause, subclinical history, and clinical history for the group can be assessed. An individual cow history can be read in the rows and the indices viewed in the columns. Cows defined as relapsed can be considered for management recommendations. The inclusion of remarks for the previous (MASRB) and current (MASRM) cases of clinical mastitis allows comparisons of severity, quarters affected, and treatment choice for consecutive cases. For other abbreviations, refer to **Fig. 3**.

ID	LACT	TMAST	DOOT	MASRM		MASRB		Quart	MINT	PRMLG	POML1	POML2	SCURM
====	=====	======	=====	======	===	======	===	======	=====	======	======	======	=====
1	1	2	20	SERFRRTO		MILF	NT	DIFF	42	1.0	2.1	2.5	CURE
2	1	2	1	MILR	NT	MIRR	NT	DIFF	23	2.0	3.7	3.1	CURE
3	1	2	4	MILF	NT	MIRR	NT	DIFF	43	3.0	4.4	5.9	FAIL
4	1	2	13	MORR	SP	SELRLFSP		DIFF	32	3.8	4.4	1.5	CURE
5	1	2	7	MORR	SP	MOLR	SP	DIFF	24	7.0	4.1	2.8	CURE
6	1	2	8	MORF	SP	SC ALL		SAME	117	1.9	1.1	1.1	CURE
7	3	2	8	MOALL	SP	MIRRRFNT		SAME	77	3.4	2.0	1.1	CURE
8	1	2	1	MIRR	NT	MIRR	NT	SAME	34	4.2	4.8	4.5	FAIL
9	3	2	2	MIRF	NT	MIRF	PI	SAME	156	4.5	6.4	4.8	FAIL
10	2	3	5	MIRR	SP	MIRR	NT	SAME	42	4.5	4.0	2.4	CURE
11	3	2	5	MOLF	SP	MOLF	SP	SAME	41	4.9	1.2	1.8	CURE
12	1	4	8	MILF	SP	MILRLFSP		SAME	86	6.1	4.7	8.6	FAIL
13	1	2	8	MILR	NT	MOLR	SP	SAME	32	6.6	6.4	6.4	FAIL
14	1	2	5	MILR	NT	MORRLRSP		SAME	40	7.4	7.5	5.3	FAIL
15	4	2	7	MORR	SP	MORR	PI	SAME	90	8.2	3.3	3.8	CURE
16	4	2	7	MOLRLFSP		MOLF	SP	SAME	46	0	4.1	4.7	FAIL
17	1	2	1	MILF	NT	MILF	NT	SAME	23	0	2.3	7.4	CURE
18	1	3	3	MIALL	NT	MIRRLRSP		SAME	29	0	4.5	5.3	FAIL
19	1	2	9	MORR	SP	MIRR	NT	SAME	19	0	2.6	2.5	CURE

Fig. 6. Subset of cows that had multiple cases of clinical mastitis and are still in the herd for measuring the treatment outcomes of days out of tank, proportion of relapses, and SCC response (cure = either post-mastitis linear score <4.14). For abbreviations, refer to **Fig. 3**. POML1, linear score 30 to 60 days post-mastitis; POML2, linear score 60 to 90 days post-mastitis; PRMLG, pre-mastitis linear score. Quart is an indication if the subsequent clinical case occurred on the same or different quarters. SCURM is a stored indication of cure or fail to cure (based on measuring SCC post-mastitis).

of animals and are useful for managing herd health, and for evaluation of treatment protocols, environmental risk factors, and milking performance.

The structure for each report is similar in that individual animals in the cohort are listed. The items included in each report are relevant information that can be used for either oversight of previously treated cows or allow for monitoring performance indexes of the group. The reports can be evaluated relative to CM SOP to determine compliance with protocols. Animals that do not appear to be progressing can be detected and identified for reexamination. The reports integrate information from cases of both SM and CM and other useful productive indexes of the cows such as fertility status and production. Cohorts can be defined by the specific interest groups of cows (eg, parity, level of milk production, and pathogen). The history of each animal is included and the data can be sorted or exported to spreadsheets (such as Excel; Windows) for determination of KPIs. It is important to note that the KPIs used are generally farm-specific and depend on the milk quality goals of the mastitis control program. General KPIs for controlling SM and CM have been described elsewhere.[16]

Cohort of First Cases of Clinical Mastitis

A cohort of cows with their first case of CM (in the current lactation) in a predetermined time window is demonstrated in **Fig. 3**. Review of individual animals included in this report allows the detection of cows that need reevaluation, but the primary purpose of this report is to monitor the epidemiology of first cases. The time period used should be determined by herd size so that an adequate numbers of cases are presented to result in a large enough number of cases to have confidence that the proportions are representative of the current situation. The data can be exported and summarized to compare KPI with herd and industry benchmarks. This report summarizes the following specific data:

- *Parity (LACT):* Parity is a proxy for age and has been considered an important factor associated with the incidence of CM[10,11] and also the likelihood of a successful outcome for CM.[12]
- *Stage of lactation (DIM):* Identifies high-risk periods for infection and gives guidance relative to therapeutic decisions.
- Pathogen (CULTR = remark of last mastitis culture): Knowledge about the proportions of specific pathogens responsible for cases is used in developing and modifying protocol decisions, prevention strategies, biosecurity plans, and our expectations about outcomes from current treatments.
- *SM data* (SCCTX = days in milk at subclinical work; SCREM = remark from subclinical work) are present in order to have culture and quarter information from previous subclinical work available with the CM data.
- *Severity* (MASRM = mastitis remark includes severity): the distribution of severity has value in monitoring pathogen shifts in virulence and types. For example, for a herd where most cases are caused by gram-negative pathogens, a greater proportion of severe cases are expected. Proportions of mild cases also have value in assessing the competency of detecting mild cases at milk harvest and the attitude by either parlor or management personnel toward treatment of mild cases.
- *Additional CM data* (MASTX = days in milk at first case, and PRMLG = pre-mastitis LS) are important information about the pattern of cases detected on the dairy.
- *Subclinical history:* CM and SM should be integrated into our mastitis management plan. The presence of endemic pathogens, the detection plan for CM, and the relationship between CM and SM are all significant for interpreting the SM history on a dairy. These data are also valuable as an indicator for the expectation of successful resolution of CM.[13]

As epidemiology patterns change with time, the decision to further investigate or modify the SOP or protocols can be considered. In the field, we are responsible for managing the ever changing balance between cows, the environment, the pathogens, the facility, the management practices in place, and the application of those to animals. The most accurate understanding of the interplay between all these comes from understanding accurate cow data. Production medicine is really understanding clinical medicine and then using the recordings of health events to interpret the application of management practices to achieve the intent of the care package offered by the dairy. The SOP for handling a case on the dairy (detection, examination, treatment decision, assessment of convalescence, and completion) can be monitored within the records gathered. The compliance and competency for carrying out the written protocol can be monitored and the accountability of appropriate usage is within the recordings from each cohort.

The report shown in **Fig. 3** lists 20 cows out the cohort of cows with their primary case. Cow 3 demonstrates noncompliance with farm protocols since the milk culture results was *Streptococcus* spp (remark of culture, CULTR = STREP) while no treatment was given (contrary to the written protocol for this farm). In this case, the treatment decision for cow 3 can be considered as a teachable moment for the veterinarian. Identification of protocol drift indicates that either a mistake has occurred (which merely needs to be discussed) or there is dissatisfaction by personnel with the protocol (which needs to be investigated). Cows 4 and 5 are high producing cows (milk = 113 and 115 lb, respectively) and may require special interventions to ensure that the rest of the lactation is not affected by mastitis or by treatments.

Cows 14, 16, and 18 are all late lactation cows with severe CM caused by gram-negative pathogens (remark of culture, CULTR = G–). This history should be reviewed when these cows freshen again so that poor early lactation production is not erroneously attributed to other risk factors such as the transition program.

Cohort of Cows That Have Had Multiple Cases of Clinical Mastitis in the Current Lactation

A cohort of 20 cows with multiple cases of CM (in the current lactation) is demonstrated in **Fig. 5**. Monitoring the epidemiology of multiple cases is possible as was done with the cohort of primary cases, but the primary purpose here is to review of individual animal to detect of cows that need a management decision.

A relapse has been defined by researchers as a subsequent case of CM within a broad range of time intervals (8–90 days after the previous case) that occurs in the same cow, or the same quarter, or caused by the same pathogen.[17–19] For practical purposes, producers often define relapses as repeated cases in the same cow, regardless of quarter or pathogen. As veterinarians serving a dairy, this cohort of cows with multiple cases can be monitored for recognizable subsets needing a management recommendation.

Any information considered valuable by management for either evaluating an individual cow or monitoring for manageable subsets can be included. In **Fig. 5**, the ID, age as lactation number, DIM, PRMLG, MASRM, MASRB, TMAST, MINT, and MILK (current production) are shown.

Notice the number of cases that were mild (MASRM = MI) that are no treatment decisions (MASRM = NT) and the 3 cows that have had mastitis 4 times (cows 7, 13, and 15). Two of them have been removed from the breeding pool (cows 7 and 13), and cow 15 has been bred and her fourth case of mastitis was treated. These kinds of individual cow management decisions can be made when adequate history is present and used.

Using Records to Evaluate Treatment Outcomes

Monitoring outcomes is essential for assessing the efficacy of antibiotic therapy and for economical evaluation of the treatment program. The short-term aim of most dairy producers who treat mild or moderate CM is to return the appearance of milk to normal so that it can be legally sold. In addition to clinical cure, different indicators of therapeutic efficacy are used. Short-term indicators of efficacy include bacteriologic cure and number of days milk is not saleable (days out of tank).[20,21] Long-term outcomes have also been evaluated and include CM relapses, post-treatment SCC, milk production, and the time interval between CM and death or removal from the herd.[17–19]

Data from farm records have been the cornerstone for making treatment decisions, assessing convalescence, evaluating the epidemiology of the primary cases, and monitoring for subsets of cows that have had multiple cases requiring management intervention. The records can also be used to measure outcomes of the treatments. When data entry has been sufficient (as described earlier), analysis for 4 outcomes can be performed: (1) average days out of tank, (2) proportion of cows with multiple cases, (3) SCC levels post-mastitis, and (4) retention in the herd after mastitis.

Fig. 6 demonstrates a report that has been generated to measure treatment outcomes. This report has been generated for cows that had multiple cases of CM, but the same report can be generated for other cohorts of interest such as cows that did not receive antibiotics, cows with specific severity scores (such as severe cases), cases of CM caused by a specific pathogen, or cows sold within 60 days of the case.

The oversight of the cows currently under treatment and monitoring of cows with recent primary or multiple cases has allowed watching outcomes as they occurred. The recording system has the data stored for analysis of the outcomes for the variety of subsets of mastitis that may be of interest on a specific dairy. Expectations of achieving KPI goals and level of successful outcomes all need to be specific for a dairy and depend on management decisions.

Reduction of SCC is an indication of bacteriologic cure and is a desirable post-treatment outcome. Reduction of SCC can be defined based on either of the 2 post-CM DHI tests in the 30-to-60 or 60-to-90 day window being less than 200,000 (failure can be defined as neither test being <200,000 cells/mL).[13] SCC reduction has been associated with age, pathogen, pre-mastitis SCC, and stage of lactation.[13] Summarizing KPIs from multiple herds has value, but the individual herd needs to have their own goals planned based on management practices that impact them and use the herd's own pattern of KPIs to measure them through the records.

From **Fig. 6** we can see that as a group we have an acceptable proportion of satisfactory SCC levels after mastitis for this most troublesome cohort (11 of 19 had at least 1 of 2 SCC counts <200,000 cells/mL post-mastitis). Cows 2 and 3 are both first calf heifers whose CM examinations called for no treatment. SCC for cow 2 was less than 200,000 post-mastitis, but greater than 200,000 cells/mL for cow 3. It would be logical to reexamine cow 3 to determine if therapeutic intervention should be considered. Cow 11 is an example of a cow that experienced a desirable SCC reduction post-mastitis.

Occurrence of SM and CM are well known to increase the likelihood of culling. In a study including herds in New York, cows diagnosed with CM caused by environmental mastitis pathogens were 5 times more likely to be culled as were uninfected cows.[22] Thus, retention in the herd after mastitis has been used as a measurable mastitis outcome.[12]

Days out of tank measures the number of days that milk is not saleable and has to be diverted from the bulk tank, and this is one of the main sources of economic losses attributable to CM.[3] This period of milk discard may include the number of days milk has an abnormal appearance but has not been treated with antimicrobials and the number of days that cows were treated with antimicrobials, in addition to the withholding period of the specific drug. It can be seen in **Fig. 6** that cows 1 and 4 remained for long periods in the hospital pen (20 and 13 days of milk discard, respectively), but most cows had expected periods of milk discard for the farm.

SUBCLINICAL MASTITIS

SM is the most prevalent disease on most dairies, is often undetected unless individual cows are specifically screened, and has the greatest economic consequence because of long term reduction in milk yield.[3,4] Detection of cows with SM is dependent on the use of individual cow SCC testing. If individual cow SCC testing is not performed, this disease cannot be appropriately managed. For many larger herds, SM is detected when new SCC data are downloaded after monthly DHI tests. Many DHI centers provide comprehensive reports that focus on analysis of SCC data for individual cows or groups of cows. Dairy veterinarians should understand how to interpret these reports and spend part of their consultative time reviewing them with clients. When using dairy management software, individual reports that address specific characteristics of SM can be generated for each herd. The group of cows diagnosed with SM can be divided into cohorts (eg, by lactation, stage of lactation, age, and location of the dairy) that can be analyzed to diagnose mastitis problems, implement corrective actions, and assess management practices used as part of the mastitis control program. The individual cow SM plan is to identify cows appropriate for individual cow management decisions such as segregation, culling, milk culturing, and treatment.[16]

Monthly review of SCC at the cow and herd levels can be highly diagnostic for troubleshooting mastitis problems.[9,16] Analyzing monthly patterns of these selected cohorts can offer insight into areas needing investigation or management recommendations: A series of KPIs for SM (based on SCC) can be used to monitor SM.[2,9,16] Examples of such indices include (1) prevalence of SM for first lactation and older cows; (2) dynamics of intramammary infections across the dry period; (3) rate of new infections during lactation; and (4) percent of cows chronically infected.

A variety of KPIs are provided by DHI centers using test day information. SM indices can be further assessed using computer management programs to monitor subsets significant to the dairy (such as animals in a specific environment, dry cow strategy, or CM strategy). Industry-summarized KPIs are available from a variety of references and DHI associations,[9,16] but the most significant KPI is the pattern on the dairy itself. If monitoring herd KPIs is to be effective and valuable, it should stimulate actions and recommendations. We then need to monitor the results of these actions and recommendations.

Individual Cow Actions

The use of SCC records for individual cows can result in a number of actions:

- Selection of cows that can be further examined to gain additional knowledge and improve decision making when costly intervention such as treatment or culling are being considered:
  1. Use of a diagnostic test (such as California Mastitis Test) to identify affected quarters
  2. Milk culturing to identify bacteria cause
  3. Examination of teat end to evaluate physical issues
- Watching of infected cows until a more appropriate time for action
- Segregation of infected from uninfected animals when the pathogen is contagious or to reduce the risk of exposure from chronically infected to uninfected cows
- Culling or removal from the breeding pool
- Treating the bacterial infection with an antibiotic.

Just as with CM, the management decisions ultimately need to be based on an awareness of medical history, diagnostic examination, knowledge of scientific information relative to potential cure of a cow subclinically infected (either spontaneously or therapeutically), and the relative value of the individual within the herd. The cow information needs to be used in conjunction with background knowledge that is available in the cows' records.

One of the most useful applications of cow-level SCC records is the production of action lists, which allow the identification of cows to which management practices can be targeted.[2,9,16] Examples of customized lists (**Fig. 7**) are:

- List of cows chronically infected (sorted by milk production) that could be culled
- List of infected fresh heifers to identify individuals for further examination
- List of cows that were infected during the dry period or pre-test fresh period to identify causative bacteria

ID	LACT	DIM	DRYLG	MASTX	MASRM	CULTR	SCC	MILK
====	====	=====	=====	=====	========	========	======	======
1	2	21	7.6	9	MORFS5	STREP	6341	41
2	4	22	5.4	0	-	-	1150	64
3	2	26	5.1	0	-	-	2576	59
4	3	27	5.5	7	MOLRRRS5	STAPH	650	87
5	2	28	4.4	0	-	-	774	123
6	2	30	7.2	0	-	-	1871	105
7	5	35	4.5	0	-	-	3940	81

Fig. 7. Cohort of cows that had a high SCC on both the last test day of the previous lactation and the first test of the subsequent lactation listed to screen for SM cows to make a management decision. DRYLG, linear score for the last test day of the previous lactation; SCC (×1000 cells/mL) for the most current test day. For other abbreviations, refer to **Fig. 3**.

- List of cows that had high SCC on both tests across the dry period to identify cows at greater risk of CM during early lactation to determine if examination of cause would aid in a CM decision if or when they develop CM[11]
- List of open cows chronically infected to consider removal from the breeding pool.

The number of lists and qualifiers for a potential list is herd dependent based on the pattern of SM on the dairy and the size of the dairy. Also, it is important to know that the KPI determinations are based on the definition that an infected cow has SCC greater than 200,000 cells/mL (or LS >4). In the field, the qualifier for inclusion into an action list is based on the goal of the mastitis control program. Examples of KPIs for SM can be found elsewhere.[16] The size of the dairy is significant only for creating an action list of a manageable size. A 100-cow herd with 30% prevalence has 30 infected cows and a single list is not overwhelming, but in a 1000-cow dairy with the same infection rate, a single list is difficult to manage and fractionating the list into the cohorts identified earlier makes the work more manageable.

Fig. 7 is an example of the cohort of recently fresh cows that maintained high SCC during the dry period (>200,000 pre-dry and >200,000 cells/mL on the first DHI test). The list was limited to those with greater than 400,000 cells/mL (an arbitrary decision). The objective of such a cohort is to decide if they should be removed from the breeding pool, cultured to determine the causative pathogen, or considered for therapy. These are individual cow management decisions that are best made with ample individual cow history, which in this case also includes a review of the records of past lactations. **Fig. 7** demonstrates integrating CM history, SM history including last lactation, and cow information valuable for making a management decision.

SUMMARY

Developing a records plan useful for managing the complex relationships between environment, personal application of SOP, and protocols that integrates clinical and subclinical udder requires planning the data entry and data reports that interpret the herd without abandoning the individual cow. Then use the data regularly.

REFERENCES

1. Hogeveen H, Kamphuis C, Steeneveld W, et al. Sensors and clinical mastitis-the quest for the perfect alert. Sensors 2010;10:7991–8009.
2. Schukken YH, Wilson DJ, Welcome F, et al. Monitoring udder health and milk quality using somatic cell counts. Vet Res 2003;34:579–96.

3. Hortet P, Seegers H. Calculated milk production losses associated with elevated somatic cell counts in dairy cows: review and critical discussion. Vet Res 1998;29:497–510.
4. Huijps K, Lam T, Hogeveen H. Costs of mastitis: facts and perception. J Dairy Res 2008;75:113–20.
5. American Veterinary Medical Association. Principles of veterinary medical ethics of the AVMA. Available at: http://www.avma.org/issues/policy/ethics.asp#VIII. Accessed March 24, 2012.
6. Pol M, Ruegg PL. Treatment practices and quantification of antimicrobial drug usage in conventional and organic dairy farms in Wisconsin. J Dairy Sci 2007;90:249–61.
7. Wenz JR, Barrington GM, Garry FB, et al. Use of systemic disease signs to assess disease severity in dairy cows with acute coliform mastitis. J Am Vet Med Assoc 2001;218:567–72.
8. Wenz JR. Practical monitoring of clinical mastitis treatment programs. In: Proceedings of the 43rd NMC Annual Meeting. Charlotte (NC). National Mastitis Council: Verona (WI); 2004, p. 41–6.
9. Ruegg PL. Investigation of mastitis problems on farms. Vet Clin North Am Food Anim Pract 2003;19:47–73.
10. Steeneveld W, Hogeveen H, Barkema HW, et al. The influence of cow factors on the incidence of clinical mastitis in dairy cows. J Dairy Sci 2008;91:1391–402.
11. Pantoja JCF, Hulland C, Ruegg PL. Somatic cell count status across the dry period as a risk factor for the development of clinical mastitis in subsequent lactations. J Dairy Sci 2009;92:139–48.
12. Pinzón-Sánchez C, Ruegg PL. Risk factors associated with short-term post-treatment outcomes of clinical mastitis. J Dairy Sci 2011;94:3397–410.
13. Lago A, Rhoda D, Cook NB. Using DHIA recorded individual cow somatic cell counts to determine clinical mastitis treatment cure rates. In: Proceedings of the 43rd NMC Annual Meeting. Charlotte (NC). National Mastitis Council: Verona (WI); 2004, p. 290–1.
14. Constable PD, Morin DE. Treatment of clinical mastitis using antimicrobial susceptibility profiles for treatment decisions. Vet Clin North Am Large Anim Pract 2003;19:139–55.
15. Bradley AJ, Green MJ. Factors affecting cure when treating bovine clinical mastitis with cephalosporin-based intramammary preparations. J Dairy Sci 2009;92:1941–53.
16. Ruegg PL. Managing mastitis and producing quality milk. In: Risco CA, Melendez P, editors. Dairy production medicine. Hoboken (NJ): John Wiley & Sons; 2011. p. 207–32.
17. Wenz JR, Garry FB, Lombard JE, et al. Efficacy of parenteral ceftiofur for treatment of systemically mild clinical mastitis in dairy cattle. J Dairy Sci 2005;88:3496–9.
18. Schukken YH, Hertl J, Bar D, et al. Effects of repeated Gram-positive and Gram-negative clinical mastitis episodes on milk yield loss in Holstein dairy cows. J Dairy Sci 2009;92:3091–105.
19. Bar D, Gröhn YT, Bennett G, et al. Effect of repeated episodes of generic clinical mastitis on milk yield in dairy cows. J Dairy Sci 2007;90:4643–53.
20. Guterbock WM, Van Eenennaam AL, Anderson RJ, et al. Efficacy of intramammary antimicrobial therapy for treatment of clinical mastitis caused by environmental pathogens. J Dairy Sci 1993;76:3437–44.
21. Hoe FGH, Ruegg PL. Relationship between antimicrobial susceptibility of clinical mastitis pathogens and treatment outcome in cows. J Am Vet Med Assoc 2005;227:1461–8.
22. Gröhn YT, Gonzalez RN, Wilson DJ, et al. Effect of pathogen-specific clinical mastitis on herd life in two New York State dairy herds. Prev Vet Med 2005;71:105–25.

The Role of Communication in Improving Udder Health

Jolanda Jansen, MSc, PhD[a],*, Theo J.G.M. Lam, DVM, PhD[b,c]

KEYWORDS

- Udder health • Communication • Motivation • Mindset

KEY POINTS

- To be effective, a mastitis control program should do more than distributing technical information about best management practices to dairy farmers. Prevention of complex diseases such as mastitis requires customized communication strategies as well as an integrated approach.
- Two factors of farmer mindset are the most important behavioral determinants for mastitis management: believing there is a mastitis problem in the herd and belief in the effectiveness of mastitis management to solve that problem.
- Veterinary practitioners can be important intermediaries in communication about udder health, provided that they are aware of their role as advisor and apply the accompanying communication skills.
- It is important to segment communication strategies. Most farmers are interested in improving udder health if you approach them in the right way and offer the services they want.
- The most important step in creating demand for veterinary services is to offer them.

This article aims to help understanding dairy farmers' behavior and mindset regarding udder health management and to describe the efficacy of various communication strategies. Our findings are based on experience gained during the execution of a national udder health improvement program in the Netherlands. These experiences involve the relation between the farmer and the veterinary practitioner but also imply changes in the way national or regional udder health programs should be executed.

The article starts with describing farmers' mindset toward mastitis and the way it relates to farm management and mastitis incidence. Subsequently, the role of communication as an intervention instrument is evaluated, including the role of veterinary

The authors have nothing to disclose.
[a] Wageningen UR Livestock Research, PO Box 65, 8200 AB Lelystad, The Netherlands; [b] Dutch Udder Health Centre UGCN, GD Animal Health Service, PO Box 9, 7400 AA Deventer, The Netherlands; [c] Department of Farm Animal Health, Faculty of Veterinary Medicine, Utrecht University, Yalelaan 1, PO Box 80163, 3508 TD Utrecht, The Netherlands
* Corresponding author.
E-mail address: jolanda.jansen@wur.nl

practitioners (eg, veterinarians). The article concludes by summarizing the main findings in our national program and the implications for future mastitis control programs.

FARMERS' MINDSET TOWARD MASTITIS

From a historical perspective, agricultural extension specialists, researchers, and veterinarians assumed that agriculture was an activity executed by an individual farmer, based primarily on rational, technical, and economic considerations.[1,2] Although such rational choices play an important role in farm management, we have learned that farmers' decision making about mastitis management is not always clear and understandable.[3] Why some farmers, even though it would benefit their results, do not implement effective mastitis management practices is not always known,[4] but it is often assumed that, besides these deliberate rational considerations, other farmer mindset factors play a role.[1,3–14]

The farmer mindset comprises a variety of social psychology constructs such as the farmer's personality, attitudes, beliefs, values, intentions, skills, knowledge, perceived norms, and perceived self efficacy (see, eg, the Theory of Planned Behavior[15–17] and the Health Belief Model,[18–20] which are both frequently used to explain people's health behavior[21–23]). All of these factors, and probably more, comprise the "human factor," which, for the sake of convenience, is summarized as "mindset."

In an extensive study on self-reported attitudes, behavior, and mastitis incidence conducted on 336 Dutch dairy farms, it was found that mastitis can be explained to a certain extent by farmer mindset and behavior.[24] In this study, elements of farmer mindset explain 17% of the variance in clinical mastitis incidence and 47% of the variance in bulk milk somatic cell count (BMSCC), while farmers' self-reported behavior explains, respectively, 12% and 14% of the variance of these parameters. Our findings are supported by studies by Bigras-Poulin and colleagues[25] and Tarabla and Dodd[10] that also showed the effect of farmer mindset on farm performance.

For a mastitis control program, it is important to influence elements of farmer mindset in order to change farmers' management practices to improve udder health. **Fig. 1** is a visual representation of our advancing insight into the relationship between a mastitis control program and the udder health status on a farm, and it explains why only a part of the variance in udder health can be explained by surveys and models.[24] The figure shows that a mastitis control program can affect elements of farmer mindset and therefore behavior and udder health. It also shows that institutional factors, such as

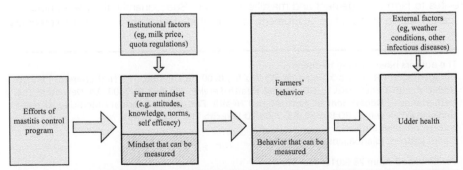

Fig. 1. Advancing insight into the potential efficacy of mastitis control programs to improve udder health and the limitations of evaluative surveys.

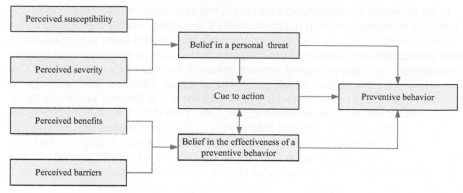

Fig. 2. The Health Belief Model.

quota regulations, influence farmers' decision making. Additionally, external factors, such as hot and humid weather, have a direct effect on udder health. This makes it difficult to explain 100% of the variance in udder health between herds. Although feedback loops are not shown in this figure, it should be taken into account that the past udder health status and external factors also affect farmer mindset and behavior.

Based on the results of our studies,[24,26–29] 2 factors of farmer mindset seem to be the most important behavioral determinants for mastitis management: belief in a personal health threat (influenced by perceived susceptibility to, and perceived severity of, mastitis problems) and belief in the effectiveness of mastitis management (influenced by perceived benefits from, and perceived barriers to, execution of mastitis management). Interestingly, these factors are also known to be indispensable in motivating people to work on their own health and are included in the so-called Health Belief Model, as presented in **Fig. 2**.[18–20,30,31]

The mechanisms behind the Health Belief Model correspond to important behavioral determinants such as attitudes, norms, and perceived self-efficacy from the Theory of Planned Behavior[15–17,19,20] and seem to apply to mastitis management as well. For example, farmers who think that their herd will not have big problems (their herd is "not susceptible") or who think that mastitis is not a severe animal health or economic problem do not think of mastitis as a "personal threat" and probably are less motivated to change their mastitis management. In addition, if required mastitis management measures are perceived as difficult or as hardly resulting in animal health or economic benefit, farmers may not be motivated to change their mastitis management either.[32–34]

Perceived threat and perceived effectiveness were found to be important parts of farmer mindset regarding mastitis management. Regarding the perceived threat of mastitis problems, the normative frame of reference (ie, When is mastitis a problem?) varies among farmers, is associated with farmers' interest in working on mastitis, and explains a substantial part of the variance in mastitis incidence.[24] Farmers' perception on the effectiveness of management measures is strongly associated with mastitis incidence.[24] Additionally, it was shown that farmers' interest in mastitis prevention is associated with the expected efficacy of recommended management tools in improving udder health.[26] Jansen and colleagues[27] showed that nonmotivated farmers either believe that the mastitis problem is not serious enough or are not convinced of the efficacy of the proposed management measures on their farms.

In 32 extended semistructured interviews, the relevance of the constructs of the Health Belief Model in relation to farmer mindset regarding mastitis management was further explored.[28] During the interview, farmers were asked open questions about their perceptions on mastitis and their reasons for working or not working on mastitis management, in order to explore farmers' reasons for improving udder health. The interviews were transcribed in full and were analyzed following the Health Belief Model.[18] The results are presented in **Fig. 3** and show that farmers' perceived threat and perceived efficacy of recommended measures indeed are the main arguments for working or not working on mastitis management. This corresponds with findings on farmers' entrepreneurial behavior change in general[35] and with findings on farmers' response to information on economic losses associated with BMSCC levels.[36] It is important to note that farmers perceive clinical mastitis and subclinical mastitis as 2 different problems associated with different management measures.[24]

The results of the 32 interviews presented in **Fig. 3** suggest that farmers have ambivalent perceptions toward their intention to work on udder health and their actual behavior. It seems that some farmers are in a state of cognitive dissonance[37,38] and use several social-psychological coping strategies to reduce the dissonance between their perceptions and their actual behavior.[39] For example, the interviewed farmers proposed many internal barriers (eg, lack of time or disruption of established routines) and external barriers (eg, limitations of the current housing, lack of support) to defend why they are not doing what they ought to do. These proposed barriers match with barriers to the implementation of zoonotic control programs.[40] Interestingly, when a farmer perceives serious mastitis problems, general measures to improve udder health will be implemented and thus, at the herd level, are used mostly curatively rather than preventively. This implies that when the problem is perceived as important enough, the benefits outweigh the barriers.

Although the interviewed farmers in this study voice a strong demand for simple, short-term, effective solutions, they know that mastitis is a multifactorial and complex disease and that a simple panacea does not exist.[41] This seems to reinforce farmers' beliefs that preventive measures are neither effective nor practical. This perception is one of the main reasons why recommended measures are not always adopted.[34,42–44]

Message for the veterinary practitioner:

- When farmers do not believe in the solution offered, the problem itself is less relevant.
- When farmers don't think they have a problem, the solution offered is not relevant.

Stop telling farmers they have a problem when they do not believe in the offered solutions or are not able to execute them. Try to focus perceived benefits and remove or reduce barriers. To be able to do that, you need to know what benefits and barriers a farmer perceives. Thus, ask questions like 'What is your goal, when will you be satisfied?', 'What do you like about this measure?', 'What stops you from implementing this?'

COMMUNICATION STRATEGIES AS INTERVENTION INSTRUMENT

The Dutch Udder Health Centre (Uier Gezondheids Centrum Nederland [UGCN]) was established to improve udder health in the Netherlands. In the national mastitis control program, several communication strategies were used to change farmers' behavior. In a study in which we evaluated the effect of the program on farmer mindset,[29] we found that elements of farmer mindset did change during the course of the program.

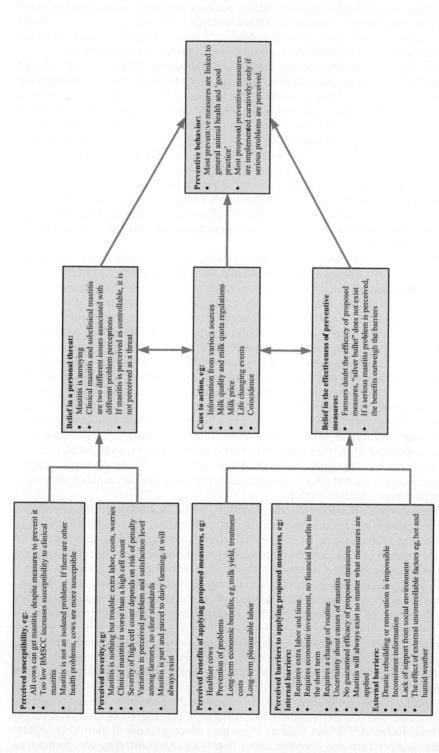

Fig. 3. Dairy farmers' perceptions toward management measures to improve udder health, based on analyses of 32 in-depth interviews by applying constructs of the Health Belief Model.

In particular, it seems that important factors such as perceived threat and perceived efficacy of management measures changed favorably. This is important because, as stated earlier, normative values and self-efficacy are strongly associated with the actual BMSCC[24] and influence farms' udder health status in the long term.

In relation to the efficacy of the various communication strategies, our findings suggest that, in order to reach as much farmers as possible, various strategies need to be deployed.[26,27,45,46] We evaluated 2 strategies[26] that are potentially effective in reaching dairy farmers and changing their behavior using the Elaboration Likelihood Model.[47,48] The effect of the traditional central route, which uses comprehensive, rational, science-based educational tools in, for example, study group settings, is highly dependent on farmers' internal motivation to decrease mastitis.[47,48] Our findings show that farmers' familiarity with the tools and their interest in using the tools are associated with aspects of farmer mindset, such as the perceived importance of improving udder health and the perceived economic benefits of udder health improvement.[26] This suggests that for farmers who are less internally motivated, such communication strategies are less effective and other ways to reach these farmers need to be explored.

Peripheral communication strategies, as used in the milking glove campaign, without using science-based argumentation, were found to be useful.[26] For this strategy to be successful, farmers' internal motivation is a less important prerequisite.[47,48] It was shown that a relatively short peripheral campaign on a single management practice can be quite effective in changing farmers' behavior. The results show that not only the use of milking gloves changed from 21% to 42%, but also the opinion of farmers about the usefulness of wearing milking gloves changed, even though no such arguments were employed in the campaign.[26] In contrast to the central route, communication using peripheral change is generally considered to be temporary, susceptible to counter persuasion, and unable to predict future behavior.[48] Surprisingly, this was not the case for the milking glove campaign. Even though there was a stronger effect on attitudes right after the campaign, the use of milking gloves increased further after the end of the initial campaign. A substantial and increasing number of farmers continued to buy milking gloves, even when extrinsic cues such as free samples were no longer present.[26] These findings suggest internalization of new behavior is possible as a profound and sustainable effect of a peripheral communication strategy.

Using peripheral communication strategies,[47,48] multifaceted goals of decreasing a complex disease like mastitis will not be met in the short term.[49] However, single management practices (eg, wearing milking gloves during milking) and short-term behavior change can be communicated using a peripheral route, because they are more easily adopted than a combination of multiple actions to achieve a certain goal.[49] Thus, a step-by-step approach to changing farm management using peripheral communication strategies can be effective. It should be taken into account that ongoing efforts of our national mastitis control program, including central route communication strategies such as the development of educational tools and the implementation of study groups, created a basic awareness among farmers. This may have resulted in an increased efficacy of the peripheral campaigns and suggests that a combination of both peripheral and central communication strategies is most beneficial.

Obviously, not all farmers are reached in udder health programs. We described the results of in-depth interviews with farmers who were considered by their veterinarian to be hard-to-reach.[27] Those findings show that although most of them do consider mastitis as a problem and perceive udder health as important, they vary in the way they use information sources and approach mastitis on their farms. These farmers do not perceive a lack of information on mastitis and they do not have more mastitis problems than other Dutch dairy farmers, which contrasts with veterinarians' perceptions.[27] It appears that one specific characterization of a hard-to-reach farmer cannot be made; it was found to be a heterogeneous group. These farmers differ in the way they trust external information and the way they are open toward information from the outside world. Like every farmer, they are part of a social network and receive information from different sources. Thus, it should be possible to reach them through these channels via, for example, local events, coaching by trusted persons, or articles published in farm journals. However, whether they will apply the available information depends on their mindset and the way that their mindset is affected by these strategies.[27]

The provided information has to be considered as relevant by farmers in order for them to process and apply it.[50] If farmers have aspirations other than improving udder health, they may not be interested in reading the message in the first place. One should also take into account that changes in farm management entail a long-term process and are much influenced by contextual and institutional factors[1] such as milk price, quota regulations, or other infectious disease outbreaks. Fluctuating milk prices and uncertainty about quota regulations probably influence farmer mindset (see **Fig. 1**) and act as cues for action (see **Fig. 3**). Milk quota utilization, for example, has been described in several countries as an important factor in farmers' decision making regarding the treatment of mastitis.[3] If, instead of mastitis, other issues are the focus of an advice, farmers may be more motivated to adopt a certain desired management practice, because the information may relate better to their needs, goals, and demands.[51] Thus, there are several reasons mastitis does not necessarily need to be the point of departure for communication strategies to improve udder health.

Message for the veterinary practitioner:

Can veterinarians develop communication strategies within their own practice? Yes, they can!

First find a common mission and vision as a practice. The goals of the individual vets have to be taken into account, find the common denominator. For a communication strategy to be successful, you all have to send the same message. Do you actually want this?

If so: subsequently: set a goal for the practice and make a plan to reach that goal. There is much information on how to make a communication and a marketing plan. The most important questions to be answered are: why? what? who? when? where? how? Some other issues to consider:

- Consider stakeholders to cooperate with
- Involve some of your best clients in the plan, if they think your plan is good, they can become your ambassadors
- Segment communication strategies
- Make sure the timing fits with other issues

CREATING DEMAND AND SUPPLY FOR ADVICE

If communication strategies are implemented to change mastitis management, farmers' demand for advice and the supply of that advice need to be taken into account. Working with the right intermediaries is important,[52–54] because dealing with the complexities of cause and effect in farming systems, and learning to apply practices to a whole farming system, requires strong interaction between advisor and farmer.[55,56] Regular veterinarian–farmer contacts are a potentially powerful way to achieve this because of (1) the high frequency of service contacts, (2) familiarity with each others' context, personal characteristics, preferences, beliefs, aspirations, and competencies that builds up over the years, and (3) the relationship of trust that develops.[1,57] This interaction can be shaped in several ways, depending on the positions farmer and veterinarian take in the process of knowledge construction.[58] In our studies, farmers perceive the veterinarian as an appreciated, important, and frequently contacted information source concerning mastitis.[24,59,60] In addition, study groups on udder health for farmers organized by their veterinarian have been successful in decreasing mastitis.[45,46,61] Although veterinarians' regular advisory contacts play an important role in optimizing farm management, there are also several constraints.[54,56,58,62] These constraints relate to advisory competencies and to the room for addressing mastitis management in a commercial, demand-driven, farmer–veterinarian relationship.[54,56,58,62]

In view of these constraints, a number of measures can be proposed to improve the interaction between the demand and supply side of the market for advisory services.[51,54,63] Important measures are to (1) improve social skills; best practice exchange about how to convey mastitis management messages in an interactive facilitative way; and (2) raise farmer awareness about the importance of mastitis management in order to stimulate demand for services that address the issue.

On a larger scale, improving linkages between research and practice, and in general a more coordinated research and extension system in support of mastitis management advice, is advisable.[54,56,62] These local and regional measures can be applied to strategies to be used in mastitis programs. As a guideline, **Table 1** displays the different components of the measures adopted in the Netherlands to promote the provision of mastitis management advice.[64] With respect to the first measure to support advisors, the Dutch mastitis program developed free-of-charge educational materials for veterinarians to use during study group meetings and when giving individual advice, and veterinarians had the opportunity to attend study group facilitation workshops. Despite the intention to empower veterinarians in individual advisory encounters, most of the educational materials were mainly used in contacts with internally motivated farmers.[26] Veterinarians seem to be less successful in reaching farmers that they presume to be nonmotivated to work on mastitis. Veterinarians were found to have difficulties in being proactive advisors and applying essential communication skills.[65] Our findings suggest that veterinarians seem to be persistent in their curatively oriented, prescriptive, and reactive expert role that prevails in veterinarian–farmer contacts. Instead of being mere technical experts, veterinarians should take on the role of coach, sparring partner, and facilitator from a reflexive and adaptive position.[1,62,66–68] This indicates that opportunities exist to improve the professional education of veterinarians on communication skills.[62,67,69]

With respect to the second measure, to increase farmer awareness to stimulate demand for advice, our results[24,29] show that farmers' awareness about mastitis hardly changed during the course of the Dutch program; most farmers disliked mastitis in 2009 as they did in 2004. The longitudinal study, however, did show an increase in farmers' feeling of control, suggesting that awareness of the efficacy of preventive measures had improved. Thus, in order to stimulate application of mastitis management measures, one should focus on the awareness of the effectiveness and feasibility of practical measures rather than addressing the importance of the problem.

Table 1
A selection of measures applied by UGCN to promote the provision of udder health advice

Factors to Support Demand and Supply of Advice	
Supporting advisors in providing udder health advice	• Lectures for veterinarians and other advisors • Providing supporting materials for successful organization of study groups • Free-of-charge distribution of educational materials to veterinary practices and other advisors • Regular contact with veterinarians and farmers on UGCN advisory panels
Raising farmer awareness of the importance of mastitis	• Study groups facilitated by veterinarians • UGCN as information source with database on udder health management and prevention of mastitis • Articles in farming magazines, newsletters, calendars, posters • Mass media campaigns on, eg, the use of milking gloves and the use of a standardized treatment plan • Udder health workshops, open farm days, symposia
Financial incentive to create demand	• Indirect incentive: decrease mastitis and therefore fewer costs and higher milk production • Indirect incentive: helping to comply with somatic cell count norms, thus preventing fines
Optimizing knowledge system linkages between extension and research	• (Coordinated) exchange between research projects, associated veterinary practices, and professional education for veterinarians and farmers • Central advisory service, including technical information and practical tools on website • Research results are used to optimize communication strategies

The third measure to create demand for advice is to use financial incentives. In our mastitis control program, as is the case for veterinary practitioners, direct financial incentives could not be applied as a policy measure. Therefore we tried to use indirect incentives. The most important indirect financial incentive for farmers was the decrease in mastitis incidence, as clinical mastitis costs on average $276 per case.[70] The baseline survey in 2004 showed that 95% of farmers perceived mastitis as a costly disease and that 69% of farmers worried about the cost of mastitis.[59] However, when farmers were asked about the most annoying aspects of mastitis, the economic cost was mentioned in third place (20%), after the additional required labor to treat the animal (24%) and the uncertainty about a cow's recovery after treatment (31%).[59] Thus, although economic cost of mastitis is important, there are also other factors that are important for the adoption of mastitis management measures.[36]

Another important financial measure is the penalty level for BMSCC. We found that, if the existing level would hypothetically be decreased from 400,000 cells/mL to 350,000 cells/mL, 65% of farmers said they would try to improve udder health, and 67% said they would treat cows with mastitis sooner. The perception on the importance of penalties was found to be associated with the herds' udder health status. Our findings are supported by other research, showing that penalties in relation to milk quality seem to have more impact on behavior than bonuses.[33] Further lowering the penalty level in the Netherlands is difficult due to the lack of support within the dairy sector and the perceived need for compatibility with European threshold levels.

The fourth measure includes the optimization of the connection between research and extension activities. The findings in research projects were implemented as much as possible in communication strategies in order to optimize the program. Furthermore, national campaigns to influence farmers' behavior in relation to mastitis management measures (eg, wearing milking gloves and developing mastitis treatment protocols) were developed in cooperation with important stakeholders such as suppliers of, for example, pharmaceuticals, feed, and farm management systems. The network of stakeholders coordinated by the UGCN supported the distribution of knowledge from science to practice. Our findings show that although several measures were included in our mastitis control program, mastitis is such a complex disease that it is difficult to optimize the intervention by using only one communication strategy. A mastitis control program needs to be supported by a full mix of policy instruments including regulations, subsidies, and penalties to optimize the efficacy of changing farmer mindset and behavior,[63,71] provided that such policy measures are clear, integrated, and stable.[1,72]

Message for the veterinary practitioner:

The most important step in creating demand for veterinary services is to offer them! Offering these services should be part of the communication strategy.

Again: it is important segment communication strategies. Most farmers are interested in improving udder health if you approach them in the right way and offer the services they want. To be able to reach that, it is crucial to ask questions. Ask what they want, what their goals are and how you can help them achieve it. Do not think for them, if they think your proposal is too expensive, they are very well able to tell that. Some farmers will not be interested, but be sure of that before you delete an opportunity to sell your services.

IMPLICATIONS FOR MASTITIS CONTROL PROGRAMS

In the design of effective mastitis control programs, essential communication principles to change people's behavior, as described in **Table 2**, need to be implemented.[50,73–76] First, it should be taken into account that a farmer is not a passive absorber of knowledge. Originally, agricultural extension had a strong supply-driven character employing a downstream transfer-of-technology (TOT) approach, in which farmers were seen as passive recipients of information that they should uniformly adopt and apply.[1] As the presented material shows, communication strategies need to take into account the complexity of farmer mindset and decision making in order to understand underlying motivations for behavior and to find opportunities for communication strategies. To motivate farmers to improve udder health, one should acknowledge that farmers are part of a wide social context. Attention should be given to cues for action, such as life-changing events,[77] and perceived barriers should be taken into account. Arguments on the efficacy of measures, using economic arguments and arguments on practical feasibility, should be used consistently by all stakeholders to stress the profitability and benefits of preventive measures.

A second important principle is the segmentation of target audiences, which is needed to customize communication strategies to farmer mindset.[43,50,76,78,79] Our findings show that different types of farmers, such as information seekers, do-it-yourselfers, wait-and-see-ers, and reclusive traditionalists, have different ways of using information sources.[27] Thus, they should be approached differently and with different strategies; for example, the central and peripheral routes of the Elaboration

Table 2	
Seven principles for designing an effective mastitis control program	
1	*The receiver is an active processor of information* A message will be received differently by different people; the individual mindset affects the way a person attends to, interprets, and accepts a message. Campaigns should include not only a downstream transfer-of-technology approach, but also an upstream approach, taking into account social determinants of people's mindset and behavior.
2	*Different target audiences may respond to different messages differently* Target audiences must be segmented into meaningful subgroups based on important characteristics such as demographic and mindset variables, before the development of targeted messages.
3	*Formative research, including message pretesting and process evaluation is essential* Research (focus groups/interviews) is needed to understand the target audience. The target audience needs to pretest the messages to ensure that they are both appropriate and effective. Continuous monitoring and evaluation of outcomes is necessary to study the efficacy of the chosen strategies.
4	*A theoretical framework increases likelihood of success* Campaigns using theoretical frameworks such as the Health Belief Model, the Theory of Planned Behavior, or the Elaboration Likelihood Model are more likely to be successful than those that do not. Theories suggest important determinants around which to develop messages and help ensure that the chosen strategy supports the processes of behavioral change.
5	*Comprehensive, coordinated interventions are most successful* Successful campaigns are comprehensive and coordinated together with other stakeholders, including a variety of strategies and policy measures to support the communication campaign.
6	*Multiple delivery channels and multiple sources increase likelihood of success* Communication campaigns involving a number of message delivery channels and more than one source appear to be more successful than those that do not.
7	*Campaigns must be sustained over time* Communication campaigns need time to achieve and maintain sustainable success. The end of the campaign needs to be flexible depending on monitoring and evaluation of outcomes and should not have a predetermined deadline.

Likelihood Model[47,48] should be used to reach farmers with different levels of internal motivation.

A third important principle of effective large-scale strategies is to include formative research as a fundamental theme within the program design. As the Dutch program shows, cooperation between scientists from different disciplines can lead to new insights. This can lead to a new normative frame of reference on mastitis and to the development of mastitis management measures that are perceived as effective in improving udder health. Additionally, it is important to monitor and evaluate the progress being made.[50]

The fourth principle of effective mastitis control programs is the use of theories such as models from social psychology. These theories provide insight into important behavioral determinants[21–23]; see, for example, the Theory of Planned Behavior,[15–17] the Health Belief Model,[18–20] and the Elaboration Likelihood Model.[47,48] Our findings show that such theories can have added value in understanding farmer mindset and can therefore contribute to the development of effective communication strategies.

The fifth and sixth principles of effective mastitis control programs are the development of comprehensive interventions, preferably with multiple channels and multiple approaches. Currently, most animal health programs still focus on influencing farmers' behavior according to the traditional TOT approach. This approach, however, has become increasingly criticized because it ignores the highly interactive and locally specific nature of knowledge construction. Nowadays, it is recognized that to achieve more sustainable agricultural practice, advisors and farmers, as well as other stakeholders, need to engage in a process of joint experiential learning to which all parties equally contribute knowledge.[1,80,81] Our findings show that when a complex disease such as mastitis is being addressed, an approach integrating different disciplines as well as provisions and policy instruments is needed. This also has consequences for the way a mastitis control program is designed. By addressing different stakeholders as equal partners instead of informative consultants, communication strategies can be designed that are more effective in changing farmers' behavior than traditional TOT strategies that reach only the internally motivated farmers. This implicates that veterinarians should not be the only intermediary in disease control programs. Cooperation with other advisors may be the cue to make steps forward. Efforts should be made to build networks among stakeholders to tailor and to customize communication strategies to farmer mindset.[43,50,76,78,79]

A last principle for designing effective mastitis control programs is the need for sustainment over time. Sustainable behavioral change needs a long-term approach and therefore complex interventions should not aim to finish within a certain limited time frame. Consistent rehearsal of the same message and follow-up on previous activities is needed over longer periods, sometimes even generations, including continuous monitoring and evaluation of the progress being made.[50] A sudden end of disease control programs would suggest that the disease is no longer considered to be an important issue. It can also result in a lack of trust among stakeholders about cooperating with new initiatives in the future, because of uncertainty about the longevity of these initiatives and supporting policies.[1,72] This implicates that mastitis control programs need to be institutionalized to be most effective in improving udder health in the long run.

Message for the veterinary practitioner:

For veterinary practices to develop and implement a mastitis control program it is important to:

- Have a plan on practice level
- Take communication serious
- Make sure everyone communicates the same message
- Cooperate with other stakeholders
- Use and harmonize all communication channels to reach the farmer

---

SUMMARY

Our findings provide insight into Dutch dairy farmers' behavior and mindset toward mastitis management, and into the way these can be affected by communication strategies. They may differ from those of North American dairy farmers, but probably many findings are comparable. Elements of farmer mindset are important determining factors in mastitis control, including the perceived threat (ie, "Do I have a problem?") and the perceived efficacy of mastitis management measures (ie, "Can I solve the problem easily?"). These issues need to be addressed in communication strategies. Veterinarians can be important intermediaries in communication about udder health, provided that they are aware of their role as proactive advisor and apply the accompanying communication skills.

To be effective, a mastitis control program should do more than distributing technical information about best management practices to dairy farmers. Prevention of complex diseases such as mastitis requires customized communication strategies as well as an integrated approach between various stakeholders and different scientific disciplines. Because farmers are part of, and are influenced by a wide institutional context, such programs need to be supported by a combination of several policy measures to change farm management in the long run.

REFERENCES

1. Leeuwis C. Communication for rural innovation. Rethinking agricultural extension. 3rd edition. Oxford (UK): Blackwell Science; 2004.
2. Burton RJF. Reconceptualising the 'behavioural approach' in agricultural studies: a socio-psychological perspective. J Rural Stud 2004;20:359–71.
3. Vaarst M, Paarup-Laursen B, Houe H, et al. Farmers' choice of medical treatment of mastitis in Danish dairy herds based on qualitative research interviews. J Dairy Sci 2002;85:992–1001.
4. Barkema HW, Van der Ploeg JD, Schukken YH, et al. Management style and its association with bulk milk somatic cell count and incidence rate of clinical mastitis. J Dairy Sci 1999;82:1655–63.
5. Seabrook MF. The psychological interaction between the stockman and his animals and its influence on performance of pigs and dairy-cows. Vet Rec 1984;115:84–7.
6. Van der Ploeg JD. Bedrijfsstijlen als socio-technische netwerken. De virtuele boer. 1st edition. Assen (Netherlands): Van Gorcum & Cromp BV; 1999. p. 110–56.
7. Beaudeau F, Van der Ploeg JD, Boileau B, et al. Relationships between culling criteria in dairy herds and farmers' management styles. Prev Vet Med 1996;25:327–42.
8. Andersen HJ, Enevoldsen C. Towards a better understanding of the farmer's management practices: The power of combining qualitative and quantitative data. In: Andersen HJ, editor. Radgivning, Bev aegelse mellem data og dialog. Aarhus (Denmark): Mejeriforeningen; 2004. p. 281–301.
9. Reneau JK. Milk quality mind set. Proceedings of the Great Lakes Dairy Conference. Oregon (OH) April 30–May 2, 2002.
10. Tarabla H, Dodd K. Associations between farmers' personal characteristics, management practices and farm performance. Br Vet J 1990;146:157–64.
11. Barnouin J, Chassagne M, Bazin S, et al. Management practices from questionnaire surveys in herds with very low somatic cell score through a national mastitis program in France. J Dairy Sci 2004;87:3989–99.
12. Wenz JR, Jensen SM, Lombard JE, et al. Herd management practices and their association with bulk milk somatic cell count on United States dairy operations. J Dairy Sci 2007;90:3652–9.
13. Dohoo IR, Martin SW, Meek AH. Disease, production and culling in Holstein-Friesian cows. VI. Effects of management on disease rates. Prev Vet Med 1984;3:15–28.
14. Nyman AK, Ekman T, Emanuelson U, et al. Risk factors associated with the incidence of veterinary-treated clinical mastitis in Swedish dairy herds with a high milk yield and a low prevalence of subclinical mastitis. Prev Vet Med 2007;78:142–60.
15. Ajzen I, Madden TJ. Prediction of goal-directed behavior:attitudes, intentions and perceived behavioral control. J Exp Soc Psychol 1986;22:453–74.
16. Ajzen I. The theory of planned behavior. Organ Behav Hum Decis Proc 1991;50:179–211.

17. Fishbein M, Yzer MC. Using theory to design effective health behavior interventions. Commun Theory 2003;13:164–3.

18. Janz N, Becker MH. The health belief model: A decade later. Health Educ Q 1984;11:1–47.

19. Sun X, Guo Y, Wang S, et al. Predicting iron-fortified soy sauce consumption intention: application of the theory of planned behavior and health belief model. J Nutr Educ Behav 2006;38:276–85.

20. Garcia K, Mann T. From 'I Wish' to 'I Will': social-cognitive predictors of behavioral intentions. J Health Psychol 2003;8:347–60.

21. Armitage CJ, Conner M. Efficacy of the theory of planned behaviour: a meta-analytic review. Br J Soc Psychol 2001;40:471–99.

22. Painter JE, Borba CP, Hynes M, et al. The use of theory in health behavior research from 2000 to 2005: a systematic review. Ann Behav Med 2008;35:358–62.

23. Noar SM, Chabot M, Zimmerman RS. Applying health behavior theory to multiple behavior change: considerations and approaches. Prev Med 2008;46:275–80.

24. Jansen J, Van den Borne BHP, Renes RJ, et al. Explaining mastitis incidence in Dutch dairy farming:the influence of farmers' attitudes and behaviour. Prev Vet Med 2009; 92:210–23.

25. Bigras-Poulin M, Meek AH, Martin SW, et al. Attitudes, management practices, and herd performance: a study of Ontario dairy farm managers. II. Associations. Prev Vet Med 1985;3:241–50.

26. Jansen J, Renes RJ, Lam TJGM. Evaluation of two communication strategies to improve udder health management. J Dairy Sci 2010;93:604–12.

27. Jansen J, Steuten CDM, Renes RJ, et al. Debunking the myth of the hard-to-reach farmer: effective communication on udder health. J Dairy Sci 2010;93:1296–306.

28. Jansen J, Steuten CDM, Renes RJ, et al. Mastitis control programs: farmers'reasons for action. In: Hillerton JE, editor. Mastitis research into practice. Proceedings of the 5th IDF Mastitis Conference. Christchurch (New Zealand). Wellington (New Zealand): Dunmore Publishing Limited; 2010. p. 664.

29. Jansen J, Van Schaik G, Renes RJ, et al. The effect of a national mastitis control program on the attitudes, knowledge and behavior of farmers in the Netherlands. J Dairy Sci 2010;93:5737–47.

30. Rogers RW. Cognitive and physiological processes in fear appeals and attitude change: a revised theory of protection motivation. In: Cacioppo JT, Petty RE, editors. Social psychology: a source book. New York: Guilford Press; 1983. p. 153–76.

31. Griffin RJ, Dunwoody S, Neuwirth K. Proposed model of the relationship of risk information seeking and processing to the development of preventive behaviors. Environ Res Sect A 1999;80:S230–45.

32. Huijps K, Lam TJGM, Hogeveen H. Costs of mastitis: facts and perception. J Dairy Res 2008;75:113–20.

33. Valeeva NI, Lam TJGM, Hogeveen H. Motivation of dairy farmers to improve mastitis management. J Dairy Sci 2007;90:4466–77.

34. Garforth C, Mc Kemey K, Rehman T, et al. Farmers' attitudes towards techniques for improving oestrus detection in dairy herds in South West England. Livestock Sci 2006;103:158–68.

35. Gielen PM, Hoeve A, Nieuwenhuis LFM. Learning Entrepreneurs: learning and innovation in small companies. Eur Educ Res J 2003;2:90–106.

36. van Asseldonk MAPM, Renes RJ, Lam TJGM, et al. Awareness and perceived value of economic information in controlling somatic cell count. Vet Rec 2010;166:263–7.

37. Festinger L. A theory of cognitive dissonance. Stanford (CA): Stanford University Press; 1957.

38. Cameron KA. A practitioners guide to persuasion: an overview of 15 selected persuasion theories, models and frameworks. Patient Educ Counsel 2009;74: 309–17.

39. Carver CS, Scheier MF, Weintraub JK. Assessing coping strategies: a theoretically based approach. J Personal Soc Psychol 1989;56:267–83.

40. Ellis-Iversen J, Cook AJC, Watson E, et al. Perceptions, circumstances and motivators that influence implementation of zoonotic control programs on cattle farms. Prev Vet Med 2010;93:276–85.

41. Bradley AJ. Bovine mastitis: an evolving disease. Vet J 2002;164:116–28.

42. Rehman T, McKemey K, Yates CM, et al. Identifying and uderstanding factors influencing the uptake of new technologies on dairyfarms in SW England using the theory of reasoned action. Agri Syst 2007;94:281–93.

43. Chase LE, Ely OL, Hutjens MF. Major advances in extension education programs in dairy production. J Dairy Sci 2006;89:1147–54.

44. Armitage CJ, Conner M. The theory of planned behaviour: assessment of predictive validity and 'perceived control.' Br J Soc Psychol 1999;38:35–54.

45. Lam TJGM, Jansen J, Van Gent RJM, et al. Directions for national mastitis control programs: experiences from The Netherlands. In: Hillerton JE, editor. Mastitis research into practice. Proceedings of the 5th IDF Mastitis Conference. Christchurch (New Zealand). Wellington (New Zealand): Dunmore Publishing Limited; 2010. p. 142–6.

46. Lam TJGM, Jansen J, Van den Borne BHP, et al. What veterinarians need to know about communication to optimise their role as advisor on udder health in dairy herds. N Z Vet J 2011;59:8–15.

47. Petty RE, Cacioppo JT. The elaboration likelihood model of persuasion. Adv Exp Soc Psychol 1986;19:123–205.

48. Petty RE, Wegener DT. The elaboration likelihood model: Current status and controversies. In: Chaiken S, Trope Y, editors. Dual-process theories in social psychology. New York: Guilford Press; 1999. p. 41–72.

49. Sheeran P. Intention-behavior relations: a conceptual and empirical review. Eur Rev Soc Psychol 2002;12:1–36.

50. Noar SM. A 10-year retrospective of research in health mass media campaigns: where do we go from here? J Health Commun 2006;11:21–42.

51. Klerkx L, de Grip K, Leeuwis C. Hands off but strings attached: the contradictions of policy-induced demand-driven agricultural extension. Agri Hum Values 2006;23: 189–204.

52. Garforth C, Angell B, Archer J, et al. Fragmentation or creative diversity? Options in the provison of land management advisory services. Land Use Policy 2003;20: 323–33.

53. Nagel UJ, Von der Heiden K. Germany: privatizing extension in post-socialist agriculture-the case of Brandenbug. In: Rivera WM, Alex G, editors. Privatization of extension systems. Case studies of international initiatives. Washington DC: World Bank; 2004. p. 30–4.

54. Botha N, Coutts J, Roth H. The role of agricultural consultants in New Zealand in environmental extension. J Agri Educ Extens 2008;14:125–38.

55. Leeuwis C. Learning to be sustainable. Does the Dutch agrarian knowledge market fail? J Agri Educ Extens 2000;7:79–92.

56. Ingram J, Morris C. The knowledge challenge within the transitions towards sustainable soil management: an analyisis of agricultural advisors in England. Land Use Policy 2007;24:100–17.

57. Sligo FX, Massey C. Risk, trust and knowledge networks in farmers' learning. J Rural Stud 2007;23:170–82.
58. Ingram J. Agronomist-farmer knowledge encounters: an analysis of knowledge exchange in the context of best management practices in England. Agri Hum Values 2008;25:405–18.
59. Jansen J, Kuiper D, Renes RJ, et al. Report on baseline survey mastitis: knowledge, attitude and behaviour [Nulmeting kennis, houding en gedrag]. Communication and Innovation Studies. Wageningen University, Wageningen; September 2004.
60. Jansen J, Renes RJ, Lam TJGM. Mastitis control: seize the opportunity. The role of veterinarians as effective udder health advisors. Proceedings of the 47th Annual Meeting of the National Mastitis Council. New Orleans (LA). Verona (WI): National Mastitis Council; 2008.
61. Lam TJGM, Jansen J, Van den Borne B, et al. A structural approach of udder health improvement via private practitioners: ups and downs. Proceedings of the 46th Annual Meeting, National Mastitis Council. San Antonio (TX). Verona (WI): National Mastitis Council; 2007.
62. Mee JF. The role of the veterinarian in bovine fertility management on modern dairy farms. Theriogenology 2007;68(Suppl 1):S257–65.
63. Van Woerkum C, Kuiper D, Bos E. Communicatie en innovatie. Een inleiding. Alphen aan de Rijn (Netherlands): Samsom; 1999.
64. Klerkx L, Jansen J. Building knowledge systems for sustainable agriculture: support-ing private advisors to adequately address sustainable farm management in regular service contacts. Int J Agri Sustain 2010;8:148–63.
65. Jansen J, Klinkert H, Renes RJ, et al. Effective communication of veterinary advice: interaction between the veterinarian and the farmer. In: Hillerton JE, editor. Mastitis research into practice. Proceedings of the 5th IDF Mastitis Conference. Christchurch (New Zealand). Wellington (New Zealand): Dunmore Publishing Limited; 2010. p. 185–91.
66. Nettle R, Paine M. Water security and farming systems:implications for advisory practice and policy making. J Agri Educ Extens 2009;15:147–60.
67. Noordhuizen JPTM. Changes in the veterinary management of dairy cattle: threats or opportunities. Vet Sci Tomorrow 2001;2:1–9.
68. Cannas da Silva J, Noordhuizen JPTM, Vagneur M, et al. Veterinary dairy herd health management in Europe. Constraints and perspectives. Vet Q 2006;28:23–32.
69. Noordhuizen JPTM, Van Egmond MJ, Jorritsma R, et al. Veterinary advice for entrepreneurial Dutch dairy farmers. From curative practice to coach-consultant:what needs to be changed? Tijdschrift Voor Diergeneeskunde 2008;133:4–8.
70. Huijps K, Lam TJGM, Hogeveen H. Costs of mastitis: facts and perception. J Dairy Res 2008;75:113–20.
71. Snyder LB, Hamilton MA, Mitchell EW, et al. A meta-analysis of the effect of mediated health communication campaigns on behavior change in the United States. J Health Commun 2004;9:71–96.
72. Valentine I, Hurley E, Reid J, et al. Principles and processes for effecting change in environmental management in New Zealand. J Environ Manage 2007;82:311–8.
73. Henley N, Donovan R, Francas M. Developing and implementing communication messages. In: Doll L, Bonzo S, Mercy J, et al . editors. Handbook of injury and violence prevention. New York: Springer; 2007. p. 433–47.
74. Henley N, Raffin S. Social marketing to prevent childhood obesity. In: Waters E, Swinburn B, Seidell J, et al, editors. Preventing childhood obesity: evidence, policy and practice. West Sussex (UK): Wiley-Blackwell; 2010. p. 243–52.

75. Koelen MA, Van den Ban AW. Health education and health promotion. Wageningen (Netherlands): Wageningen Academic Publishers; 2004.

76. Noar SM, Benac CN, Harris MS. Does tailoring matter? Meta-analytic review of tailored print health Behavior change interventions. Psychol Bull 2007;133:673–93.

77. Osler M. The life course perspective: a challenge for public health research and prevention. Eur J Public Health 2006;16:230.

78. Bergevoet RHM, Ondersteijn CJM, Saatkamp HW, et al. Entrepreneurial behaviour of Dutch dairy farmers under a milk quota system: goals, objectives, attitudes. Agri Syst 2004;80:1–21.

79. Hawkins RP, Kreuter M, Resnicow K, et al. Understanding tailoring in communicating about health. Health Educ Res 2008;23:454–66.

80. Eshuis J, Stuiver M. Learning in context through conflict and alignments:farmers and scientists in search for sustainable agriculture. Agri Hum Values 2005;22:137–48.

81. Bouma J. Implications of the knowledge paradox for soil science. Adv Agron 2010; 106:143–71.

Index

Note: Page numbers of article titles are in **boldface** type.

A

Anti-inflammatory drugs
  in clinical mastitis management, 277
  nonsteroidal
    in cattle
      with mastitis, 298–301
      use of, 296–298
Antibiotic(s)
  in clinical mastitis management, 275–277
  in dairy cows
    alternatives to, 176–177
    cessation of use of
      impact on antimicrobial resistance, 173–175
    for mastitis
      issues related to, 166–167
    nonuse of
      consequences of, 175–176
  for mastitis, 166–167
    in dairy cows
      issues related to, 166–167
    in dry cow, 166
    prudent use of, 177–181
  resistance to. *See* Antimicrobial resistance
Antimicrobial resistance
  of mastitis pathogens, **165–185**
    from conventional or organic dairy farms, 170–173
    in dairy cows
      cessation of antibiotic use effects on, 173–175
      resistance patterns, 167–168
    trend studies over time, 168–170
Arcanobacterium pyogenes
  clinical mastitis due to
    management of, 283

B

Bacillus spp.
  clinical mastitis due to
    management of, 283
Bacteria
  gram-negative
    mastitis due to, **239–256**. *See also specific types and* Mastitis, causes of, gram-negative bacteria

Vet Clin Food Anim 28 (2012) 381–390
http://dx.doi.org/10.1016/S0749-0720(12)00040-0
0749-0720/12/$ – see front matter © 2012 Elsevier Inc. All rights reserved.

vetfood.theclinics.com

Behavior(s)
    voltage exposure effects on
        research on, 324–341
Between-herd biosecurity
    in *S. aureus* and *S. agalactiae* infections management, 211–212
Biosecurity
    between-herd
        in *S. aureus* and *S. agalactiae* infections management, 211–212
    within-herd
        in *S. aureus* and *S. agalactiae* control in mastitis management, 206–207
Bulk tank culture
    in mastitis diagnosis, 192–194

C

Clinical mastitis
    after experimental challenge
        management of
            NSAIDs in, 299
    dairy cows with
        pain in
            assessment and management of, **289–305**. See also Pain, in dairy cows
    endotoxin-induced
        management of
            NSAIDs in, 298–299
    management of, **271–288**
        anti-inflammatory drugs in, 277
        antibiotics in, 275–277
        culture-based therapy in, 273–274
        fluids and electrolytes in, 275
        FMO in, 284
        homeopathy in, 283
        oxytocin in, 284
        pathogen-related, 277–283
            Arcanobacterium pyogenes, 283
            Bacillus spp., 283
            environmental streptococci, 278–280
            gram-negative, 280–281
            S. aureus, 280
            staphylococci, 282
            yeast/prototheca, 282
        polymyxin B in, 283
    records related to, 349, 352–358
        cohort of cows having had multiple cases in current lactation, 357
        cohort of first cases, 355–357
        cow-side reports, 352–354
        herd-level reports for interpretation of mastitis management plan, 354–355
        treatment outcomes–related, 357–358
Communication
    in udder health, **363–379**
        creating demand and supply for advice, 369–372
        as intervention instrument, 366–369

Corral(s)
  dry
    in environmental mastitis management, 220
Culling
  in *S. aureus* and *S. agalactiae* infections management, 211
Culture-based therapy
  in clinical mastitis management, 273–274
Current
  basic concepts of, 322–323

D

Dairy cattle
  antibiotics in. *See* Antibiotic(s), in dairy cows
  antimicrobial resistance in. *See* Antimicrobial resistance
  clinical mastitis in
    pain associated with, **289–305**. *See also* Pain, in dairy cows
  illness in
    physiological and behavioral characteristics associated with, 293–294
  mastitis in
    physiological and behavioral characteristics associated with, 293–294
  pain in. *See* Pain, in dairy cows
Dry cow therapy
  for *S. aureus* and *S. agalactiae* infections, 211
Dry lots and corrals
  in environmental mastitis management, 220

E

Electrolyte(s)
  in clinical mastitis management, 275
ELISA milk testing
  in mastitis diagnosis, 198–200
Endotoxin(s)
  clinical mastitis due to
    management of
      NSAIDs in, 298–299
Enterobacter spp.
  mastitis due to, 251–252
Enterobacteriaceae
  mastitis due to, 240–242
Environmental mastitis, 150–154
  diagnosis of
    issues related to, 154–159
  management of, **217–224**
    control programs in
      diagnostic microbiology in, 198
    described, 217–218
    dry lots and corrals in, 220
    grazing systems in, 220
    issues related to, 154–159

during maternity, 220
milking hygiene in, 220–221
monitoring in, 221–222
seasonality in, 219
stall bedding in, 218–219
seasonal effects on, 219
streptococci and
clinical mastitis due to
management of, 278–280

F

Fluids and electrolytes
in clinical mastitis management, 275
FMO. See Frequent milk-out (FMO)
Frequent milk-out (FMO)
in clinical mastitis management, 284

G

GNCABs. See Gram-negative "core-antigen" bacterins (GNCABs)
Gram-negative bacteria
mastitis due to, **239–256**. See also specific types and Mastitis, causes of,
gram-negative bacteria
Gram-negative "core-antigen" bacterins (GNCABs)
for mastitis, 260–261
strategies for use, 262–266
Gram-negative pathogens
clinical mastitis due to
management of, 280–281
Grazing systems
in environmental mastitis management, 220

H

High-frequency voltage, 325
Homeopathy
in clinical mastitis management, 283

K

Klebsiella spp.
mastitis due to, 242–247
outbreaks of, 244–245
prevention of, 246–247
treatment of, 245–246
vaccination for, 245–246

L

Lipopolysaccharide(s)
mastitis due to, 240–242

Lot(s)
  dry
    in environmental mastitis management, 220

M

Mastitis
  bovine
    MRSA and, 171–173
  causes of
    gram-negative bacteria, **239–256**. *See also specific types*
      described, 239–240
      Enterobacter spp., 251–252
      enterobacteriaceae, 240–242
      immune response patterns, 242
      Klebsiella spp., 242–247
      lipopolysaccharides, 240–242
      Raoultella spp., 251
      Serratia spp., 247–251
  classification of, 150, 271–273
  clinical. *See* Clinical mastitis
  control of, 149, 166
    milking machine in, **307–320**. *See also* Milking machine, in mastitis control
    programs for
      diagnostic microbiology in, **187–202**. *See also* Mastitis control programs, diagnostic microbiology in
  defined, 165–166
  described, 149, 347–348
  diagnosis of
    zero tolerance in, 197
  environmental. *See* Environmental mastitis
  farmers' mindset toward, 364–366
  management of
    antibiotics in, 166–167
      prudent use of, 177–181
    "5-point plan" in, 150
    records in. *See* Mastitis, records related to
    S. aureus and *S.agalactiae* control in, **203–216**. *See also Staphylococcus aureus* infection; *Streptococcus* spp., *S. agalactiae* infection
    vaccines in, **257–270**. *See also* Vaccination(s), for mastitis
  mild, 272
    management of, 274–277
  moderate, 272–273
    management of, 274–277
  Mycoplasma, **225–237**. *See also Mycoplasma* mastitis
  naturally occurring
    management of
      NSAIDs in, 299–301
  pathogens causing, 149–150
    antimicrobial resistance of, **165–185**. *See also* Antimicrobial resistance
    changing distribution of, 150, 151

environmental, 150–154
    diagnostic and treatment issues in era of, 154–159
prevention of, 257. *See also* Vaccination(s), for mastitis
records related to, **347–361**
    culture results, 349–350
    described, 348
    exit remark, 351
    for monitoring drug use
        importance of, 348–349
    somatic cell count data, 350–351
    udder health data, 349–352
    veterinarian-client-patient relationship, 348–349
S. aureus
    immunization for, 264–266
seasonal effects on, 219
severe, 273
    management of, 274–277
stray voltage and, 325–341
subclinical
    records related to, 358–360
S.uberis
    immunization for, 266
vaccination strategies for, **257–270**. *See also* Vaccination(s), for mastitis
Mastitis control programs
    decision to use, 196
    diagnostic microbiology in, **187–202**
        bulk tank culture, 192–194
        considerations related to, 188–189
        environmental mastitis, 198
        mile ELISA, 198–200
        on-farm testing, 196–197
        PCR, 198–200
        scope of service, 194–196
        shedding pattern effects on, 189–192
        zero tolerance, 197
    implications of, 372–374
Maternity
    dry lots during
        in environmental mastitis management, 220
Methicillin-resistant *Staphylococcus aureus* (MRSA)
    bovine mastitis due to, 171–173
Milk
    quality of
        stray voltage effects on, **321–345**. *See also* Stray voltage
Milking hygiene
    in environmental mastitis management, 220–221
Milking machine
    in mastitis control, **307–320**
        contamination prevention, 315–316
        described, 307–308
        discussion of, 313–315

mechanisms of, 308–313
    changing numbers of pathogens on teat skin or teat orifice, 308
    changing resistance of teat canal to invasion by mastitis pathogens, 309–310
    dispersing pathogens within udder, 312
    frequency and/or degree of udder evacuation, 313
    providing forces to overcome resistance of teat canal to bacterial invasion,
       310–312
    RPGs, 312
Milking practices
  in reducing incidence of *S. aureus* and *S. agalactiae* infections, 207–208
MRSA. *See* Methicillin-resistant *Staphylococcus aureus* (MRSA)
Mycoplasma mastitis, **225–237**
  carriage of, 228–230
  control of, 232–233
  epidemiology of, 226–230
  introduction to, 225–226
  prevalence of, 226–227
  transmission of, 227–228
Mycoplasma spp.
  pathogenic
    characteristics of, 230–231

N

Nerve stimulation
  biomechanics of, 323–324
Nonsteroidal anti-inflammatory drugs (NSAIDs)
  in cattle, 296–298
    with mastitis, 298–301
NSAIDs. *See* Nonsteroidal anti-inflammatory drugs (NSAIDs)

O

Organic bedding
  in environmental mastitis management, 218–219
Oxytocin
  in clinical mastitis management, 284

P

Pain
  in dairy cows
    with clinical mastitis
      assessment of, **289–305**
        introduction to, 289–290
        objective, 294–296
      management of, **289–305**
        NSAIDs in, 298–301
     perceptions of, 291–293
      dairy producers', 291
      public, 292–293
      veterinary practitioners', 291–292
    research on, 293
  defined, 290

PCR. *See* Polymerase chain reaction (PCR)
Polymerase chain reaction (PCR)
  in mastitis diagnosis, 198–200
Polymyxin B
  in clinical mastitis management, 283
Prototheca
  clinical mastitis due to
    management of, 282

R

Raoultella spp.
  mastitis due to, 251
Resistance
  basic concepts of, 322–323
Reverse pressure gradients (RPGs)
  in machine milking in mastitis control, 312
RPGs. *See* Reverse pressure gradients (RPGs)

S

Sand bedding
  in environmental mastitis management, 218
Segregation
  in control of *S. aureus* and *S. agalactiae* infections in mastitis management, 209
Serratia spp.
  mastitis due to, 247–251
    outbreaks of, 248–249
    prevention of, 249–251
    treatment of, 249
Shedding pattern
  effect on bacterial detection in mastitis, 189–192
Somatic cell count data, 350–351
Stall bedding
  in environmental mastitis management, 218–219
    organic bedding, 218–219
    sand bedding, 218
Staphylococcus(i)
  coagulase-negative
    clinical mastitis due to
      management of, 282
  coagulase-positive
    clinical mastitis due to
      management of, 282
Staphylococcus aureus
  clinical mastitis due to
    management of, 280
  control of
    in mastitis management
      introduction to, 203–204
  methicillin-resistant
    bovine mastitis due to, 171–173

Staphylococcus aureus infection
  control of
    in mastitis management, **203–216**
      segregation, 209
  detection of, 205
  epidemiology of, 204–205
  incidence of
    milking practices in reducing, 207–208
  management of
    between-herd biosecurity in, 211–212
    culling in, 211
    dry cow therapy in, 211
    lactational, 210
    within-herd biosecurity in, 206–207
  presentation of, 204–205
  prevalence of, 205–206
    reducing of, 209–210
  public health consequences of, 206–207
Staphylococcus aureus mastitis
  immunization for, 264–266
Stray voltage. *See also* Voltage
  defined, 321
  introduction to, 321–322
  mastitis related to, 325–341
  milk quality effects of, **321–345**
  research on, 325–341
  stress related to, 325–341
Streptococcus(i)
  environmental
    clinical mastitis due to
      management of, 278–280
Streptococcus spp.
  S. agalactiae infection
    control of
      in mastitis management, **203–216**
        introduction to, 203–204
    detection of, 205
    epidemiology of, 204–205
    incidence of
      milking practices in reducing, 207–208
    management of
      between-herd biosecurity in, 211–212
      culling in, 211
      dry cow therapy in, 211
      lactational, 210
      segregation in, 209
      within-herd biosecurity in, 206–207
    presentation of, 204–205
    prevalence of, 205–206
      reducing of, 209–210
    public health consequences of, 206–207
Streptococcus spp. mastitis
  immunization for, 266

Stress
   stray voltage and, 325–341

T

Transient voltage, 325

U

Udder health. *See also* Mastitis
   communication in, **363–379**. *See also* Communication, in udder health
   data related to, 349–352
   management of
      new perspectives in, **149–163**
      programs in
         implementation of, 159–160
   molecular methodologies in
      in era of environmental pathogens, 150–154

V

Vaccination(s)
   described, 258
   for *Klebsiella* spp., 245–246
   for mastitis, **257–270**
      efficacy of, 258–260
      GNCABs, 260–261
         strategies for use, 262–266
      immunology of, 258–260
      protocols for
         strategies for use, 262–266
Voltage
   basic concepts of, 322–323
   exposure to, 325–341
      behavioral responses to
         research on, 324–341
   high-frequency, 325
   stray
      milk quality effects of, **321–345**. *See also* Stray voltage
   transient, 325

W

Within-herd biosecurity
   in *S. aureus* and *S. agalactiae* control in mastitis management, 206–207

Y

Yeast
   clinical mastitis due to
      management of, 282

Z

Zero tolerance
   in mastitis diagnosis, 197

Printed and bound by CPI Group (UK) Ltd, Croydon, CR0 4YY

03/10/2024

01040461-0009